Understanding Youth Mental Health

Perspectives from Theory and Practice

Understanding Youth Mental Health

Perspectives from Theory and Practice

Eilis Hennessy, Caroline Heary and Maria Michail

Open University Press

Open University Press
McGraw Hill
Unit 4,
Foundation Park
Roxborough Way
Maidenhead
SL6 3UD

email: emea_uk_ireland@mheducation.com
world wide web: www.openup.co.uk

First edition published 2022

A catalogue record of this book is available from the British Library

ISBN-13: 9780335250530
ISBN-10: 033525053X
eISBN: 9780335250547

Library of Congress Cataloging-in-Publication Data
CIP data applied for

Typeset by Transforma Pvt. Ltd., Chennai, India

Praise page

"The mental health of young people has become a global crisis over the past two decades, a crisis worsened by megatrends and major global shocks in society, including financial crises and pandemics. The US Surgeon General Dr Vivek Murthy acknowledged this in late 2021, confirming what the pioneering authors of this timely book have known for many years. Mental ill health is the greatest contributor to the burden of disease in emerging adults, as they enter puberty and this threat builds through the many years of transition until mature adulthood is reached. Mental ill health delays this maturation process, undermines the achievement of full potential, causes enormous suffering and disability, and all too often threatens or tragically ends the lives of young people. This is not a case of "medicalising the human condition". It is a top public health priority which demands a comprehensive response in every single society on the globe.

'Understanding Youth Mental Health' covers the full spectrum of what is needed. Firstly, we need to understand why the mental health of young people is steadily declining form an already fragile base. This means determining the relative contribution of powerful megatrends in our society, notably climate change, financial insecurity, social media and other forces, notably war and pandemics. Insecurity is the common thread here. Secondly, we need to be able to recognise early on when there is a need for professional care and to create safe and welcoming primary care cultures in partnership with young people and families for this to occur. This is a major global construction project which is already underway and a number of the builders are included among the authorship. This already represents a paradigm shift which is gaining momentum in many parts of the world, and depends upon a new workforce being created with special skills and a deep affinity for working with young people, plus the assembly of a scientific evidence base to guide this reform. Finally there is a need to design and scale up a more specialised multidisciplinary back up system for the primary or entry level services to offer recovery focused interventions to the substantial proportion of young people with more complex and sustained forms of mental ill health and illness. All this adds up to building a new and diverse field of scholarship, professional identity and skills, and culture, which adds value to current paradigms of child psychiatry and psychology and adult mental health but ultimately transcends these approaches to become a holistic new field in its own right. Young people deserve no less and will be central contributors in this historic construction project. 'Understanding Youth Mental Health' is a welcome and important building block."

Patrick McGorry, Professor of Youth Mental Health,
University of Melbourne, Executive Director,
Orygen: National Centre for Youth Mental Health

Seen and Heard – a creative piece by young people (18–25 years old),
as part of the work of the YOULEAD Research Group,
National University of Ireland, Galway, Ireland, and
Fregoli Theatre Company, Galway, Ireland in
collaboration with SpunOut.ie

To be seen.
To be heard.
To be seen as you are.
To be heard and know the listener is trying to understand.
To be seen as you are and accepted.
To be heard and understood.

Available at: https://www.youtube.com/watch?v=Wuz-XE8hCao&feature=youtu.be

Contents

Acknowledgements

Many people helped in the production of this book. Thanks in particular to the authors of individual chapters who responded so eagerly to our invitation to write about their research work. Through their research they have made a significant contribution to our understanding of the value of focusing on young people's mental health and it is gratifying to see the diversity of this work combined in a single book. Thanks to our many graduate students who have approached the study of youth mental health with such enthusiasm and from whom we learned about the need to bring this collection of topics together. Particular thanks to Cal McDonagh, Lynn McKeague and Daráine Murphy who allowed us to use quotations from the participants in the research that formed part of their doctoral dissertations – and of course thanks to the research participants from whom we have learned so much about the experience of having a mental health difficulty or about parenting a young person with a mental health difficulty. We are also very grateful to the young people who worked with the YOULEAD Research Group, and Fregoli Theatre Company, Galway, Ireland to produce *Seen and Heard* from which we have drawn quotations throughout the book. Their full production can be found at https://www.youtube.com/watch?v=Wuz-XE8hCao&feature=youtu.be. Finally, thanks to Roisin McNamara who did so much work to bring a greater level of consistency to the many ways in which the different chapters referred to mental health and mental health difficulties.

Editors and contributing authors

Eilis Hennessy PhD is a professor in the UCD School of Psychology. Her research addresses stigma, bias and discrimination experienced by children and adolescents with chronic health problems with a particular focus on those who have mental health and behavioural problems. She is particularly interested in processes of help-seeking by adolescents and parents.

Caroline Heary PhD is a senior lecturer in Developmental Psychology at the National University of Ireland, Galway. Her research focuses on experiences of living with mental health difficulties during childhood and adolescence (with a specific focus on stigma-related experiences), barriers to accessing services, and experiences of seeking help.

Dr Maria Michail is a Marie Curie Global Fellow and an Associate Professor in the Institute for Mental Health, University of Birmingham, UK. Maria is a leading expert in the field of self-harm and suicide prevention, and is co-chair of the International Association for Suicide Prevention Special Interest Group 'Suicide Prevention in Primary Care'. Her work has had demonstrable impact on improved clinical practice across primary care in the UK through the development of good-practice guidelines in managing suicide risk in consultations with young people.

Alan Bailey is a research assistant and PhD candidate at Orygen and the Centre for Youth Mental Health, University of Melbourne Australia. His research interests include physical activity, youth depression and anxiety.

Andrew Baxter has worked as a clinician in school-based and community mental health for over 18 years. He has provided direct treatment for students and consultation for their families and teachers. Andrew currently serves as the team lead for mentalhealthliteracy.org and the Alberta Mental Health Literacy Project.

Karen Butler (BA Psychology (Int), MSc Health Psychology) is a former research assistant and Youth Advisory Panel member at Jigsaw: The National Centre for Youth Mental Health, Ireland. Her dual experience provides unique insight into the experience and impact of youth participation in mental health services and research.

Dr Wendy Carr is an emerita professor in language and literacy education in the Faculty of Education at the University of British Columbia, Canada. She has co-created a mental health literacy curriculum for pre-service teachers and has led system-wide teacher professional development in mental health literacy.

Dr Samantha Dockray is a senior lecturer in Applied Psychology at University College Cork, Ireland. Her research examines the interactions of biological processes, such as puberty and the stress response, experience and psychological well-being during adolescence.

Professor Barbara Dooley is Acting Registrar, Deputy President and Vice-President for Academic Affairs at University College Dublin. Her research focuses on the application of psychological theory and methodology to a range of priority mental health areas such as risk and protective factors in youth mental health, body-image research, alcohol and eating disorders.

Professor Gary Donohoe is the Established Professor and Chair of Psychology at National University of Ireland, Galway and an internationally recognised expert in the cognitive neuroscience of psychosis. His research, supported by major fellowships and grants from the European Research Council and the Irish Health Research Board (HRB), has led to publication of more than 250 peer-reviewed articles and resulted in over 27,000 citations of his work. Gary is currently a HRB Research Leader in the area of early interventions for psychosis, in partnership with the National Early Intervention for Psychosis Service in Ireland.

Snigdha Dutta PhD contributes to the enhancement of inclusive educational initiatives at the University of Cambridge, UK, to support students' mental health and well-being. She has a background in psychology, and her research has focused on university students' resilience from a socio-ecological perspective.

Emmanuelle Godeau is a public health medical doctor and holds a PhD in social anthropology. She is currently a senior researcher at EHESP School of Public Health in Rennes, in charge of the national training for school doctors. Her research focuses on health behaviour of adolescents, with a specific interest on students with chronic conditions.

Dr Sarah Hetrick is the Associate Professor of Youth Mental Health, University of Auckland, New Zealand. Sarah's research focuses on youth depression and suicide and self-harm prevention. She is a co-ordinating editor for the Cochrane Common Mental Disorders Group and is a clinical psychologist.

Dr Emma Howard is an assistant professor with the UCD School of Mathematics and Statistics. Her research interests include youth mental health, learning analytics, mathematics education and aiding student support services through the use of data analytics.

Melissa Keller-Tuberg: Since recovering from her lived experience of mental illness, Melissa Keller-Tuberg became involved in youth advocacy and consultancy roles across various organisations and settings; she is on Orygen's Youth Research Council (YRC) and Research Review Committee (RRC).

Dr Stan Kutcher is a psychiatrist and emeritus professor at Dalhousie University, who has helped young people successfully manage major mental illnesses. His appointment to the Senate of Canada allows him to put his decades of medical, academic and policy expertise at the service of all Canadians.

Siobhán McGrory (B.Ed. and M.A. Health Promotion) is Director of Education and Community at Jigsaw: The National Centre for Youth Mental Health, Ireland. Siobhán leads Jigsaw's Youth Mental Health Promotion Department and oversees Jigsaw's Youth Voice and Engagement framework and practice. Her area of expertise is in mental health promotion.

Dr Nadine Messerli-Bürgy is an associate professor of Clinical Child and Adolescent Psychology at the University of Lausanne, Switzerland. Her research focuses on the underlying mechanisms of psychopathological processes in children, adolescents and young adults.

Michal Molcho PhD is a professor in Children's Studies in the School of Education at the National University of Ireland, Galway. Her research focuses on inequalities in child and adolescent health. She is particularly interested in the health of under-represented children and adolescents.

Daráine Murphy's research interests are in the areas of help-seeking, stigma and how to support families of adolescents who have mental health problems. Her PhD research focused on how parents seek help for adolescents who have mental health problems.

Dr Christine Musyimi, PhD promotes excellence in community-based mental health research with a focus on depression, intimate partner violence and dementia, and improving maternal and child mental health to increase mental health care access in remote settings.

Victoria Mutiso, a PhD clinical psychologist at Africa Mental Health Research and Training Foundation, has an interest in mental health with underserved and marginalised populations in Kenya. She has served as PI and Co-I in mental health and substance-abuse projects.

David M. Ndetei is Professor of Psychiatry in the University of Nairobi; Director of Africa Mental Health Research and Training Foundation (AMHRTF); and Director of the World Psychiatric Association Collaborating Centre for Research and Training, Kenya. He is also a member of various professional mental health and psychiatry bodies across the globe.

Professor Alexandra (Alex) Parker is the Executive Director, Institute for Health and Sport (IHES), Victoria University. Alex leads a multidisciplinary research group that aims to measure, understand and promote physical activity to optimise mental well-being and prevent and treat mental health problems and is a practising clinical psychologist.

Karen O'Connor is a consultant psychiatrist and the National Clinical Lead for the Early Intervention in Psychosis Clinical Programme. Dr O'Connor is a medical graduate of University College Cork, Ireland. She completed most of her postgraduate training in psychiatry in Dublin but also spent one year on a fellowship at Orygen Youth Mental Health Service in Melbourne, Australia. Dr O'Connor has a Medical Doctorate in Early Intervention in Psychosis with RCSI and is the Clinical Lead of the RISE service, an Early Intervention in Psychosis service in South Lee, Cork, Ireland.

Dr Aileen O'Reilly is Research and Evaluation Manager at Jigsaw: The National Centre for Youth Mental Health, Ireland, and adjunct Assistant Professor in the School of Psychology, University College Dublin (UCD). Her research/evaluation work has played a critical role in the development of youth mental health services.

Susan Preece has worked in the mental health Lived Experience workforce for 15 years. Currently Susan works at Orygen, Australia as senior family/carer consultant, as well as being a consultant for the Lived Experience Workforce nationally and internationally. She believes passionately in hope and recovery for both young people and their families.

Debra Rickwood (PhD) is Professor of Psychology at the University of Canberra, Australia; Chief Scientific Advisor for *headspace*, Australia's National Youth Mental Health Foundation; and Fellow of the Australian Psychological Society. Her research focuses on help-seeking behaviour for mental health issues.

Dr Magenta Simmons is a senior research fellow at Orygen and the Centre for Youth Mental Health at The University of Melbourne, Australia. She has expertise in youth involvement, including shared decision-making, peer support and youth partnerships in research.

Lorraine Swords PhD is an assistant professor in child and adolescent psychology at Trinity College Dublin. She has particular research interest in peer interactions in the context of physical or mental health conditions, focusing on children's help-seeking, help-giving and stigmatising responses.

Dr Yifeng Wei is an expert in school-based mental health literacy. She is currently an assistant professor with the Department of Psychiatry, Faculty of Medicine and Dentistry at the University of Alberta, Canada. Dr Wei's research interests focus on promoting mental health literacy and improving the quality of referral between systems.

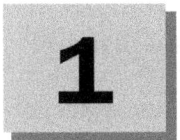

1 Introduction and overview

Eilis Hennessy
University College Dublin, Ireland

Caroline Heary
National University of Ireland, Galway, Ireland

Maria Michail
University of Birmingham, UK

Introduction

The last decade has seen the growth of a significant movement to rethink and reshape mental health services that are offered to young people around the world. Publications like the The International Declaration on Youth Mental Health (Coughlan et al. 2013) and the World Economic Forum report on youth mental health (WEF, 2020) represent significant milestones in bringing international attention to the importance of young people's well-being as well as the challenges that must be addressed to ensure that it remains a priority in countries around the world. These publications highlight key principles that place the needs and perspectives of young people at their core: awareness of the context of adolescent development; rapid, easy and affordable access to mental health services; youth-specific care; early intervention; youth partnership; family engagement and support; continuous improvement; and prevention. These are explored in more detail below. The theory that underpins each of these principles as well as research providing evidence to support their importance has been growing in recent years.

Led by service providers and researchers in Australia, Ireland and the UK (McGorry et al. 2013), this new approach to youth mental health services has taken a developmental perspective on mental health in adolescence and emerging adulthood, highlighting the significance of this period of development and drawing attention to the distinctive challenges that young people face in the 21st century. This new model of care has contributed to the redesign of services in some contexts, through processes of consultation with young people and communities in order to ensure that services are accessible, meeting the needs of service users and are non-judgemental and non-stigmatising.

In addition, within this movement significant emphasis is placed on evidence-based approaches promoting young people's mental health and improving mental health literacy. Schools and colleges are ideal venues for such educational interventions; evidence for their value is emerging (Barry et al. 2013) although more robust data is required (Reis et al. 2021).

What characterises the youth mental health approach to service delivery?

Research evidence, professional leadership, grassroots movement and the wider policy context have long now supported the need for transformational change in how we respond to the global youth mental health crisis. The need for 'fit for purpose' mental health systems and services for young people has been at the forefront of key initiatives across the globe including *The Global Strategy for Women's, Children's and Adolescents' Health (2016–30)* (Every Woman Every Child, 2015); as well as the previously mentioned International Declaration on Youth Mental Health (Coughlan et al. 2013) and more recently the Global Framework for Youth Mental Health (WEF, 2020). These initiatives adopt a life-course approach to a young person's health and well-being, physical and mental, while providing the roadmap for global service reform and innovation at the heart of which are young people themselves.

A youth mental health approach to service reform and delivery is one which acknowledges, respects and embraces the unique, complex and ever-changing needs of young people by designing systems and services that are developmentally, socially and culturally sensitive and appropriate (McGorry et al. 2013). The key principles underlying such an approach, as outlined in the WEF Global Framework for Youth Mental Health (2020), are listed below.

- **Youth participation** across all levels of service reform, redesign and delivery to ensure services are safe, feasible and acceptable to young people and their families.
- **Enhanced and integrated primary and community-based services** where young people can seek and receive support for any health issues including mental health, physical health and social care. A prime example of this is the *headspace* model in Australia designed to offer multidisciplinary youth-friendly services, including primary care, mental health, substance use and vocational, to young people aged 12–25 (McGorry et al. 2013). Such a service model allows for inclusive, personalised and coordinated care for young people and their families while capitalising on the skills and expertise of a diverse workforce working collaboratively.
- **Focus on early intervention and prevention** through the provision of developmentally appropriate and personalised care in order to reduce long-term mortality and morbidity (McGorry & Mei, 2018). Seventy-five per cent of all mental health problems develop before the age of 25; and are associated with significant impairment and relapse in adulthood (Patel et al. 2007). The basic principle of early intervention is the early identification of young people who might be at risk for the development of future mental health problems. Intervening at the right time through the provision of appropriate and personalised care can support successful outcomes (McGorry & Mei, 2018). Young people often seek help early for anxiety, low mood, distress and poor functioning from various sources including primary care (Rickwood et al. 2007). At that time, access to care and service provision should focus on their needs rather than crude diagnostic criteria.
- **Continuity of care and accessibility** eliminating arbitrary boundaries between child and adult mental health services, thus ensuring a smooth transition

during developmental periods when risk for experiencing mental health difficulties is elevated.

These key principles have guided service innovation across many high-income countries including Australia, the UK and Ireland. It is important, however, to highlight that the implementation of a youth mental health approach to service reform needs to take into account key contextual factors including cultural, socio-economic, religious, infrastructure and resources. In countries, for example, where suicide remains illegal, young people are likely to be hesitant to seek help and access care for fear of consequences (International Association for Suicide Prevention, 2021). Understanding the impact that the wider context can have on young people's willingness to seek help will ensure that any service reform is culturally sensitive, meaningful and acceptable to local context (WEF, 2020).

The voice of young people

As we have already noted, youth participation is at the core of recent efforts to reimagine youth mental health services. In countries and states where this approach is being implemented it has resulted in a notable shift in policy, practice and service provision with efforts to strengthen and support the voice of our youth in shaping policy and service development. The benefits of youth participation on health, well-being and self-development have increasingly been recognised. Many countries have signed up to the UN Convention of the Rights of the Child (1990) which gives children and young people the right to be involved in matters that affect their lives. Creating sustainable mechanisms to support the meaningful engagement of young people at a research, service and policy level remains critically important (Efuribe et al. 2020).

Recognising the expertise of young people and valuing their lived experiences can create opportunities for shared understanding of their needs, experiences and preferences. Understanding the needs and experiences of young people is important when developing or tailoring interventions and supports for their needs. For example, Thabrew et al. (2018) report on three different co-design projects to develop e-health supports for young people's mental health; they note the importance of the use of appropriate settings and techniques to ensure meaningful engagement and participation from these groups. Actively listening to the voices of diverse groups of young people can also help to contextualise efforts to support youth mental health and address local needs in local communities.

Supporting youth involvement in the design and development of services is key to creating services that are fit for purpose. New models of service delivery are emerging, involving enhanced user participation and shared decision-making. These developments place the young person at the centre of decisions on their care and treatment and provide more person-centred models of care. However, to date most research on shared decision-making and the development of collaborative care plans has been conducted in adult mental health settings (Bjønness et al. 2020).

Increased support has also been garnered for the involvement and meaningful participation of young people in all aspects of youth mental health research (Mei et al. 2020). Public patient involvement is increasingly required from funders, with the potential to change the research landscape. The involvement of young people as advisors or 'authors' of the research, can help shape research agendas and the design and dissemination of individual projects (Wilson, 2020). There is emerging consensus on the importance of meaningful inclusion of young people, to ensure research is consequential and relevant (Sharma et al. 2021). Qualitative research has been found to be particularly important in capturing the narratives of young people with lived experiences. However, there is still some way to go as Fazel and Hoagwood (2021) recently commented on the absence of the student voice from much school-based mental health research.

Throughout the planning and writing of this textbook, we have incorporated the perspectives of young people in a variety of different ways. At the planning and design stage of the book, we sought input from the Youth Advisory Group of the YOULEAD Doctoral Training Programme in the National University of Ireland, Galway, on what should be included in this textbook. Authors of individual chapters were encouraged to highlight examples of youth participation, where possible, as well as identifying where gaps remain in young people's involvement. For example, in Chapter 4 the authors make a clear call for involving young people as co-creators in the development of mental health promotion programmes. In Chapter 11, which is co-authored with youth advocates, models of youth participation are introduced and a series of recommendations are presented as to how services can facilitate meaningful youth participation. The chapter also highlights two international case studies in order to provide insight into youth participation in action at a service level. Chapter 13 emphasises the importance of meaningful engagement of young people and their families in the design and delivery of services.

One of the recommendations that emerged from our consultation with the Youth Advisory Group was to provide readers with direct accounts of the experiences of young people, in their own words. In order to do this, we have drawn from our own research programmes and engagement activities to include insights from young people and parents on their experiences of seeking and accessing mental health support as well as their experiences of living with mental health difficulties. These quotations from young people and parents are interspersed throughout the book. For examples see pages 11, 43, 60, 91, 122, 148, 181, 197 and 213. These quotes illustrate the challenges young people and their families faced when reaching out for help, the concerns and fears some had around sharing stories about their mental health difficulties with others, but also some of the positive aspects of their experiences, as reported by young people and their families.

What we set out to do

Despite world-wide interest in this new approach to youth mental health, the academic literature of relevance is scattered across journals in psychiatry, clinical psychology, social science and developmental psychology, among other disciplines. A student trying to develop a cohesive picture of the nature of this approach to youth mental health would have difficulty linking the disparate

publications and making sense of them in the context of the much larger literature on traditional approaches of clinical psychiatry and psychology. Our plan
for this book is to provide students with a conceptual map of the approach as
well as detailed introductions to each of its key elements. Collectively the chapters provide students with a foundation for developing their understanding of
individual topics while allowing them to see how the various elements fit
together.

In writing the book we set out to be as inclusive as possible. We started by
focusing on being geographically inclusive and invited authors from around the
world and are delighted to have contributors from eight different countries with
disparate research and clinical experience. Our authors are from Australia, Canada, France, Kenya, Ireland, United Kingdom, New Zealand and Switzerland.
You will also see that, where possible, the chapters draw on research findings
from around the world and not just from high-income countries. In addition,
Chapter 8 provides a specific focus on youth mental health service provision
in Kenya. Our YOULEAD Youth Advisory Group also advised at the outset on
the importance of representing young people from a diverse array of
backgrounds.

There are many more topics that we could usefully have considered in the
book. For example, we do not have a chapter on the economic argument for
investing in prevention, support and treatment for young people. This is despite
the fact that there is growing evidence that investment in these services makes
economic sense (Le et al. 2021; McDaid et al. 2019). Another topic that is not considered in the book is the gap between research evidence and its implementation
in practice. Unfortunately, demonstrating that an intervention is effective is not
the end of the road and it cannot be assumed that this will automatically result in
implementation (Langley et al. 2010). However, we believe that the breadth of
topics that we have included will give the reader an introduction to a much wider
range of topics critical to understanding youth mental health than other books on
the market and will ignite interest in pursuing other related issues. While an argument could be made for the inclusion of many other topics in this textbook, given
the relative novelty of the youth mental health approach we have chosen to focus
on bringing together a selection of key topics and to leave the interested reader
to follow up on these issues. To this end, each chapter includes a list of further
suggested readings.

The language that we use in the book

There is much semantic confusion associated with mental health and mental ill-
health and a plethora of terms are in use. There can also be disagreements regarding the preferred terminology to use. Bolinger (2021) argues that reliance on
generic terms such as *mental health challenges* to refer to the gamut of mental
health experiences, may trivialise the impact that mental health disorders can
have on individuals. Malla and colleagues (2020) discuss an emerging trend to
identify newly emerging youth mental health services, as 'wellness centres' for
example. The authors however, argue that while the concept of wellness may be
more semantically attractive, it may not subsume the range of treatments and

supports required for youth with mental health disorders. Throughout this book, we will adopt the World Health Organization definition of mental health: 'Mental health is a state of well-being in which an individual realises his or her own abilities, can cope with the normal stresses of life, can work productively and is able to make a contribution to his or her community.'

The authors of the mental health literacy programme *The Guide* argue for the importance of clarity in the language that we use and the need to distinguish, on one hand, between day-to-day fluctuations in mood and, on the other hand, mental health disorders that have been diagnosed by a mental health professional using an internationally recognised system of classification (Kutcher & Wei, 2017).

Within this textbook, we use the terms 'mental health problem/difficulty' interchangeably to refer to the experience of mental distress and/or specific symptoms identified by responses to standardised questionnaires but which do not necessarily refer to a formal diagnosis. Thus, a young person may have a high score on a questionnaire that measures anxiety/depression, which signals that they are experiencing distress, but this does not mean that they have a diagnosed 'disorder'.

Throughout this textbook, we also will use the term 'disorder' to identify a clinical diagnosis according to DSM or ICD criteria. The WHO in their *Comprehensive Action Plan* (2013–30) use the term 'mental disorders' to denote a range of mental and behavioural disorders that fall within the *International Statistical Classification of Diseases and Related Health Problems, Tenth revision* (ICD-10). These include disorders that cause a high burden of disease such as depression, bipolar affective disorder, schizophrenia, anxiety disorders, substance-use disorders, intellectual disabilities and developmental and behavioural disorders with onset usually occurring in childhood and adolescence, including autism. The recent Global Framework for Youth Mental Health (WEF, 2020) also uses this term. While we understand that this terminology may not appeal to all readers of our book and it was not the first preference of many chapter authors, there is as of yet no universally agreed alternative terminology.

Throughout this textbook, we seek to adopt person-based terminology. The intention of this is to reflect the 'disorder or illness is only one aspect of a person's life, not the defining characteristic' (Volkow et al. 2021 p. 2).

Definitions of the terms 'adolescence' and 'youth' also vary. We reviewed several authoritative sources to arrive at our definitions of adolescent age groups (e.g. Arnett et al., Žukauskienė & Sugimura, 2014; Sawyer et al. 2018). We have also taken into account the widespread use of the word 'youth' in the description of mental health services specifically designed to meet the needs of young people. Our chosen terms are a compromise but we hope that they will serve the purpose of allowing consistency across chapters in the book.

- Adolescence: 10–19 years old
- Early adolescence/younger adolescents: 10–14 years old
- Late adolescence/older adolescents: 15–19 years old
- Youth: 15–24 years old
- Young people: 10–24 years old
- Emerging adulthood: 18–24 years old

How the book is structured

As we noted in the introductory paragraphs to this chapter, the aim of the book is to provide the reader with a single source of up-to-date theory, research and practice on the range of topics relevant to this new approach to youth mental health. A key feature of the book is that it does not have the diagnosis of mental disorders as its primary focus. Instead, the book takes the key principles of a developmental approach to adolescence and emerging adulthood. It structures the chapters around aspects of the environment, neurological development, understanding of mental health, help-seeking and stigma, as well as including chapters on the epidemiology of mental health difficulties and service development and provision, all of which are critical to understanding the context of mental health in adolescence.

Chapter 2 introduces the reader to the developmental context of adolescence and emerging adulthood as a time of significant physical and neurological changes that precipitate changes in cognition (increased analytic ability), emotional maturity (growing independence from parents) and social role expectations. In order to fully understand youth mental health, it is necessary to understand the nature of these changes and their impact on the developing person and their relationships with their family and their peer group.

Although the relationship between social context and mental health is well established in adulthood there has been much less research with young people. However, there is now a growing body of research evidence on the influence of social context beyond family on the mental health and well-being of young people. Chapter 3 explores the evidence of the associations between different social determinants of health and the mental health of young people. The chapter focuses on key aspects of young people's lives such as socio-economic status, race and social media.

Chapter 4 links mental health and well-being and identifies their critical importance for individuals and communities in all cultures. Evidence from a wide range of school- and community-based mental health interventions for young people indicates that well-designed programmes can achieve a wide range of positive outcomes including positive behavioural change, increased self-confidence and self-esteem as well as reduced symptoms of depression and anxiety. The chapter introduces the topic of mental health promotion, which seeks to elevate levels of positive mental health and protect against its loss.

Stigma has long been regarded as a central feature of the experience of having a mental health problem and although it has been studied more in adults than in adolescents and emerging adults there is a growing body of research showing that high levels of stigma or the fear of stigma are powerful forces that are associated with lower levels of help-seeking and self-blame among young people who have or suspect that they may have a mental disorder. Chapter 5 introduces the concept of mental health stigma and synthesises research findings on the forms that mental health stigma can take during adolescence and emerging adulthood and what we can do to address these changes.

International research reports that only a minority of young people in need of professional help have accessed it. This is a cause for concern as problems that are treated quickly are more likely to be alleviated and less likely to persist over time (Hooven et al. 2010). Chapter 6 explores the factors associated with help-seeking and considers how to overcome the obstacles faced by young people and their families as well as the role of emerging digital technologies in supporting young people's help-seeking.

Chapter 7 introduces the concept of mental health literacy, providing examples of such interventions and an analysis of their impact on young people's mental health and well-being. The chapter also considers schools' wider role in supporting young people's mental health and how schools – as communities – may differ from one another in the extent to which they work collectively to promote a sense of well-being, address the emotional needs of young people (e.g. through provision of pastoral care) and have adequate structures for addressing mental health promotion.

The great majority of studies on youth mental health are carried out in countries with high incomes, despite the fact that the great majority of young people in the world live in low- and middle-income countries (LMIC; Kieling et al. 2011). Taking the example of Kenya, in Chapter 8 the authors explore the mental health needs of young people and consider the challenges associated with delivering youth-focused mental health interventions. They provide examples of good practice in the development and implementation of interventions and family-focused youth-friendly services.

Adolescence and emerging adulthood are developmental periods during which many will experience mental health difficulties and when most adult mental disorders initially present. Chapter 9 introduces the international epidemiological data on the emergence and prevalence of mental health problems during these life stages. The authors also present evidence on changes in prevalence over time, and the challenges posed by the wide variety of different measures and sampling strategies used by researchers.

Chapter 10 describes the development of early intervention services and their underpinning theories. The authors emphasise the importance of 'hitting the right target' by reducing the duration of untreated illness, reducing symptoms and improving function. The authors also discuss pharmacological and psychological treatments.

A focus on involving young people and families in the design of services is one of the key differences between new youth mental health service models and the older CAMHS services. Involving adolescents and emerging adults in the design of all features of a youth mental health service model has many potential advantages: consultation with young people in the context of their developing autonomy and independence can result in empowerment and great lifelong engagement; engagement with young people ensures that services are designed to meet their needs and avoids the potential for alienation. Chapter 11 explores the ways in which young people have been involved in mental health service development and the research evidence on the benefits of this engagement.

Family support is critical for the well-being of the majority of young people and this is true whether a young person has no mental health problem or has been diagnosed with a serious mental disorder. Chapter 12 explores the ways in which family engagement in the professional services offered to young people who have diagnosed mental disorders can support recovery and help to maintain functioning.

The chapter also notes the fact that these families will also have support needs and considers how these can be provided.

In the last decade, several models of youth mental health service delivery have emerged in different parts of the world that enshrine the key elements of the International Declaration on Youth Mental Health. Chapter 13 briefly introduces three of these new models to give the reader an insight into the workings of these models and the diversity that can exist when services respond to the needs of local communities and health services.

Summary

There is growing international awareness of the importance of taking young people's mental health seriously and ensuring that the appropriate preventive supports and clinical services are in place to enable optimal development and early intervention when needed. The chapters that follow develop on each of the issues considered in this introduction and present the reader with a starting point for further enquiry on each of the important topics.

References

Arnett, J. J., Žukauskienė, R., & Sugimura, K. (2014). The new life stage of emerging adulthood at ages 18–29 years: Implications for mental health. *The Lancet Psychiatry, 1*(7), 569–576.

Barry, M. M., Clarke, A. M., Jenkins, R., & Patel, V. (2013). A systematic review of the effectiveness of mental health promotion interventions for young people in low and middle income countries. *BMC Public Health, 13*(1), 1–19.

Bjönness, S., Viksveen, P., Johannessen, J.O., & Storm, M. (2020). User participation and shared decision-making in adolescent mental healthcare: A qualitative study of healthcare professionals' perspectives. *Child Adolescent Psychiatry Mental Health, 14, 2.* https://doi.org/10.1186/s13034-020-0310-3

Bolinger, R.J. (2021). The Language of Mental Illness. In J. Khoo & R. Sterken (Eds). *The Routledge Handbook of Social and Political Philosophy of Language.* Routledge.

Coughlan, H., Cannon, M., Shiers, D., Power, P., Barry, C., Bates, T., Birchwood, M., Buckley, S., Chambers, D., Davidson, S., Duffy, M., Gavin, B., Healy, C., Healy, C., Keeley, H., Maher, M., Tanti, C., & McGorry, P. (2013). Towards a new paradigm of care: The international Declaration on Youth Mental Health. *Early Intervention in Psychiatry, 7*(2), 103-108. DOI: 10.1111/eip.12048

Efuribe, C., Barre-Hemingway, M., Vaghefi, E., & Suleiman, A.B. (2020). Coping with the COVID-19 crisis: A call for youth engagement and the inclusion of young people in matters that affect their lives. *Journal of Adolescent Health, 67,* 16–17.

Every Woman Every Child. (2015). *The Global Strategy for Women's, Children's and Adolescents' Health (2016–2030).* https://globalstrategy.everywomaneverychild.org/

Fazel, M., & Hoagwood, K. (2021). School mental health: Integrating young people's voices to shift the paradigm. *Lancet Child & Adolescent Health, 5,* 156–157. DOI: 10.1016/S2352-4642(20)30388-6. Epub 2021 Jan 21. PMID: 33484659.

Hooven, C., Herting, J. R., & Snedker, K. A. (2010). Long-term outcomes for the Promoting CARE Suicide Prevention Program. *American Journal of Health Behavior, 34*(6), 721–736. https://doi.org/10.5993/AJHB.34.6.8

International Association for Suicide Prevention. (2021). Decriminalising Suicide: Saving Lives Reducing Stigma. https://unitedgmh.org/sites/default/files/2021-09/UNITEDGMH%20Suicide%20Report%202021%C6%92.pdf October 17, 2021

Kieling, C., Baker-Henningham, H., Belfer, M., Conti, G., Ertem, I., Omigbodun, O., Rohde, L. A., Srinath, S., Ulkuer, N., & Rahman, A. (2011). Child and adolescent mental health worldwide: Evidence for action. *The Lancet, 378*(9801), 1515–1525. DOI:10.1016/S0140-6736(11)60827-1

Kutcher, S. & Wei, Y. (2017). Mental Health and High School Curriculum Guide (Guide v.3). Mental Health & High School Curriculum Guide. Understanding mental health and mental illness. Canada: Teenmentalhealth.org

Langley, A. K., Nadeem, E., Kataoka, S. H., Stein, B. D., & Jaycox, L. H. (2010). Evidence-based mental health programs in schools: Barriers and facilitators of successful implementation. *School Mental Health, 2*(3), 105–113.

Le, L. K. D., Esturas, A. C., Mihalopoulos, C., Chiotelis, O., Bucholc, J., Chatterton, M. L., & Engel, L. (2021). Cost-effectiveness evidence of mental health prevention and promotion interventions: A systematic review of economic evaluations. *PLoS Medicine, 18*(5), e1003606.

Malla A., Frampton A., & Mansouri B.I. (2020). Youth mental health services: Promoting wellness or treating mental illness? *The Canadian Journal of Psychiatry, 65*(8):531–535. DOI: 10.1177/0706743720920033

McDaid, D., Park, A.L., & Wahlbeck, K. (2019). The economic case for the prevention of mental illness. *Annual Review of Public Health, 40*, 373–389. https://doi.org/10.1146/annurev-publhealth-040617-013629

McGorry, P.D., & Mei, C. (2018). Early intervention in youth mental health: Progress and future directions. *Evidence-Based Mental Health, 21*, 182–184.

McGorry, P., Bates, T., & Birchwood, M. (2013). Designing youth mental health services for the 21st century: Examples from Australia, Ireland and the UK. *The British Journal of Psychiatry, 202*(s54), s30–s35.

Mei, C., Fitzsimons, J., Allen, N., Alvarez-Jimenez, M., Amminger, G.P., Browne, V., Cannon, M., Davis, M., Dooley, B., & Hickie, I.B. (2020). Global research priorities for youth mental health. *Early Intervention in Psychiatry, 14, 3*–13.

Patel, V., Flisher, A. J., Hetrick, S., & McGorry, P. (2007). Mental health of young people: A global public-health challenge. *The Lancet, 369*(9569), 1302–1313.

Reis, A.C., Saheb, R., Moyo, T. *et al.* (2021). The impact of mental health literacy training programs on the mental health literacy of university students: A systematic review. *Prevention Science.* https://doi.org/10.1007/s11121-021-01283-y

Rickwood, D. J., Deane, F. P., & Wilson, C. J. (2007). When and how do young people seek professional help for mental health problems? *Medical Journal of Australia, 187*(S7), S35–S39.

Sawyer, S. M., Azzopardi, P. S., Wickremarathne, D., & Patton, G. C. (2018). The age of adolescence. *The Lancet Child & Adolescent Health, 2*(3), 223–228.

Sharma, U., Sokal, L., Wang, M., & Loreman, T. (2021). Measuring the use of inclusive practices among pre-service educators: A multi-national study. *Teaching and Teacher Education, 107*, 103506, https://doi.org/10.1016/j.tate.2021.103506.

Thabrew, H., Fleming, T., Hetrick, S. & Merry, S. (2018). Co-design of eHealth interventions with children and young people. *Frontiers in Psychiatry, 9*: 481. DOI: 10.3389/fpsyt.2018.00481

United Nations. (1990). *Human rights: The rights of the child.* Fact Sheet No. 10. Geneva: United Nations.

Volkow, N., Gordon, J., & Koob, G. (2021). Choosing appropriate language to reduce the stigma around mental illness and substance use disorders. *Neuropsychopharmacology.* DOI: 10.1038/s41386-021-01069-4

Wilson, E. (2020) Where next for youth mental health? Reflections on current research and considerations for the future, *Journal of Mental Health, 29*(4), 371–375, DOI: 10.1080/09638237.2020.1766001

World Economic Forum. (2020). *A Global Framework for Youth Mental Health: Investing in Future Mental Capital for Individuals, Communities and Economies.* https://www.weforum.org/reports/a-global-framework-for-youth-mental health-db3a7364df

World Health Organization. (2021). Comprehensive mental health action plan 2013–2030. Geneva: World Health Organization. Licence: CC BY-NC-SA 3.0 IGO.

Quotation from a young person who participated in Lynn McKeague's (2013) Doctoral Dissertation, University College Dublin.

'In secondary school, more so than any place else, your place in the school is defined by how normal you seem to everyone. [...] If you've got something that sticks you out [sic], and you can't do anything to change it, it makes you different, it makes you weird. And in secondary school, that's not allowed.'

2 Biological, cognitive, social and emotional development

Samantha Dockray
University College Cork, Ireland

Nadine Messerli-Bürgy
University of Lausanne, Switzerland

Introduction

The second and third decades of life are periods of great transformation, during which there is profound development of the biological, cognitive, social and emotional aspects of the person. The period of early adolescence, considered to be from 10–14 years old, is developmentally distinctive, in part as it encompasses the processes of puberty and brain maturation. The person continues this process of biopsychosocial development in late adolescence (15–19 years old) and emerging adulthood (18–24 years old) (Arnett et al. 2014; Sawyer et al. 2018) and these are remarkable changes the young person experiences within a specific social and cultural context. Adolescence and emerging adulthood are sensitive periods for mental health, partly due to the direct effects of biological change on thoughts and feelings, and in part via indirect pathways of changes in the expectations of others about the capacities of the person. During this period of youth the person's understanding of themselves and their world develops iteratively, via introspection and interactions with others. Mostly, these changes are experienced without extreme difficulty or distress, but for some people, these biopsychosocial transitions may activate a pre-existing vulnerability or create a risk for mental health disorder.

During adolescence and emerging adulthood the capacity for abstract and analytical thinking improves, and greater introspection and meta-cognitive processes are possible. There are changes in the emotional and social aspects of the person, including the development of emotion-regulation skills, and the ability to take another person's perspective is enhanced. During youth there is an increasing value placed on peers and friends as a source of emotional support, and adolescents develop independence from their families; developing bonds with friends that can support positive youth development. In early adolescence, between the ages of 10–14 years old, people are acutely sensitive to evaluations by peers, and in seeking peer approval, may engage in greater risk-taking however this is developmentally normative and can contribute to an emerging sense of self as a competent, confident person at late adolescence and emerging adulthood.

Biopsychosocial models of well-being during adolescence and emerging adulthood indicate the complexities of interactions at all levels of the person, and within the wider cultural context (Sawyer et al. 2012). More recent theoretical and empirical work evidence that these interactions are more intricate, time-sensitive and impactful on youth mental health than previously conceptualised. Developmentally sensitive models of mental health difficulties must incorporate a multi-faceted approach inclusive of the neurological, neuroendocrine, cognitive, social and emotional changes to adequately represent the complexity of youth development, which begins in late childhood and extends through to emerging adulthood.

Biological development

Puberty

Puberty encompasses myriad physical and biological changes and is a central component in theories of adolescent well-being (Dorn et al. 2019; Viner et al. 2017; Worthman et al. 2019). Typically, puberty occurs during early adolescence (10–14 years old) but some people may continue pubertal development into late adolescence (15–19 years old). Puberty and adolescence are different yet interactive processes; biological changes shape experience, development and behaviour and in turn, experiences and behaviour have the potential to alter biological processes. There is considerable evidence which demonstrates that puberty is associated with mental health difficulties (Angold et al. 1998; Byrne et al. 2017; Costello et al. 2011; Mendle et al. 2020) including anxiety, depression, conduct problems, substance misuse and eating disorders (Beltz et al. 2014; Rudolph, 2014), and although puberty tends to occur in early adolescence, the effects may play out across late adolescence and into emerging adulthood. Puberty and mental health are associated via two pathways:

1. directly, via the effects of hormones on brain activity and development, resulting in changes to patterns of thinking and emotions
2. indirectly, via changes in social experiences in response to changes in the person's physical appearance, which prompt changes in self-perceptions and the perceptions of others (Rudolph, 2014; Susman and Dorn, 2013).

Puberty has overlapping phases:

1. adrenarche, when the adrenal glands are 'awakened' with a subsequent rise in adrenal androgens
2. gonadarche, when the ovaries and testes begin to grow and the production of sex steroids increases. Both adrenarche and gonadarche have been related to adolescent development mental health (Byrne et al. 2017; Ladouceur et al. 2012). Despite long-standing evidence of an association between adrenarche and mental health, there has been a greater focus on the relationship of gonadarche, and emotional and behavioural problems. This may be partially explained by considering the research methods used, as the effects of gonadarche (e.g. changes in breast size) are more visible than those of adrenarche. Pubertal processes develop on individual timelines, with differences in personal and social meanings and subsequently, effects on psychosocial development and mental health (Negriff & Susman, 2011; Rudolph & Troop-Gordon, 2010).

Puberty may affect mental health through an indirect pathway, as the pubertal transition may be inherently stressful, and stress may activate a vulnerability to mental health problems (Conley & Rudolph, 2009; Ge & Natsuaki, 2009). There is evidence for this hypothesis although emotional difficulties during puberty do not always arise, and an alternate explanation is biologically based, explaining internalising symptoms (e.g. depression, anxiety) and externalising symptoms (e.g. antisocial behaviours) in relation to a rapid increase in hormones (Brooks-Gunn & Warren, 1989; Schulz et al. 2009; Schulz & Sisk, 2016), or when pubertal processes begin. Pubertal timing, the age at which puberty begins, and pubertal tempo, the rate at which a person progresses through puberty, are closely linked to youth mental health (Mendle et al. 2020; Negriff & Susman, 2011). Explanations for the consequences of being pubertally 'off-time' in comparison to peers emerges from two theoretical perspectives: maturational deviance and developmental readiness. The maturational deviance hypothesis posits vulnerability to mental health difficulty arises from the stress of being different from what is expected by adults, or from same-age peers. The developmental readiness hypothesis is more relevant to early pubertal timing. It highlights the risk of asynchronous physical, social, emotional and cognitive maturity, when the person is not sufficiently psychologically mature to appropriately respond to social expectations and behavioural norms that are shaped by the appearance of physical maturity (Graber, 2013; Negriff & Susman, 2011). The early timing of puberty, particularly in girls, is one of the most studied and well-replicated predictors of mental health difficulties in adolescence and emerging adulthood, independent of the cultural background (Deng et al. 2011; Joinson, et al. 2011; Ullsperger & Nikolas, 2017), and has been linked to antecedents such as adverse childhood experience (Belsky, 2019). These 'off-timing' hypotheses should be considered in relation to culture, ethnicity and gender role expectations, as these may influence the association of pubertal timing and mental health (Deardorff et al. 2021; Rudolph & Troop-Gordon, 2010).

Brain development

The brain is a complex system of connected structures, each with specific and general functions, and the structural and functional changes which occur in the brain during adolescence and emerging adulthood have a profound effect on the social and cognitive well-being, and mental health of the person. Neurons, the cells of the brain, form the bulk of the cerebral cortex and have grey cell bodies that are closer to the surface, layered over axonal 'tails' that are insulated with myelin. The number of, and connections between, the neurons in the prefrontal cortex are changed via processes of synaptic pruning and myelination during adolescence. Changes in the density of the cell's grey matter occur sequentially across brain regions, and the sensory and motor brain regions mature first, followed by the remainder of the cortex, with a 'back-to-front' pattern (see Figure 2.1) (Casey et al. 2008; Fuhrmann et al. 2015; Gogtay et al. 2004). The sequence of maturation maps onto the development of abilities; areas that are responsive to social and other rewards develop before the areas that contribute to self-regulation of emotions and behaviour, and to executive functioning (Casey et al. 2008; Giedd, 2004). The factors which determine the timing of brain development are not fully known, however it is likely a combination of several internal and external factors. Furthermore, there is a difference in the timing of this maturation in girls and boys, with the brains of girls maturing slightly earlier than boys (Wierenga et al. 2018).

Changes in the insulating myelin and in the number and strength of neural connections typify brain development and enable new abilities of the adolescent, beginning in early adolescence, with maturation of some form continuing into emerging adulthood. Just before puberty, there is a proliferation of new synapses – the space between neurons that enable transmission of electrochemical signals from one neuron to another – leading to an overabundance of neuronal connections (Casey et al. 2008). During late adolescence and into emerging adulthood, these connections can be reinforced or pruned away. The lived experiences of the youth contribute to this process; the neural pathways that are activated more frequently get reinforced, and are more likely to remain through adulthood, while those accessed less frequently are weakened and ultimately removed in the process of synaptic pruning. This pruning has been framed as a type of 'use it or lose it' rationalisation of the total number of synapses and connections between brain regions (Giedd, 2004; Goddings et al. 2019), as well as the strengthening of connections throughout the brain (Lerner, Scherf et al. 2019; Stevens et al. 2009). These processes contribute to a reorganisation of the brain, directly influencing a person's cognitive, emotional and social development, and in turn, their mental health.

Processes of synaptic pruning and myelination during adolescent development contribute to brain maturation (see Figure 2.1). Brain maturation is complete at approximately 25 years old, that is during emerging adulthood. The maturation of the prefrontal cortex **(indicated by the darker grey colour)** occurs in an ordered sequence, with the final developments in areas related to executive functions.

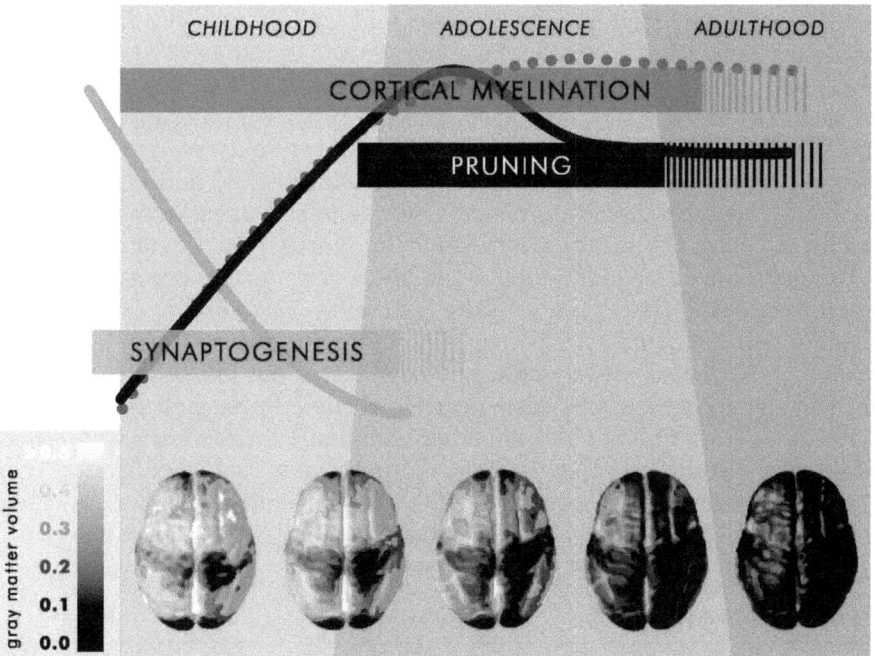

Figure 2.1 Parietal cortex to frontal cortex

Source: Adapted from Gogtay, et al. 2004, Copyright (2004) National Academy of Sciences, U.S.A.

The mid-adolescent brain has a maturational imbalance between the prefrontal cortex and the limbic system. The limbic system – an area which is involved in emotional responses and social sensitivity – begins to develop before the prefrontal regions which support emotion regulation, meta-cognition and the ability to think about one's thoughts. This difference in maturational timing of these brain structures provides a biological explanation for the increased inclination towards risk-taking, and heightened sensitivity to socio-emotional stimuli and rewards (Fuhrmann et al. 2015; Galván, 2017; Goddings et al. 2019). The person's emotional responsivity is further influenced by the changes in levels of neurotransmitters (such as dopamine and serotonin) in the limbic system and prefrontal cortex (Galván, 2017) which contribute to increased sensation-taking, and increased drive for immediate rewards, increased impulsivity and increased risk for substance misuse in young people (Geier, 2013; Guyer et al. 2016; Van Duijvenvoorde et al. 2016). The development of social cognitive processes, such as regulating emotions and considering other people's perspectives, support positive mental health and are reliant on the brain maturation that occurs during adolescence and emerging adulthood (Crone & Dahl, 2012; Fuhrmann et al. 2015), indicating that youth is a sensitive period for mental health.

Plasticity of the adolescent brain

The development of the brain can be influenced by the experiences of the person themselves, as neural connections are considered plastic and adaptive to the individual's patterns of thoughts and experiences. This brain plasticity may be affected by synaptic pruning, as the areas and amount of neuronal pruning are partially related to the repetition of experience and thoughts (Blakemore & Mills, 2014; Spear, 2013). There is relatively limited relevant research in human populations, however there is some evidence that the process of axonal myelination is partially determined by situational experiences (Fandakova & Hartley, 2020). This consolidates neural connections in late adolescence and emerging adulthood, making certain thought processes more likely to occur in the future. Brain plasticity indicates the salience of biological processes that occur during adolescent to mental health, as individual experience can literally change the ways in which the brain will function across the life course. The unique pattern of neural connections in the brain of a person, known as the connectome, is shaped by individual experiences and thought patterns across the life course, and is especially sensitive to experiences during early and late adolescence (Kaufmann et al. 2017). Brain plasticity provides some explanation for individual differences in mental health (Tymofiyeva et al. 2017) and represents remarkable opportunities for positive development (Lerner et al. 2009) as enriching experiences can alter pruning and myelination (Chavez & Heatherton, 2015; Whittle et al. 2014).

Cognitive development

Pubertal maturation and brain development support youth cognitive development. Brain maturation contributes to improved decision-making about the balance of risk and reward, and changes in emotional arousal and motivation, which are also mediated by pubertal processes. The capacity to be self-reflective, self-directed and self-regulated relies on the maturation of the prefrontal cortex and the range of cognitive processing it supports. The maturation of cognitive abilities is not synchronous with social and emotional abilities, but this asynchrony is typical, and not inherently a risk for mental health difficulties among young people, although may become so in certain contexts (Galván, 2017; Geier, 2013).

During youth, executive functions, the set of cognitive processes that are necessary for the management of behaviour, such as self-monitoring and self-control, begin to assume 'control' over the emotional and social regulatory systems and this allows developments in self-regulation skills. This process is extended, over several years, however young people have already begun to experience heightened emotional arousal, and encounter emotionally charged situations, which may contribute to mental health vulnerabilities to mood disorders (Galván, 2017) and/or behavioural problems such as conduct disorders (Geier, 2013).

The brain continues to mature through to the mid-20s and this supports the development of higher-level cognitive functioning during emerging adulthood. During early adolescence, young people typically progress from concrete logical operations and problem solving to acquiring the ability to analyse and synthesise information about themselves and their experiences. Engagement with complex concepts increases and young people are enabled to think reflectively and develop meta-cognition (Konrad et al. 2013). With brain maturation comes an improved ability to consider the future and to develop personal goals at emerging adulthood. The increased capacity for analytical thought and reflection, including the development of moral and ethical thinking, exemplifies youth cognitive development (Larsen & Luna, 2018). The person in late adolescence and emerging adulthood may develop a more relativistic moral thinking, and more expert thinking linked to higher education and/or workplace experiences. The young person is developing autonomy, may have increasing goal-directed behaviours (for example completing college, establishing themselves in a workplace) and greater use of executive functions. Further, some facets of social cognition are continuing to develop throughout late adolescence and into emerging adulthood, for example increased sensitivity to other's perspectives (Taylor, 2015).

Emotional development during adolescence

Emotions serve as indicators that prompt the person to respond to a situation, with a coordinated set of physiological, experiential and behavioural response tendencies (John & Gross, 2007). Emotions impact on the individual's thought patterns, and the intensity and duration of an emotion determines the impact on an individual's well-being (Grusec & Hastings, 2014). Emotions can be experienced as overwhelming, and the skills of managing emotions are typically acquired during childhood and consolidated during adolescence and emerging adulthood. The experience of intensity, as well as frequency and valence of emotion (negative or positive) changes across youth. Negative emotions are more frequently experienced in late adolescence and emerging adulthood than during early adolescence, whereas positive emotions are experienced both less frequently, and

Table 2.1 Indicative changes in emotional, social and cognitive domains over the developmental stages of early, mid and late adolescence

	EARLY ADOLESCENCE	MID ADOLESCENCE	LATE ADOLESCENCE
EMOTIONAL	Peak emotional intensity. Increased emotional lability. Increased frequency of positive emotions.	Increased emotional clarity. Increased emotional awareness. Increasingly efficient emotion regulation.	Increased empathy. Increased frequency of negative emotions. Establishing efficient emotional regulation.
SOCIAL	Social support derived from peers. Increased sharing of feelings with peers. Increased sensitivity to social evaluation.	Increased risk-taking. Increased capacity for mentalising. Increased romantic & sexual interest.	Continuing identity formation. Development of social autonomy. Establishing intimate, secure relationships.
COGNITIVE	Development of formal operations. Increased attentional control & memory. Development of abstract & logical thinking.	Increased cognitive flexibility. Increased speed of thought-processing. Increased capacity for abstract reasoning.	Maturation of executive function. Capable of complex abstract reasoning. Maturation of introspection & metacognition.

less intensely from early to late adolescence and into emerging adulthood (Frost et al. 2015; Larson et al. 2002). Young people are more likely to experience mixed emotions, that is, concurrent emotions with opposite valence (Burkitt et al. 2019; Wintre & Vallance, 1994) and more rapidly changing emotions, especially at the onset of puberty (Larson et al. 2002; Maciejewski, 2015), which contributes to a change in emotionality and stress during adolescence. When the person enters emerging adulthood (at about 18 years old) these mixed emotions are more tolerable, and may actually contribute to measured decision-making, by guiding the consideration of the consequences for situations that have emotional weight.

Emotions are determined by the appraisal processes of an individual, where a person interprets a situation as beneficial or threatening, and as manageable or overwhelming, and this appraisal results in positive or negative emotions. Emotion regulation, the strategies used to manage emotions to modulate the intensity and/or duration of positive and negative emotions (Cicchetti et al. 1995; Gross, 1998), develops over childhood and youth (Zeman et al. 2006). The growth and maturation of the brain supports the increasing capacity for emotional awareness and improvement in emotional clarity (i.e. the ability to identify, label and characterise emotions). This enhances the efficiency of emotion-regulation strategies (i.e. reducing and limiting negative emotions), which in turn impacts on an individual's social functioning during adolescence and emerging adulthood, and supports positive social relationships.

The development of emotional competence in youth is represented by high levels of efficient emotion regulation, the ability of an individual to be aware of, and understand their own, and other people's emotions, and by empathy (Lau & Wu, 2012). The development of emotional competence is influenced by internal and external factors, for example, previous experiences of a person, understanding of emotion-relevant appraisal processes, personality and emotional socialisation (Morris et al. 2007). Peer interactions, especially friendships, can support this development in young people (Brown & Larson, 2009), for example one's own feelings can be validated through the perspective of a peer, and peers can model emotion regulation. The converse is also true, as friends may model inefficient strategies, or direct the child or adolescent towards more negative emotions, such as engaging in co-rumination which contributes to mental health problems (Rose et al. 2007). A broad range of mental health difficulties have been related to emotion regulation, as ineffective emotion regulation can result in high, prolonged distress, increasing the likelihood of mental health problems in adolescence and emerging adulthood.

Social development

Youth is a time of significant changes in social behaviour and improvement in social skills. During youth, social relationships with peers become increasingly important. Peer interactions typically become more frequent and intense (e.g. increased sharing of feelings) (Cairns et al. 1995) during early adolescence time spent with parents and family reduces, as young people prioritise social interactions with similarly aged peers. Although parental influence on social development continues, it is now in combination with the influence of peers who model and shape young people's expression and management of emotions and behaviour (Zeman et al. 2006). Developing social capital, including quality and access to supportive peer relationships, is an important predictor of youth mental health and, as such, the socialisation context (e.g. the education environment, work and new living environments in emerging adulthood or extracurricular activities in adolescence and emerging adulthood) is important (Adams & Berzonsky, 2008).

Social connections grow and often diversify in late adolescence and emerging adulthood, with increased complexity of individual and group relationships (Lerner & Steinberg, 2009), and peers provide an important social and emotional support during new or difficult challenges (Zimmer-Gembeck & Skinner, 2010). These peer interactions shape enduring relationship patterns for the person, providing a context to practice social communication, develop insight into the emotions, behaviours and experiences of others (i.e. mentalising), and providing and receiving emotional support in intimate and non-intimate relationships in late adolescence and emerging adulthood. Peer interactions and friendships can, however, amplify risk for mental health difficulties as young people have a strong desire for peer acceptance and value group belonging. Young people are sensitively attuned to the social evaluations of peers, and alert to signals of social exclusion (Somerville, 2013). This sensitivity to social feedback peaks in early adolescence (Silvers et al. 2012), and individuals become more vulnerable to peer rejection and victimisation (Reijntjes et al. 2011; Somerville, 2013). Negative peer experiences, and the increased risk to perceived peer rejection, can impact on the development of adolescents' emotion-regulation skills (Herd & Kim-Spoon, 2021) and result in increased risk-taking and mental health problems during adolescence and emerging adulthood. The heightened sensitivity to social evaluation in early adolescence tapers during late adolescence.

The development of a personal identity is a critical development task of adolescence and emerging adulthood (Arnett, 2007). During adolescence and emerging adulthood, people aim to achieve independence and social autonomy, and this development of identity also incorporates the development of moral values (Hardy et al. 2020) and identity. In sum, limited social competencies in youth cause difficulties in social relationships and social adaptability, and put adolescents at risk for low school achievement, low prosocial behaviour and high levels of mental health problems (Laceulle et al. 2019) which may continue into emerging adulthood. The consequences of limited social competencies may be more pronounced at emerging adulthood when major goals are sought, for example completion of education, stable work and financial independence, moving out and living on one's own as well as being in an intimate relationship or establishing a family.

Developmental processes and mental health

Explanatory models of young people's mental health must be developmentally-sensitive and consider the changes in cognitive, social and emotional aspects of the person. These psychosocio-emotional changes are unique to youth, prompted by the maturation of biological structures and processes, and mediated by social and cultural contexts. These changes can confer risks to youth and life-span mental health in several ways, for example, if the young person experiences the biopsychosocial transition as stressful, or by the activation of an existing vulnerability by biological or social processes. During early and late adolescence there is a maturational mismatch between brain regions responsible for emotional arousal and social sensitivity, and regions that guide higher-level thinking, introspection and meta-cognition may confer risk. However, this asynchronous development is experienced by all young people, but not all of them experience effects on their mental health. Individual differences in social and emotional developmental processes, and the individual's social environment may explain why some young people can fully leverage opportunities for positive growth, and some become more vulnerable to mental health difficulties such as anxiety, depression or eating disorders (Angold et al. 1998; Bakalar et al. 2015; Mendle et al. 2020).

Young people's mental health may also be affected by changes in others' expectations of the young people's behaviour and abilities. Adults, peers and others may perceive the young person as younger or older than they actually are, influenced by the stage of physical development, and expect the adolescent to have attained certain milestones of cognitive and psychosocial maturation. This is significantly less likely during emerging adulthood when there is greater concordance between perceptions of a person's physical, cognitive and social maturation. Increases in reflective self-evaluation and in the process of identity formation have also been associated with changes in emerging adults' mental health (Berzonsky & Kinney, 2019; Luyckx et al. 2008). Furthermore, the pace at which young individuals progress through developmental stages (e.g. some adolescents move through puberty faster than others) and pattern of identity formation (i.e. differences in the social-cognitive processes used to construct and maintain a sense of identity), may be salient to mental health (Berzonsky & Kinney, 2019). Furthermore, there may be additional risk for adolescents who are in minority groups (Meeus, 2011).

Anxiety in youth serves as an exemplar of how unique developmental processes can interact to predict onset, duration and symptomology of anxiety. Adolescence is a particularly high-risk period for the onset and intensification of several types of anxiety, for example social anxiety (Angold et al. 1998; Mendle et al. 2020). Pubertal stage and timing have both been associated with adolescent-onset anxiety, explained by the direct effects of hormones on brain activity, or by indirect pathways, via changes in social experiences in youth (Forbes & Dahl, 2010; Graber, 2013). The increased likelihood of experiencing anxiety during youth has also been linked to the activation of neural circuits related to emotion regulation, and an increased sensitivity to social processes, (Galván, 2017; Lockhart et al. 2018). Epidemiological studies have also shown that anxiety is also highly prevalent in emerging adulthood (Arnett et al. 2014) although the age of onset is most often in adolescence.

The risk of developing anxiety may be increased in stressful peer relationships, conversely, positive relationships may protect against increases in symptoms (Markovic & Bowker, 2017). Developing emotional regulatory processes, amplified by increased emotional reactivity and increasingly sophisticated social evaluation processes, which develop in early adolescence, have also been associated with adolescent onset anxiety (Young et al. 2019). These social, emotional and cognitive changes are mediated by the maturation of brain networks and by biological processes of puberty, but none are the sole effector of increased risk for onset or persistence of anxiety in youth. The tempo and timing of pubertal processes, and of brain maturation, may activate existing vulnerabilities, or create additional risk for mental health issues in youth. However, it is through the multiple interactions of each which provides the most comprehensive explanation of why anxiety is most likely to emerge at adolescence, and further exemplifies the unique developmental context of adolescence. Anxiety may be more likely to occur during early adolescence but can persist into emerging adulthood. There is a high prevalence of anxiety and depression during emerging adulthood, which has been explained with reference to feelings of being less 'adult' than expected (Arnett et al. 2014) and with consideration of the contextual factors such as economic climate (Ranta et al. 2020).

Furthering the understanding of youth development

Youth is a psychological, socio-emotional and biological maturational phase, and complex conceptual models are needed to fully articulate how it can influence mental health. As mental health is determined by multiple processes, experiences and individual differences operating within social, cultural and other contexts, interdisciplinary, multi-method approaches, are necessary to understand this unique transitionary period. However, there have been relatively few dedicated research efforts to examine the intricacies of the relationships between brain, puberty, and social and emotional changes of youth (Worthman et al. 2019) and there remain challenges in fully describing the dynamics of individual differences in development during adolescence and emerging adulthood (Currie, 2019). Large-scale, international studies of youth development and methodological advances can transform developmental science, but there remain significant opportunities to refine and apply models of youth development to support positive development. This could be achieved by interdisciplinary collaborations and transdiagnostic approaches and plaiting together theory and practice to understand the multidimensional aspects of mental health, fully articulating youth as an exceptional period of potential and vulnerability. Collaborations of young people during adolescence and during emerging adulthood, researchers, practitioners and others in participatory research projects, as well as the incorporation of ecological assessment approaches, will provide insight into the complex interplay of factors that contribute to mental health across the years of adolescence and emerging adulthood.

In recent years there has been increasing effort towards understanding mental health disorders in youth using transdiagnostic approaches. These provide a framework to understand why symptomologies may vary and have rapid onset at youth (Wichers et al. 2019). The transdiagnostic model conceives mental health as a set of six domains: positive valence systems, negative valence systems, cognitive systems, systems for social process, arousal/modulatory systems and sensorimotor systems. Each of these domains have varying units of measurement, analysis and development: genes, molecules, cells, circuits, physiology, behaviour, self-reports and paradigms (Dalgleish et al. 2020). The transdiagnostic approach may better articulate the fluctuations within and across positive and negative mental health processes and explicate why some people have trajectories of positive mental health in youth, and others have increased vulnerability to mental health difficulties.

Large-scale, longitudinal studies of adolescents' well-being have proven invaluable in understanding how mental health varies within and between adolescents, and across decades and countries, using measures and methods designed to represent the person from cellular to the social contextual level (e.g. Currie & Morgan, 2020; Zhao & Castellanos, 2016). Research-informed policy and practice that supports positive youth development should be drawn from data that is both rich in measurement type (e.g. socio-emotional and cognitive development, brain, puberty) and large in scale, fully representative of youth diversity (Berenbaum et al. 2015; Dahl et al. 2018; Lerner, Tirrell et al. 2019). Collaborative approaches to collecting big data that represents the complexity of development and mental health in youth would enable a birds-eye view of development and mental health in youth. Further, there is a need for greater focus on individual differences to adequately represent the many trajectories of young people's development (Dahl et al. 2018) which can provide opportunities to tailor preventive and interventional approaches for youth mental health. The many physical, cognitive, social and emotional changes experienced by young people may support positive development. However, some people may experience youth as a stressful and difficult period that confers or activates a vulnerability for mental health problems. These problems are caused by the interactions of biological, cognitive, social and emotional developments that make youth such a distinctive developmental period. With this exceptionalism comes increased vulnerability to mental health difficulties, and extraordinary opportunities for positive development of youth mental health.

Further reading

Blakemore, S. J., Burnett, S., & Dahl, R. E. (2010). The role of puberty in the developing adolescent brain. *Human Brain Mapping, 31*(6), 926–933.

Currie, C., & Morgan, A. (2020). A bio-ecological framing of evidence on the determinants of adolescent mental health – a scoping review of the international Health Behaviour in School-Aged Children (HBSC) Study 1983–2020. *SSM-Population Health*, 100697.

Powers, A., & Casey, B. J. (2015). The adolescent brain and the emergence and peak of psychopathology. *Journal of Infant, Child, and Adolescent Psychotherapy, 14*(1), 3–15.

Wood, D., Crapnell, T., Lau, L., Bennett, A., Lotstein, D., Ferris, M., & Kuo, A. (2018). Emerging adulthood as a critical stage in the life course. *Handbook of Life Course Health Development*, 123–143.

Young, K. S., Sandman, C. F., & Craske, M. G. (2019). Positive and negative emotion regulation in adolescence: links to anxiety and depression. *Brain Sciences, 9*(4), 76.

References

Adams, G. R., & Berzonsky, M. (2008). *Blackwell Handbook of Adolescence* (Vol. 8). John Wiley & Sons.

Angold, A., Costello, E. J., & Worthman, C. M. (1998). Puberty and depression: The roles of age, pubertal status and pubertal timing. *Psychological Medicine, 28*(1), 51–61.

Arnett, J. J. (2007). Emerging adulthood: What is it, and what is it good for? *Child Development Perspectives, 1*(2), 68–73.

Arnett, J. J., Žukauskiene, R., & Sugimura, K. (2014). The new life stage of emerging adulthood at ages 18–29 years: Implications for mental health. *The Lancet Psychiatry, 1*(7), 569–576.

Bakalar, J. L., Shank, L. M., Vannucci, A., Radin, R. M., & Tanofsky-Kraff, M. (2015). Recent advances in developmental and risk factor research on eating disorders. *Current Psychiatry Reports, 17*(6), 1–10.

Belsky, J. (2019). Early-life adversity accelerates child and adolescent development. *Current Directions in Psychological Science, 28*(3), 241–246.

Beltz, A. M., Corley, R. P., Bricker, J. B., Wadsworth, S. J., & Berenbaum, S. A. (2014). Modeling pubertal timing and tempo and examining links to behavior problems. *Developmental Psychology, 50*(12), 2715–2726.

Berenbaum, S. A., Beltz, A. M., & Corley, R. (2015). The importance of puberty for adolescent development: Conceptualization and measurement. *Advances in Child Development and Behavior, 48*, 53–92.

Berzonsky, M. D., & Kinney, A. (2019). Identity processing style and depression: The mediational role of experiential avoidance and self-regulation. *Identity, 19*(2), 83-97.

Blakemore, S. J., & Mills, K. L. (2014). Is adolescence a sensitive period for sociocultural processing? *Annual Review of Psychology, 65*(1), 187–207.

Brooks-Gunn, J., & Warren, M. P. (1989). Biological and social contributions to negative affect in young adolescent girls. *Child Development, 60*(1), 40–55.

Brown, B. B., & Larson, J. (2009). Peer relationships in adolescence. In R. M. Lerner & L. Steinberg (Eds.), *Handbook of adolescent psychology* (pp. 74–103). John Wiley & Sons.

Burkitt, E., Watling, D., & Cocks, F. (2019). Mixed emotion experiences for self or another person in adolescence. *Journal of Adolescence, 75*, 63–72.

Byrne, M. L., Whittle, S., Vijayakumar, N., Dennison, M., Simmons, J. G., & Allen, N. B. (2017). A systematic review of adrenarche as a sensitive period in neurobiological development and mental health. *Developmental Cognitive Neuroscience, 25*, 12–28.

Cairns, R. B., Leung, M. C., Buchanan, L., & Cairns, B. D. (1995). Friendships and social networks in childhood and adolescence: Fluidity, reliability, and interrelations. *Child Development, 66*(5), 1330–1345.

Casey, B. J., Getz, S., & Galvan, A. (2008). The adolescent brain. *Developmental Review, 28*(1), 62–77.

Cicchetti, D., Ackerman, B. P., & Izard, C. E. (1995). Emotions and emotion regulation in developmental psychopathology. *Development and Psychopathology, 7*(1), 1–10.

Conley, C. S., & Rudolph, K. D. (2009). The emerging sex difference in adolescent depression: Interacting contributions of puberty and peer stress. *Development and Psychopathology, 21*(2), 593.

Costello, E. J., Copeland, W., & Angold, A. (2011). Trends in psychopathology across the adolescent years: What changes when children become adolescents, and when adolescents become adults? *Journal of Child Psychology and Psychiatry, 52*(10), 1015–1025.

Crone, E. A., & Dahl, R. E. (2012). Understanding adolescence as a period of social–affective engagement and goal flexibility. *Nature Reviews Neuroscience, 13*(9), 636–650.

Currie, C. (2019). Development is not the same as ageing: The relevance of puberty to health of adolescents. *International Journal of Public Health, 64*(2), 149–150.

Currie, C., & Morgan, A. (2020). A bio-ecological framing of evidence on the determinants of adolescent mental health – A scoping review of the international Health Behaviour in School-Aged Children (HBSC) study 1983–2020. *SSM – Population Health, 12*, 100697.

Dahl, R. E., Allen, N. B., Wilbrecht, L., & Suleiman, A. B. (2018). Importance of investing in adolescence from a developmental science perspective. *Nature, 554*(7693), 441–450.

Dalgleish, T., Black, M., Johnston, D., & Bevan, A. (2020). Transdiagnostic approaches to mental health problems: Current status and future directions. *Journal of Consulting and Clinical Psychology, 88*(3), 179.

Deardorff, J., Marceau, K., Johnson, M., Reeves, J. W., Biro, F. M., Kubo, A., Greenspan, L. C., Laurent, C. A., Windham, G. C., Pinney, S. M., Kushi, L. H., & Hiatt, R. A. (2021). Girls' pubertal timing and tempo and mental health: A longitudinal examination in an ethnically diverse sample. *Journal of Adolescent Health, 68*(6), 1197–1203. https://doi.org/10.1016/j.jadohealth.2021.01.020

Deng, F., Tao, F. B., Wan, Y. H., Hao, J. H., Su, P. Y., & Cao, Y. X. (2011). Early menarche and psychopathological symptoms in young Chinese women. *Journal of Women's Health, 20*(2), 207–213.

Dorn, L. D., Hostinar, C. E., Susman, E. J., & Pervanidou, P. (2019). Conceptualizing puberty as a window of opportunity for impacting health and well-being across the life span. *Journal of Research on Adolescence, 29*(1), 155–176.

Forbes, E. E., & Dahl, R. E. (2010). Pubertal development and behavior: Hormonal activation of social and motivational tendencies. *Brain and Cognition, 72*(1), 66–72.

Frost, A., Hoyt, L. T., Chung, A. L., & Adam, E. K. (2015). Daily life with depressive symptoms: Gender differences in adolescents' everyday emotional experiences. *Journal of Adolescence, 43*, 132–141.

Fuhrmann, D., Knoll, L. J., & Blakemore, S. J. (2015). Adolescence as a sensitive period of brain development. *Trends in Cognitive Sciences, 19*(10), 558–566.

Galván, A. (2017). Adolescence, brain maturation and mental health. *Nature Neuroscience, 20*(4), 503–504.

Ge, X., & Natsuaki, M. N. (2009). In search of explanations for early pubertal timing effects on developmental psychopathology. *Current Directions in Psychological Science, 18*(6), 327–331.

Geier, C. F. (2013). Adolescent cognitive control and reward processing: Implications for risk taking and substance use. *Hormones and Behavior, 64*(2), 333–342.

Giedd, J. N. (2004). Structural magnetic resonance imaging of the adolescent brain. *Annals of the New York Academy of Sciences, 1021*(1), 77–85.

Goddings, A. L., Beltz, A., Peper, J. S., Crone, E. A., & Braams, B. R. (2019). Understanding the role of puberty in structural and functional development of the adolescent brain. *Journal of Research on Adolescence, 29*(1), 32–53.

Gogtay, N., Giedd, J. N., Lusk, L., Hayashi, K. M., Greenstein, D., Vaituzis, A. C., ... & Thompson, P. M. (2004). Dynamic mapping of human cortical development during childhood through early adulthood. *Proceedings of the National Academy of Sciences, 101*(21), 8174–8179.

Graber, J. A. (2013). Pubertal timing and the development of psychopathology in adolescence and beyond. *Hormones and Behavior, 64*(2), 262–269.

Gross, J. J. (1998). The emerging field of emotion regulation: An integrative review. *Review of General Psychology, 2*(3), 271–299.

Guyer, A. E., Silk, J. S., & Nelson, E. E. (2016). The neurobiology of the emotional adolescent: From the inside out. *Neuroscience & Biobehavioral Reviews, 70*, 74–85.

Hardy, S. A., Krettenauer, T., & Hunt, N. (2020). Moral identity development. In L. A. Jensen (Ed) *The Oxford Handbook of Moral Development: An Interdisciplinary Perspective* (pp. 128–144). Oxford University Press.

Insel, T., Cuthbert, B., Garvey, M., Heinssen, R., Pine, D. S., Quinn, K., ... & Wang, P. (2010). Research domain criteria (RDoC): Toward a new classification framework for research on mental disorders. *American Journal of Psychiatry, 167*(7), 748–751.

John, O. P., & Gross, J. J. (2007). Individual differences in emotion regulation. In J. J. Gross (Ed.), *Handbook of emotion regulation*, (pp 351–372). Guilford Publications.

Joinson, C., Heron, J., Lewis, G., Croudace, T., & Araya, R. (2011). Timing of menarche and depressive symptoms in adolescent girls from a UK cohort. *The British Journal of Psychiatry, 198*(1), 17–23.

Konrad, K., Firk, C., & Uhlhaas, P. J. (2013). Brain development during adolescence. *Deutsches Aerzteblatt International, 110*(25), 425–431. https://doi.org/10.3238/arztebl.2013.0425

Laceulle, O. M., Veenstra, R., Vollebergh, W. A., & Ormel, J. (2019). Sequences of maladaptation: Preadolescent self-regulation, adolescent negative social interactions, and young adult psychopathology. *Development and Psychopathology, 31*(1), 279–292.

Ladouceur, C. D., Peper, J. S., Crone, E. A., & Dahl, R. E. (2012). White matter development in adolescence: The influence of puberty and implications for affective disorders. *Developmental Cognitive Neuroscience, 2*(1), 36–54.

Larsen, B., & Luna, B. (2018). Adolescence as a neurobiological critical period for the development of higher-order cognition. *Neuroscience & Biobehavioral Reviews, 94,* 179–195.

Larson, R. W., Moneta, G., Richards, M. H., & Wilson, S. (2002). Continuity, stability, and change in daily emotional experience across adolescence. *Child Development, 73*(4), 1151–1165.

Lau, P. S., & Wu, F. K. (2012). Emotional competence as a positive youth development construct: A conceptual review. *The Scientific World Journal,* 975189. https://doi.org/10.1100/2012/975189

Lerner, R. M., & Steinberg, L. (2009). *Handbook of adolescent psychology, volume 1: Individual bases of adolescent development* (Vol. 1). John Wiley & Sons.

Lerner, R. M., Tirrell, J. M., Dowling, E. M., Geldhof, G. J., Gestsdóttir, S., Lerner, J. V., King, P. E., Williams, K., Iraheta, G., & Sim, A. T. R. (2019). The end of the beginning: Evidence and absences studying positive youth development in a global context. *Adolescent Research Review, 4*(1), 1–14.

Lerner, Y., Scherf, K. S., Katkov, M., Hasson, U., & Behrmann, M. (2019). *Age-Related Changes in Neural Networks Supporting Complex Visual and Social Processing in Adolescence.* Cold Spring Harbor Laboratory.

Lockhart, S., Sawa, A., & Niwa, M. (2018). Developmental trajectories of brain maturation and behavior: Relevance to major mental illnesses. *Journal of Pharmacological Sciences, 137*(1), 1–4.

Luyckx, K., Schwartz, S. J., Goossens, L., Soenens, B., & Beyers, W. (2008). Developmental typologies of identity formation and adjustment in female emerging adults: A latent class growth analysis approach. *Journal of Research on Adolescence, 18*(4), 595–619.

Maciejewski, D. F., van Lier, P. A. C., Meeus, W. H. J., Branje, S. J. T., & Koot, H. M. (2015). A 5-year longitudinal study on mood variability across adolescence using daily diaries. *Child Development, 86*(6), 1908–1921.

Meeus, W. (2011). The study of adolescent identity formation 2000–2010: A review of longitudinal research. *Journal of Research on Adolescence, 21*(1), 75–94.

Mendle, J., Beam, C. R., McKone, K. M. P., & Koch, M. K. (2020). Puberty and transdiagnostic risks for mental health. *Journal of Research on Adolescence, 30*(3), 687–705.

Morris, A. S., Silk, J. S., Steinberg, L., Myers, S. S., & Robinson, L. R. (2007). The role of the family context in the development of emotion regulation. *Social Development, 16*(2), 361–388.

Negriff, S., & Susman, E. J. (2011). Pubertal timing, depression, and externalizing problems: A framework, review, and examination of gender differences. *Journal of Research on Adolescence, 21*(3), 717–746.

Ranta, M., Punamäki, R. L., Chow, A., & Salmela-Aro, K. (2020). The economic stress model in emerging adulthood: The role of social relationships and financial capability. *Emerging Adulthood, 8*(6), 496–508.

Reijntjes, A., Kamphuis, J. H., Prinzie, P., Boelen, P. A., Van der Schoot, M., & Telch, M. J. (2011). Prospective linkages between peer victimization and externalizing problems in children: A meta-analysis. *Aggressive Behavior, 37*(3), 215–222.

Rose, A. J., Carlson, W., & Waller, E. M. (2007). Prospective associations of co-rumination with friendship and emotional adjustment: Considering the socioemotional trade-offs of co-rumination. *Developmental Psychology, 43*(4), 1019–1031.

Rudolph, K. D. (2014). Puberty as a developmental context of risk for psychopathology. In M. Lewis & K.D. Rudolph (Eds.), *Handbook of developmental psychopathology* (3rd ed., pp. 331–354). Springer.

Rudolph, K. D., & Troop-Gordon, W. (2010). Personal-accentuation and contextual-amplification models of pubertal timing: Predicting youth depression. *Development and Psychopathology, 22*(2), 433–451.

Sawyer, S. M., Afifi, R. A., Bearinger, L. H., Blakemore, S. J., Dick, B., Ezeh, A. C., & Patton, G. C. (2012). Adolescence: A foundation for future health. *The Lancet, 379*(9826), 1630–1640.

Sawyer, S. M., Azzopardi, P. S., Wickremarathne, D., & Patton, G. C. (2018). The age of adolescence. *The Lancet Child & Adolescent Health, 2*(3), 223–228.

Schulz, K. M., Molenda-Figueira, H. A., & Sisk, C. L. (2009). Back to the future: The organizational–activational hypothesis adapted to puberty and adolescence. *Hormones and Behavior, 55*(5), 597–604.

Schulz, K. M., & Sisk, C. L. (2016). The organizing actions of adolescent gonadal steroid hormones on brain and behavioral development. *Neuroscience & Biobehavioral Reviews, 70,* 148–158.

Silvers, J. A., McRae, K., Gabrieli, J. D., Gross, J. J., Remy, K. A., & Ochsner, K. N. (2012). Age-related differences in emotional reactivity, regulation, and rejection sensitivity in adolescence. *Emotion, 12*(6), 1235–1247.

Somerville, L. H. (2013). The teenage brain: Sensitivity to social evaluation. *Current Directions in Psychological Science, 22*(2), 121–127.

Stevens, M. C., Pearlson, G. D., & Calhoun, V. D. (2009). Changes in the interaction of resting-state neural networks from adolescence to adulthood. *Human Brain Mapping, 30*(8), 2356–2366.

Susman, E. J., & Dorn, L. D. (2013). Puberty: Its role in development. In R. M. Lerner, M. A. Easterbrooks, J. Mistry, & I. B. Weiner (Eds.), *Handbook of psychology: Developmental psychology* (pp. 289–320). Wiley.

Taylor, S. J., Barker, L. A., Heavey, L., & McHale, S. (2015). The longitudinal development of social and executive functions in late adolescence and early adulthood. *Frontiers in Behavioral Neuroscience, 9,* 252.

Ullsperger, J. M., & Nikolas, M. A. (2017). A meta-analytic review of the association between pubertal timing and psychopathology in adolescence: Are there sex differences in risk? *Psychological Bulletin, 143*(9), 903.

Van Duijvenvoorde, A. C. K., Peters, S., Braams, B. R., & Crone, E. A. (2016). What motivates adolescents? Neural responses to rewards and their influence on adolescents' risk taking, learning, and cognitive control. *Neuroscience & Biobehavioral Reviews, 70,* 135–147.

Viner, R. M., Allen, N. B., & Patton, G. C. (2017). Puberty, developmental processes, and health interventions. In D. A. P. Bundy, N. de Silva, S. Horton & D. T. Jamison (Eds.), *Disease control priorities, Volume 8: Child and adolescent health and development (3rd Edn,* pp. 107–118). World Bank Group. https://doi.org/10.1596/978-1-4648-0423-6_ch9

Wichers, M., Schreuder, M. J., Goekoop, R., & Groen, R. N. (2019). Can we predict the direction of sudden shifts in symptoms? Transdiagnostic implications from a complex systems perspective on psychopathology. *Psychological Medicine, 49*(3), 380–387.

Wierenga, L. M., Sexton, J. A., Laake, P., Giedd, J. N., & Tamnes, C. K. (2018). A key characteristic of sex differences in the developing brain: Greater variability in brain structure of boys than girls. *Cerebral Cortex, 28*(8), 2741–2751.

Wintre, M. G., & Vallance, D. D. (1994). A developmental sequence in the comprehension of emotions: Intensity, multiple emotions, and valence. *Developmental Psychology, 30*(4), 509.

Worthman, C. M., Dockray, S., & Marceau, K. (2019). Puberty and the evolution of developmental science. *Journal of Research on Adolescence, 29*(1), 9–31.

Young, K. S., Sandman, C. F., & Craske, M. G. (2019). Positive and negative emotion regulation in adolescence: Links to anxiety and depression. *Brain Sciences, 9*(4), 76.

Zeman, J., Cassano, M., Perry-Parrish, C., & Stegall, S. (2006). Emotion regulation in children and adolescents. *Journal of Developmental & Behavioral Pediatrics, 27*(2), 155–168.

Zhao, Y., & Castellanos, F. X. (2016). Annual Research Review: Discovery science strategies in studies of the pathophysiology of child and adolescent psychiatric disorders – promises and limitations. *Journal of Child Psychology and Psychiatry, 57*(3), 421–439.

Zimmer-Gembeck, M. J., & Skinner, E. A. (2010). Adolescents coping with stress: Development and diversity. *School Nurse News, 27*(2), 23–28.

3 Structural and social factors in adolescent and young adult mental health

Michal Molcho
National University of Ireland, Galway, Ireland

Emmanuelle Godeau
EHESP French School of Public Health, France

Introduction: Why is it important to explore structural factors in mental health?

It is easy to view mental health as an innate trait. However, like all other health matters, the mental health of an individual is, at least to some degree, determined by the societal and environmental context in which the individual is born, grows, lives, works and ages. Therefore, in order to understand mental health and to offer efficient interventions, mental health should be examined in the broader context of one's life. There is a great deal of research on the relationship between the social context and the mental health of adults, but less is known about the social context, or the social determinants of mental health among young people. To address that gap, this chapter will first introduce the concept of social and structural determinants of health, and will then explore them with respect to the mental health of young people. To do so, the chapter will explore the roles of socio-demographic background, school environment and social media as environments that can affect young people's mental health. Lastly, taking the perspective of the social determinants of health, the chapter will review some evidence of the impact of COVID-19 on the mental health of young people.

The context: social determinants of health

One of the key publications in the area of social determinants of health was the work of the World Health Organization (WHO) Commission on Social Determinants of Health (Marmot et al. 2008). The commission's report that was published in 2008 was the culmination of years of work that were dedicated to identifying what are the social determinates of health, as opposed to the causes of diseases. So, for example, while causes of disease include smoking, obesity and malnutrition among others (WHO, 2008), the work of the Commission on Social Determinants of Health aimed to identify the 'causes of causes' of ill-health. Their argument was that if ill-health is not equally distributed across all societies and subgroups in societies, then there is a need to explore what lies beneath ill-health that can explain this unequal distribution. In their work, the panel defined Social Determinants of

Health (SDH) as the conditions in which people are born, grow, live, work and age (Marmot et al. 2008). It is clear from the aforementioned definition that the work of the Commission was set out to examine every aspect of the life of people, from families, to policies, from the individual, to the environment. The recommendations of the Commission were as ambitious as the work its members undertook; they recommended improving daily living conditions, to tackle inequitable distribution of power, money and resources, and to continue to measure the problem and the impact of whatever actions were taken. It is, therefore, clear, that examining the structural, or social, determinants of health must include exploring the causes of inequalities in health. One very clear example of health inequalities is related to life expectancy at birth. Had there not been inequalities in health, it would be expected that the average life expectancy in all societies, social groups and countries would be similar, if not the same. Any diversion from the average life expectancy can be explained through the lens of health inequality. Equally, any evidence of different prevalence of mental ill-health across different social groups and countries should be viewed as inequalities in mental health that are stemming from social and structural factors (McAllister et al. 2018).

While the work of the Commission was ground breaking in scope and impact, it is by no means novel. The concept of life chances was introduced by Max Weber in the 1920s (Cockerham et al. 1993) and later in the Black Report (Black et al. 1988), with broad definitions of structural factors of health that include the economic, social, policy and organisational environment (Rhodes, 2002; Williams, 2003). But it was only later that studies investigating the social determinants of young people's health started to appear (Currie, 2008; Viner et al. 2012). These studies identified that during adolescence, the strongest determinants of adolescent health are structural factors such as socio-demographic background and access to education. More recently, it became clearer that digital environment is another key determinant of adolescent and young adult health (Hausmann et al. 2017). Therefore, this chapter will focus on these three contexts to explore the mental health of young people.

How do structural and social factors affect mental health?

Environment can be divided into the physical environment, home environment (including family environment), social environment, socio-economic environment and digital environment. As this chapter focuses on social and structural determinants of mental health, it is important to first define what 'social environment' is. For this, we chose to use Casper's definition from 2001. According to Casper, social environment includes the immediate physical surrounding, social relationships and the cultural settings in which individuals act and interact. These include, among other aspects, cultural practices, power relations, race relations and social inequalities (Casper, 2001).

The importance of social environments for health should not be overlooked. In 1994, Syme argued that if only 40 per cent of all coronary heart disease can be explained by biological factors, then the remaining 60 per cent stems from the social environment that acts as determinants of health (Syme, 1994). Other studies found associations between positive perceptions of social environment and better physical health, mental health and self-rated health (Ehsan et al. 2019). However, the mechanism behind this is not obvious. It is much easier to link health to the biology or the behaviour of the individual than to the social environment. Yet, the growing knowledge around the influence of the environment on the genetic makeup (epigenetics), brain development and the impact of stress on the endocrine and immune system, provide some possible explanations (Carmeli et al. 2021). So much so, that we now know that early life experiences of the social environment can create neurological changes in the brain. The concept of adverse childhood experiences (ACEs) has emerged as a major research theme. Research found that early-life adverse experience stemming from the social environment can change gene expression and behaviour, leading to a lifelong impact on brain development and on mental health (Turecki & Meaney, 2016), in a social-to-biological transition (Kelly-Irving & Delpierre, 2019). Indeed, it is clearer than ever that in order to fully understand mental health, it is important to also explore the social structures, and the social environments in which one is born, grows, lives, works and ages.

The associations between social environment and mental health are not limited to adults, and are also evident among adolescents (WHO, 2014). Like many other aspects of health, the social environments shape mental health and mental problems. The rest of this chapter will explore the evidence of the associations between different social determinants of health and the mental health of young people. We will do that by first looking at the socio-demographic background – a non-modifiable set of determinants; we will move on to explore the school environment, in which many interventions are conducted; and we will end by a relatively novel environment – social media.

Socio-demographic background and mental health

Across the life span, low socio-economic status and belonging to a minority group are associated with various health outcomes, including lower health literacy (Wilkinson et al. 2009), poorer self-rated health (Quercioli et al. 2009), poorer health status (Kautiainen et al. 2009), and involvement in risk behaviours (Currie, 2008; Wahn & Nissen, 2008). However, why is this the case? What is the mechanism behind social inequalities and health?

One attempt to explain health inequalities is the *Mechanisms of Health Inequalities* model that was developed by Diderichsen (Diderichsen et al. 2012). According to Diderichsen, the social environment, including the structure of society and the relations in society, creates social stratification that assigns individuals into certain social positions. This social stratification causes differential exposure to health-damaging, or health-enhancing conditions. It also creates stratification in vulnerability to health conditions, as well as stratification in the availability of material resource. In addition to the differential exposure and vulnerability, social stratification also creates differential consequences of ill-health for the more, or less, advantaged groups (Diderichsen et al. 2012). Some good, but sad, examples can be drawn from the COVID-19 pandemic. Differential socio-economic circumstances meant that some young people could not access schoolwork either due to poor connectivity or due to limited access to devices. Different levels of parental literacy meant that some could not have asked for parental support with schoolwork. Others were benefiting from free school meals, hence school closure meant even fewer resources in the household and increased food insecurity. Those more likely to experience such adversities and to fall behind on school-work are those who were already more vulnerable to begin with. At the same time, adolescents whose parents are highly educated and well paid were able to engage with schoolwork in a safe environment, with their personal devices and good connectivity. Such families are also likely to have various insurance policies that protect them if they were sick, thus limiting the impact of the consequences of the disease on the household. And here, through different education, type of job and income, the UK saw higher levels of infection and mortality among Black, Asian and other ethnic minorities that were deemed related to life circumstances rather than to health issues (Bhala et al. 2020). This illustrates how exploring the role of ethnicity and deprivation in adolescent mental health is essential.

Race, racism and mental health

To start, we need to first define the term 'race' as, according to Graves (2010), the majority of people are not clear about the meaning of this term, and are usually using it to refer to both biological and social definitions (Graves Jr, 2010). From a biological point of view, however, it is now clear that the biological differences between groups are rather small, suggesting that only one race exists: the human race. Therefore, it became clear that race is not a biological fact, but rather a social construct (Graves Jr, 2010; Williams, 1997). By saying that race is a social construct, what we mean is that race has no real existence other that what people think about it (Barkan, 2011; Bhopal et al. 2021). However, where people perceive something as real, it becomes real in its consequences (Rousseau, 2002), and so for many 'non' white, the discourse of race is very much real in its consequences.

Now that we demonstrated that race is more of a social fact than a biological fact, we need to examine to what degree race is associated with health, or, in other words, to what degree race is a social determinant of health. Much of the research on race originated in the US, where four racial groups (white, Black, Asian/Pacific Islander, and American Indian/Alaskan Native) were compared in terms of health outcomes, in one of the first studies in this area (Williams, 1997). Findings consistently demonstrated health disparities, with higher mortality and morbidity rates among Blacks and Native American (Lillie-Blanton & Laveist, 1996; Williams, 1997). Yet, despite decades of research and policies addressing racial discrimination, these disparities are still evident nowadays (Bhala et al. 2020; Bhopal et al. 2021; Krasnik et al. 2018) and not just in the US (Bhopal et al. 2021).

One of the mechanisms that explains the links between race and mental health is racism. Racism is defined as 'organized systems within societies that cause avoidable and unfair inequalities in power, resources, capacities and opportunities across racial or ethnic groups' (Paradies et al. 2015: 2). This definition can be linked to Diderichsen's model of health inequalities (Diderichsen et al. 2012), with race feeding into social stratification, and hence, a social determinant of health.

Indeed, being a victim of racism is strongly associated with poor mental health (McAllister et al. 2018), and more specifically, with lower self-esteem, lower life satisfaction, and higher risk for suicidal ideation, depression, anxiety and post-traumatic stress disorder (PTSD) (Paradies et al. 2015). This was demonstrated well by Bailey, who shared her experience as a psychiatrist working with adolescents in an inner city in the US. She found that many of her patients reported mental health concerns that were all related to social structures and to structural racism that enable racism, exclusion, and often, violence. Bailey notes that these living conditions are clearly at play, and cannot be treated through medicine, but rather through public policies (Bailey, 2020).

The impact of race and racism on adolescent health is well documented. Adolescents and young adults that experience racism are more likely to report health problems, involvement in risk behaviours and mental health problems (Pachter & Coll, 2009). In South African young people, for example, race other than white was associated with increased engagement with risk behaviour and exposure to violence, even when all other socio-demographic variables were controlled, which could be explained through marginalisation and social exclusion (Sanders-Phillips & Kliewer, 2019); these, in turn, result in a poorer mental health status. Most recent evidence points towards the effect that exposure to racism and discrimination has on the endocrine system; enhanced secretion of stress hormone can result in poor mental health and mental health problems (Carmeli et al. 2021) through a biological-to-sociological mechanism (Kelly-Irving & Delpierre, 2019).

While racism per se is difficult to measure, it is easier to measure how the perception of racial discrimination is associated with health. Racial discrimination can affect health and well-being not just through biological mechanisms, but also through restricting access to social resources, increased exposure to risk factors, increased involvement in risk behaviours, and decreased involvement in protective health behaviours (Priest et al. 2013). Indeed, studies found that perceived racial discrimination was associated with lower self-esteem and poorer mental health (Lee & Ahn, 2011; Nakash et al. 2012), and these were related to skin tone. A study from the US found that the darker the tone of the skin of adolescents, the more likely they were to report depressive symptoms or other mental disorders (Louie, 2020). However, some studies identified some moderators that could ameliorate the impact of racial discrimination, and these include stronger ethnic identity (Romero & Roberts, 2003; Umaña-Taylor & Updegraff, 2007), positive parenting and social support (Priest et al. 2013), and having at least three supportive adults in adolescent years (Kysar-Moon, 2020).

Income inequality, poverty and mental health

Again, evidence suggesting that income inequality and deprivation influence health is not new (Black et al. 1988; Cockerham et al. 1993; Whitehead & Dahlgren, 1991). Income inequality is a structural indicator that is associated with occupation status, political power and household living conditions – as well as a range of social experiences – all forming part of a social environment that affects health (Elgar et al. 2015). Therefore, to understand mental health, we need to explore the role that income inequalities and poverty play. It is important to examine both, as data suggest that income inequality plays a different role in health to that of poverty. The link between poverty and mental health is well established. Those living in poverty are more likely to experience mental health problems in general (Fryers et al. 2004), and are more likely to report anxiety and depression, more specifically (WHO, 2014). Experiencing poverty in early life is associated with suicide attempts later in life (Shim & Compton, 2018), and poverty at any age is associated with lower life satisfaction and more mental health problems (Paradies et al. 2015; Shim & Compton, 2018).

Nevertheless, poverty does not tell the whole story. Income inequality at the national level is associated with poorer life satisfaction and more frequent reporting of emotional and somatic symptoms among adolescents (Dierckens et al. 2020; Elgar et al. 2017). Such findings indicate that even if not poor, the relative socio-economic standing of adolescents affects their mental health. Irrespective of the absolute income, lower socio-economic standing is associated with mental health problems among individuals of all ages (McAllister et al. 2018), and more specifically, with increased risk for developing anxiety and depression (Lemstra et al. 2008) or engaging in risky behaviours such as drunkenness during adolescence (Sentenac et al. 2017). This further supports the importance of socio-economic standing as social determinates of mental health among young people (Viner et al. 2012).

School as a determinant for mental health

While school's main responsibility is teaching, it can also contribute to promoting the overall health and well-being of their students, as discussed in Chapter 4.

As children grow up, and especially during secondary school years, adolescents spend many hours of the day in school, making school an important environment in their lives and a key determinant of mental health. According to Viner and colleagues, access to education is one of the most important aspects of adolescent health (Viner et al. 2012), yet, as one of the main social environments during adolescence, school can also add stress to the life of adolescents, as well as provide a supportive environment for them. Pressure to do well at school tends to have negative impact on adolescent mental health (Aldridge & McChesney, 2018), especially among adolescent girls (Basu & Banerjee, 2020). Feeling a sense of belonging and attachment to school, and having good relationships with peers and teachers have a positive mental health impact on young people (Aldridge & McChesney, 2018; Gorrese & Ruggieri, 2013).

Through spending long days in school, adolescents are provided with opportunities for socialising with peers, and developing their identity away from their parents (Pfeifer & Berkman, 2018). Given that adolescence is a stage in life characterised by heightened sensitivity to social interaction (Blakemore & Mills, 2014), it is important to appreciate the social opportunities that schools provide to adolescents. However, not all social interactions are positive, as is the case with bullying. Most cases of bullying occur at school (Cosma et al. 2020), at the expense of the physical and mental health of the victims, but also of the perpetrators (Lereya et al. 2015), and of the bystanders (Callaghan et al. 2019). Bullying can include physical bullying, as well as name-calling, abuse, spreading rumours and social exclusion, and all have direct impact on the participants of these behaviours (Craig et al. 2009). The best way to prevent school bullying is through actual and perceived school safety. Adolescents who perceive their school to be a safe and positive environment also report better mental health as well as fewer mental health problems (Aldridge & McChesney, 2018).

Promoting a positive school climate and improving the health and well-being of students is one explicit goal of the Schools for Health in Europe (SHE) network[1]. SHE stems from an approach developed by the World Health Organization (WHO) in the late 1980s to bring together the sectors of education and health and achieve a better health for the whole school (WHO, 1997). The core values of SHE – equity, sustainability, inclusion, empowerment and democracy – make clear how school can have a positive impact on the mental health of the adolescents. As a learning environment, school can also contribute to this effort through programmes tailored to lower risk behaviours, but more interestingly to foster psychosocial competencies and life skills (St Leger & Young, 2009). School is also unique in that it can run some programmes that can directly or indirectly target students most at need, with the aim to lower social inequalities.

Another way of promoting and improving mental health within schools is through the employment of dedicated staff. In countries where there are school doctors or nurses, those professionals can directly work to improve the health of all students through screening for health problems and prevention of unhealthy behaviours (Michaud et al. 2021), but also through providing health services to those with limited access to care, especially regarding mental health. In this perspective, school health services can contribute to reducing health inequity, and the health implication associated with it.

Social media and mental health

The digital world, and social media more specifically, is one of the social contexts in which adolescents live their life, and as such, it is important to examine the role that social media play in mental health. Exposure to, and engagement with, social media can have both positive and negative impacts on the different aspects of mental health (Keles et al. 2020). Some studies suggest that instant messaging can boost self-esteem and relieve distress (Dolev-Cohen and Barak, 2013), as well as satisfy the need for sense of belonging and the need for social connectedness among those feeling excluded (Knowles et al. 2015). However, other studies suggest that prolonged exposure to social media or exposure to negative comments can worsen adolescents' and young adults' mood and harm self-esteem and well-being (Sagioglou & Greitemeyer, 2014; Valkenburg & Peter, 2007). Unfortunately, those feeling most socially excluded are more likely to engage in problematic social media use (Boer et al. 2020), like befriending strangers (Knowles et al. 2015).

[1] https://www.schoolsforhealth.org/

There are several domains of social media use that can be examined with relation to mental health: time spent on social media, activity on social media, investment in social media and addiction (Keles et al. 2020). There is an indication suggesting that the time spent on social media is associated with poorer mental health and increased risk for depression and anxiety (Keles et al. 2020), with one study indicating that over two hours of daily social media use are associated with mental health difficulties (Sampasa-Kanyinga & Lewis, 2015). Other determinants of poor mental health and especially depression and anxiety include having a large number of social media accounts (Barry et al. 2017), accounts that are heavy in personal information (Keles et al. 2020), and addictive social media use (Keles et al. 2020).

Much of the attention around internet use among adolescents focuses on social media use. However, as digital natives, adolescents use the internet as their main source of information on most matters, which requires us to address the issue of digital literacy. Digital literacy is defined as 'The ability to locate, understand, exchange, and evaluate health information from online environments in the presence of dynamic contextual factors and to apply the knowledge gained across ecological levels for the purposes of maintaining or improving health' (Paige et al. 2018: 9). This suggests that even if adolescents are frequent users of the internet, it does not mean that they have a sufficient level of digital literacy or e-health literacy to properly assess the reliability and credibility of information online (Livingstone et al. 2017). Training adolescents in digital literacy provides a real opportunity to empower them, and to address the existing inequities within and between countries and regions (Keeley & Little, 2017). This is particularly relevant during a pandemic, where the digital divide increases health inequalities, and where the link between time spent on screens and digital media and mental health is no more in doubt.

The impact of COVID-19 on mental health

It is impossible to address the structural factors of adolescent mental health without addressing the global pandemic that spread across the world in 2020. At the time of writing, Ireland was still experiencing the highest level of restrictions and France was experiencing curfews, partial lock-down as well as other measures of physical distancing. While by now, a number of vaccines have proven to be successful in reducing the risk for infection and severe disease, COVID-19 is still very much present in our daily lives, and its impact is likely to be felt for a very long time. We therefore feel that it is important to identify and include some of the evidence that is already published on the impact of COVID-19 on the mental health of adolescents in the context of structural determinants of mental health.

Various countries and regions employed different strategies to stop the spread of COVID-19 with differential impact on adolescent mental health. Early studies on adolescents that were quarantined due to COVID-19 in China found that about 10 per cent of those quarantined reported depression, 20 per cent reported anxiety and 7 per cent reported both (Chen et al. 2020). Another study reported an increase in experiencing of inattention, worry and irritability during the pandemic, and not only among quarantined adolescents (Jiao et al. 2020). A study from India reported that higher proportions of those quarantined experienced helplessness, worry and fear compared to non-quarantined adolescents (Saurabh & Ranjan, 2020), indicating the impact that government policies, here quarantine, can have on adolescents over and above the mental health impact of the pandemic itself.

We have established earlier the importance of school as a determinant of mental health, yet, during the pandemic, children and adolescents found themselves outside of the school system for prolonged periods, replacing school with remote schooling. It is, therefore, important to recognise that difficulties in studying from home, poor school performance and school-related social relationships that were missing during lock-downs were all associated with low self-esteem and emotional problems (Basu & Banerjee, 2020), highlighting the potential impact of school closure during COVID-19 on the mental health of adolescents. Lack of school routine is particularly difficult for adolescents who already suffer from mental health problems or have additional education needs (Lee, 2020).

As mentioned earlier, adolescence is a period of heightened sensitivity to social interaction, which means that the measures taken to curb the spread of the virus such as social distancing and school closure have a major impact on young people, depriving them of their social contacts, especially for those in low functioning families (Orben et al. 2020). Adolescence is also a period where individuals continue to develop their social cognition and learn to better understand other people's emotions, intentions and beliefs (Blakemore & Mills, 2014). Therefore, social isolation during adolescent and young adult years (a time of hormonal and brain development) can increase general stress and impact on healthy development (Orben et al. 2020), with early indications suggesting that this period of social isolation may increase adolescents' susceptibility for long-term mental disorders (de Figueiredo et al. 2020). While there is no research that examines the impact of social deprivation in otherwise normative adolescents, studies on incarcerated adolescents and animal modelling indicate that social deprivation may lead to anxiety, depression and aggressive behaviours (Orben et al. 2020). Although physical distancing imposed during the pandemic is not an extreme form of social deprivation, it is possible that the impact it had on adolescents could be far reaching, and needs to be recognised. While exposure to social media can affect mental health as we discussed earlier, it is possible that during COVID-19 social media use acted as a moderator for the impact of social deprivation. Indeed, remote schooling does not provide the same social interaction, but it can still offer some sense of connectedness to school and, for some, without the consequences of school bullying. Equally, digital communication can, to some degree, remediate the impact of social deprivation through providing some social connectedness (Knowles et al. 2015). Digital communication allows adolescents to still see their peers and interact with them in a meaningful way, especially when used for direct communication through messaging or reacting to posts, as opposed to scrolling on social media posts, activities that are negatively associated with well-being (Orben et al. 2020). However, as helpful as these connections are, they still cannot replace the role that physical interactions have in the development of adolescents (Gallace and Spence, 2010).

The impact of COVID-19 is not uniform across adolescents, considering families with medium- to high-income resources being able to provide their children with additional opportunities to interact with peers through technology, while other families cannot (de Figueiredo et al. 2020). While some adolescents have endless opportunities to learn and explore, the digital divide is such that for the most deprived adolescent it limits their opportunities, further increasing the existing impact of inequalities on mental health. It is very clear that adolescent and young adult mental health will require attention and resources when we overcome the pandemic.

Where from here?

In this chapter, we explored some structural and social factors of adolescent mental health, focusing on inequalities, education and social media. The findings are concerning. So, what is the way forward? It is important to understand that structural factors can only be addressed through a systematic approach, that requires government to develop and implement policies, systems to change and equal opportunities to truly be made available for everyone. Marmot and his colleagues suggested that the only way to address health inequality is through redistribution of power and wealth (Marmot et al. 2008; WHO, 2008) and the same applies for inequalities in mental health. Until this happens, to improve adolescents' mental health we need to increase cultural awareness, to provide universal access to care and education, to create safer schools, and to make social media companies accountable. Without these, addressing mental health issues on the individual level will continue to have limited impact on the mental health of adolescents.

References

Aldridge, J. M., & McChesney, K. (2018). The relationships between school climate and adolescent mental health and well-being: A systematic literature review. *International Journal of Educational Research, 88*, 121–145.

Bailey, A. M. (2020). Psychiatric formulation and the structural determinants of mental health. *Academic Psychiatry, 44*(6), 804–805.

Barkan, S. E. (2011). *Sociology: Understanding and changing the social world.* Flat World Knowledge, Incorporated.

Barry, C. T., Sidoti, C. L., Briggs, S. M., Reiter, S. R., & Lindsey, R. A. (2017). Adolescent social media use and mental health from adolescent and parent perspectives. *Journal of Adolescence, 61*, 1–11.

Basu, S., & Banerjee, B. (2020). Impact of environmental factors on mental health of children and adolescents: A systematic review. *Children and Youth Services Review*, 105515.

Bhala, N., Curry, G., Martineau, A. R., Agyemang, C., & Bhopal, R. (2020). Sharpening the global focus on ethnicity and race in the time of COVID-19. *The Lancet, 395*(10238), 1673–1676.

Bhopal, R., Gruer, L., Agyemang, C., Davidovitch, N., de-Graft Aikins, A., Krasnik, A., Martinez-Donate, A. P., Miranda, J. J., Pottie, K., & Segal, U. (2021). The Global Society on Migration, Ethnicity, Race and Health: Why race can't be ignored even if it causes discomfort. *European Journal of Public Health, 31*(1), 3–4.

Black, D., Townsend, P., & Davidson, N. (1988). *Inequalities in health: the Black report.* Penguin.

Blakemore, S. J., & Mills, K. L. (2014). Is adolescence a sensitive period for sociocultural processing? *Annual Review of Psychology, 65*, 187–207.

Boer, M., van den Eijnden, R. J., Boniel-Nissim, M., Wong, S. L., Inchley, J. C., Badura, P., Craig, W. M., Gobina, I., Kleszczewska, D., & Klanšček, H. J. (2020). Adolescents' intense and problematic social media use and their well-being in 29 countries. *Journal of Adolescent Health, 66*(6), S89–S99.

Callaghan, M., Kelly, C., & Molcho, M. (2019). Bullying and bystander behavior and health outcomes among adolescents in Ireland. *Journal of Epidemiology and Community Health, 73*(5), 416–421.

Carmeli, C., Kutalik, Z., Mishra, P. P., Porcu, E., Delpierre, C., Delaneau, O., Kelly-Irving, M., Bochud, M., Dhayat, N. A., & Ponte, B. (2021). Gene regulation contributes to explain the impact of early life socio-economic disadvantage on adult inflammatory levels in two cohort studies. *Scientific Reports, 11*(1), 1–11.

Casper, M. (2001). A definition of 'social environment'. *American Journal of Public Health, 91*(3), 465–470.

Chen, F., Zheng, D., Liu, J., Gong, Y., Guan, Z., & Lou, D. (2020). Depression and anxiety among adolescents during COVID-19: A cross-sectional study. *Brain, Behavior, and Immunity, 88*, 36–38.

Cockerham, W. C., Abel, T., & Lüschen, G. (1993). Max Weber, formal rationality, and health lifestyles. *Sociological Quarterly, 34*(3), 413–425.

Cosma, A., Walsh, S. D., Chester, K. L., Callaghan, M., Molcho, M., Craig, W., & Pickett, W. (2020). Bullying victimization: Time trends and the overlap between traditional and cyberbullying across countries in Europe and North America. *International Journal of Public Health, 65*(1), 75–85.

Craig, W., Harel-Fisch, Y., Fogel-Grinvald, H., Dostaler, S., Hetland, J., Simons-Morton, B., Molcho, M., de Mato, M. G., Overpeck, M., & Due, P. (2009). A cross-national profile of bullying and victimization among adolescents in 40 countries. *International Journal of Public Health, 54*(2), 216–224.

Currie, C. (2008). *Inequalities in young people's health: HBSC international report from the 2005/2006 Survey*. World Health Organization.

de Figueiredo, C. S., Sandre, P. C., Portugal, L. C. L., Mázala-de-Oliveira, T., da Silva Chagas, L., Raony, Í., Ferreira, E. S., Giestal-de-Araujo, E., Dos Santos, A. A., & Bomfim, P. O. S. (2020). COVID-19 pandemic impact on children and adolescents' mental health: Biological, environmental, and social factors. *Progress in Neuro-Psychopharmacology and Biological Psychiatry*, 110171.

Diderichsen, F., Andersen, I., Manuel, C., Andersen, A.-M. N., Bach, E., Baadsgaard, M., Brønnum-Hansen, H., Hansen, F. K., Jeune, B., Jørgensen, T., & Søgaard, J. (2012). Health inequality-determinants and policies. *Scandinavian Journal of Public Health, 40*(8_suppl), 12–105.

Dierckens, M., Weinberg, D., Huang, Y., Elgar, F., Moor, I., Augustine, L., Lyyra, N., Deforche, B., De Clercq, B., & Stevens, G. W. (2020). National-level wealth inequality and socio-economic inequality in adolescent mental well-being: A time series analysis of 17 countries. *Journal of Adolescent Health, 66*(6), S21–S28.

Dolev-Cohen, M., & Barak, A. (2013). Adolescents' use of Instant Messaging as a means of emotional relief. *Computers in Human Behavior, 29*(1), 58–63.

Ehsan, A., Klaas, H. S., Bastianen, A., & Spini, D. (2019). Social capital and health: a systematic review of systematic reviews. *SSM-Population Health, 8*, 100425.

Elgar, F. J., Gariépy, G., Torsheim, T., & Currie, C. (2017). Early-life income inequality and adolescent health and well-being. *Social Science & Medicine, 174*, 197–208.

Elgar, F. J., Pförtner, T. K., Moor, I., De Clercq, B., Stevens, G. W., & Currie, C. (2015). Socioeconomic inequalities in adolescent health 2002–2010: A time-series analysis of 34 countries participating in the Health Behavior in School-aged Children study. *The Lancet, 385*(9982), 2088–2095.

Fryers, T., Jenkins, R., & Melzer, D. (2004). *Social inequalities and the distribution of the common mental disorders*. Psychology Press.

Gallace, A., & Spence, C. (2010). The science of interpersonal touch: An overview. *Neuroscience & Biobehavioral Reviews, 34*(2), 246–259.

Gorrese, A., & Ruggieri, R. (2013). Peer attachment and self-esteem: A meta-analytic review. *Personality and Individual Differences, 55*(5), 559–568.

Graves Jr, J. L. (2010). Biological v. social definitions of race: Implications for modern biomedical research. *The Review of Black Political Economy, 37*(1), 43–60.

Hausmann, J. S., Touloumtzis, C., White, M. T., Colbert, J. A., & Gooding, H. C. (2017). Adolescent and young adult use of social media for health and its implications. *Journal of Adolescent Health, 60*(6), 714–719.

Jiao, W. Y., Wang, L. N., Liu, J., Fang, S. F., Jiao, F. Y., Pettoello-Mantovani, M., & Somekh, E. (2020). Behavioral and emotional disorders in children during the COVID-19 epidemic. *The Journal of Pediatrics, 221*, 264.

Kautiainen, S., Koivisto, A. M., Koivusilta, L., Lintonen, T., Virtanen, S. M., & Rimpelä, A. (2009). Sociodemographic factors and a secular trend of adolescent overweight in Finland. *International Journal of Pediatric Obesity, 4*(4), 360–370.

Keeley, B., & Little, C. (2017). *The State of the World's Children 2017: Children in a Digital World.* ERIC.

Keles, B., McCrae, N., & Grealish, A. (2020). A systematic review: The influence of social media on depression, anxiety and psychological distress in adolescents. *International Journal of Adolescence and Youth, 25*(1), 79–93.

Kelly-Irving, M., & Delpierre, C. (2019). A critique of the adverse childhood experiences framework in epidemiology and public health: Uses and misuses. *Social Policy and Society, 18*(3), 445–456. https://doi.org/10.1017/s1474746419000101

Knowles, M. L., Haycock, N., & Shaikh, I. (2015). Does facebook magnify or mitigate threats to belonging? *Social Psychology (Göttingen, Germany), 46*(6), 313–324. https://doi.org/10.1027/1864-9335/a000246

Krasnik, A., Bhopal, R. S., Gruer, L., & Kumanyika, S. K. (2018). Advancing a unified, global effort to address health disadvantages associated with migration, ethnicity and race. *European Journal of Public Health, 28*(suppl_1), 1–2. https://doi.org/10.1093/eurpub/cky046

Kysar-Moon, A. (2020). Childhood adversity and internalizing problems: Evidence of a race mental health paradox. *Society and Mental Health, 10*(2), 136–162.

Lee, D. L., & Ahn, S. (2011). Racial discrimination and Asian mental health: A meta-analysis. *The Counseling Psychologist, 39*(3), 463–489.

Lee, J. (2020). Mental health effects of school closures during COVID-19. *The Lancet Child & Adolescent Health, 4*(6), 421.

Lemstra, M., Neudorf, C., D'Arcy, C., Kunst, A., Warren, L. M., & Bennett, N. R. (2008). A systematic review of depressed mood and anxiety by SES in youth aged 10–15 years. *Canadian Journal of Public Health, 99*(2), 125–129.

Lereya, S. T., Copeland, W. E., Zammit, S., & Wolke, D. (2015). Bully/victims: A longitudinal, population-based cohort study of their mental health. *European Child and Adolescent Psychiatry, 24*(12), 1461–1471.

Lillie-Blanton, M., & Laveist, T. (1996). Race/ethnicity, the social environment, and health. *Social Science & Medicine, 43*(1), 83–91.

Livingstone, S., Lemish, D., Lim, S. S., Bulger, M., Cabello, P., Claro, M., Cabello-Hutt, T., Khalil, J., Kumpulainen, K., & Nayar, U. S. (2017). Global perspectives on children's digital opportunities: An emerging research and policy agenda. *Pediatrics, 140*(Supplement 2), S137–S141.

Louie, P. (2020). Revisiting the cost of skin color: Discrimination, mastery, and mental health among Black adolescents. *Society and Mental Health, 10*(1), 1–19.

Marmot, M., Friel, S., Bell, R., Houweling, T. A., Taylor, S., & Health, C. o. S. D. o. (2008). Closing the gap in a generation: Health equity through action on the social determinants of health. *The Lancet, 372*(9650), 1661–1669.

McAllister, A., Fritzell, S., Almroth, M., Harber-Aschan, L., Larsson, S., & Burström, B. (2018). How do macro-level structural determinants affect inequalities in mental health?–a systematic review of the literature. *International Journal for Equity in Health, 17*(1), 1–14.

Michaud, P. A., Vervoort, J. P., Visser, A., Baltag, V., Reijneveld, S. A., Kocken, P. L., & Jansen, D. (2021). Organization and activities of school health services among EU countries. *European Journal of Public Health, 31*(3), 502–508. https://doi.org/10.1093/eurpub/ckaa200

Nakash, O., Nagar, M., Shoshani, A., Zubida, H., & Harper, R. A. (2012). The effect of acculturation and discrimination on mental health symptoms and risk behaviors among adolescent migrants in Israel. *Cultural Diversity and Ethnic Minority Psychology, 18*(3), 228.

Orben, A., Tomova, L., & Blakemore, S. J. (2020). The effects of social deprivation on adolescent development and mental health. *The Lancet Child & Adolescent Health, 4*(8), 634–640. https://doi.org/10.1016/s2352-4642(20)30186-3

Pachter, L. M., & Coll, C. G. (2009). Racism and child health: A review of the literature and future directions. *Journal of Developmental and Behavioral Pediatrics: JDBP, 30*(3), 255.

Paige, S. R., Stellefson, M., Krieger, J. L., Anderson-Lewis, C., Cheong, J., & Stopka, C. (2018). The transactional model of electronic health (eHealth) literacy. *Journal of Medical Internet Research, 20*(10), e10175.

Paradies, Y., Ben, J., Denson, N., Elias, A., Priest, N., Pieterse, A., Gupta, A., Kelaher, M., & Gee, G. (2015). Racism as a determinant of health: A systematic review and meta-analysis. *PloS One, 10*(9), e0138511.

Pfeifer, J. H., & Berkman, E. T. (2018). The development of self and identity in adolescence: Neural evidence and implications for a value-based choice perspective on motivated behavior. *Child Development Perspectives, 12*(3), 158–16. https://doi.org/10.1111/cdep.12279

Priest, N., Paradies, Y., Trenerry, B., Truong, M., Karlsen, S., & Kelly, Y. (2013). A systematic review of studies examining the relationship between reported racism and health and well-being for children and young people. *Social Science & Medicine, 95*, 115–127.

Quercioli, C., Messina, G., Barbini, E., Carriero, G., Fanì, M., & Nante, N. (2009). Importance of sociodemographic and morbidity aspects in measuring health-related quality of life: Performances of three tools. *The European Journal of Health Economics, 10*(4), 389–397.

Rhodes, T. (2002). The 'risk environment': A framework for understanding and reducing drug-related harm. *International Journal of Drug Policy, 13*(2), 85–94.

Romero, A. J., & Roberts, R. E. (2003). The impact of multiple dimensions of ethnic identity on discrimination and adolescents' self-esteem. *Journal of Applied Social Psychology, 33*(11), 2288–2305.

Rousseau, N. (2002). *Self, symbols, and society: Classic readings in social psychology.* Rowman & Littlefield.

Sagioglou, C., & Greitemeyer, T. (2014). Facebook's emotional consequences: Why Facebook causes a decrease in mood and why people still use it. *Computers in Human Behavior, 35*, 359–363.

Sampasa-Kanyinga, H., & Lewis, R. F. (2015). Frequent use of social networking sites is associated with poor psychological functioning among children and adolescents. *Cyberpsychology, Behavior, and Social Networking, 18*(7), 380–385.

Sanders-Phillips, K., & Kliewer, W. (2019). Violence and racial discrimination in South African youth: Profiles of a continuum of exposure. *Journal of Child and Family Studies, 29*(5), 1336–1349.

Saurabh, K., & Ranjan, S. (2020). Compliance and psychological impact of quarantine in children and adolescents due to Covid-19 pandemic. *The Indian Journal of Pediatrics, 87*, 532–536.

Sentenac, M., Ehlinger, V., Napoletano, A., Spilka, S., Gariepy, G., Godeau, E., & Elgar, F. J. (2017). Relative deprivation and episodes of drunkenness among French and Canadian adolescents. *Drug and Alcohol Review, 36*(6), 788–796.

Shim, R. S., & Compton, M. T. (2018). Addressing the social determinants of mental health: If not now, when? If not us, who? *Psychiatric Services, 69*(8), 844–846.

St Leger, L., & Young, I. M. (2009). Creating the document 'Promoting health in schools: from evidence to action'. *Global Health Promotion, 16*(4), 69–71.

Syme, S. L. (1994). The social environment and health. *Daedalus, 123*(4), 79–86.

Turecki, G., & Meaney, M. J. (2016). Effects of the social environment and stress on glucocorticoid receptor gene methylation: A systematic review. *Biological Psychiatry, 79*(2), 87–96.

Umaña-Taylor, A. J., & Updegraff, K. A. (2007). Latino adolescents' mental health: Exploring the interrelations among discrimination, ethnic identity, cultural orientation, self-esteem, and depressive symptoms. *Journal of Adolescence, 30*(4), 549–567.

Valkenburg, P. M., & Peter, J. (2007). Preadolescents' and adolescents' online communication and their closeness to friends. *Developmental Psychology, 43*(2), 267.

Viner, R. M., Ozer, E. M., Denny, S., Marmot, M., Resnick, M., Fatusi, A., & Currie, C. (2012). Adolescence and the social determinants of health. *The Lancet, 379*(9826), 1641–1652.

Wahn, E. H., & Nissen, E. (2008). Sociodemographic background, lifestyle and psychosocial conditions of Swedish teenage mothers and their perception of health and social support during pregnancy and childbirth. *Scandinavian Journal of Public Health, 36*(4), 415–423.

Whitehead, M., & Dahlgren, G. (1991). What can be done about inequalities in health? *The Lancet, 338*(8774), 1059–1063.

WHO. (1997). *Promoting health through schools: Report of a WHO expert committee on comprehensive school health education and promotion*. World Health Organization.

WHO. (2008). *CSDH final report*. WHO.

WHO. (2014). *Social determinants of mental health*.

Wilkinson, A. V., Vasudevan, V., Honn, S. E., Spitz, M. R., & Chamberlain, R. M. (2009). Sociodemographic characteristics, health beliefs, and the accuracy of cancer knowledge. *Journal of Cancer Education, 24*(1), 58–64.

Williams, D. R. (1997). Race and health: Basic questions, emerging directions. *Annals of Epidemiology, 7*(5), 322–333.

Williams, G. H. (2003). The determinants of health: Structure, context and agency. *Sociology of Health & Illness, 25*(3), 131–154.

Quotation from the parent of an adolescent who participated in Daráine Murphy's (2022) Doctoral Dissertation, University College Dublin:

'I have really good friends and they have no idea what we went through last year em they would have helped but I couldn't let them help because we couldn't talk about it because then they would treat him differently and we couldn't have that because he needed to have things normal around him until he was able to normalise and not have especially when he was doing ok so it's a very I don't know it is a very difficult one I know we need to talk about things but at the same time once is out there he is forever that kid who yeah'

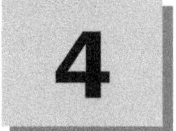

4 Promoting mental health and well-being

Snigdha Dutta
University of Cambridge, UK

Introduction

For adolescents and emerging adults across the world, their lives are marked with rapid development and for most, significant transitions to and from educational settings. It is a phase of identity exploration and competency development that involves a confluence of varied experiences that define the mental health needs of young people. The promotion of mental health and well-being of young people has come to the fore in recent times to enable successful navigation of inevitable challenges and contribute to the overall health of society (UNICEF, 2016). The former director of the World Health Organization (WHO), Brock Chisholm (1951, p. 3), famously said, 'without mental health there can be no true physical health'. Such a statement drives policies and initiatives which acknowledge and enact upon the need for lifelong approaches for the promotion of overall healthy living of individuals and communities.

The focus of this chapter is to provide an overview of the approaches to mental health promotion in young people. Considering the ambiguity surrounding the terms 'adolescence', 'youth', and 'young people', this chapter explores the provisions for mental health promotion for 'young people', which include adolescents (10–18 years old) and emerging adults (18–24 years old). The chapter clarifies the operational definitions of mental health promotion, explores the prevailing framework underlying mental health promotion, and briefly introduces some interventions for mental health promotion from the extant literature.

Mental health and mental health promotion

In recent years, the rising prevalence of mental disorders in young people has become a global cause for concern, with world-wide prevalence for mental disorders reported to range from 13.4 per cent to 26.41 per cent (Erskine et al. 2017; Polanczyk et al. 2015). Mental disorders often arise during adolescence and emerging adulthood, i.e., by 25 years old (de Girolamo et al. 2012), marking the importance of this phase to support the mental health of young people (see Chapter 9 for a detailed account of the epidemiology of mental health problems in adolescence and early adulthood).

While not all young people develop clinically poor mental health over their lifespan, they would all greatly benefit from mental health-promoting interventions and structures which support their psychological, emotional, and social well-being. Simply put, positive mental health goes beyond the absence of a mental disorder, rather the manifestation of an overall healthy state of being. Mental health is the 'state of well-being in which an individual realizes his or her [their] own abilities, can cope with the normal stresses of life, can work productively and is able to make a contribution to his or her [their] community' (WHO, 2018). The focus of this chapter is on positive mental health and 'mental health and well-being' are mentioned together to include a range of experiences as well as the emotional, social, and psychological needs of young people.

The promotion of mental health and well-being joins a continuum of care that includes prevention, treatment and recovery. Therefore, a distinction between mental health and mental disorder is important to avoid the conflation of terminologies and to recognise that the needs of young people can manifest across the spectrum between disease and health (Becker et al. 2010). The conceptual clarification of mental health and mental disorders also has implications for the provisions of care and support that are available for young people. Notably, 'traditional public mental health interventions that are effective in alleviating mental illness do not necessarily promote mental health' (Fledderus et al. 2010, p. 2372). This suggests that mental health promotion requires a shift from the psychopathological and risk-reduction models of care. Instead, mental health promotion can be described as a 'process that involves enhancing the capacities of individuals and societies to take charge of their health and thereby improve their psychological resilience, by creating supportive environments through intersectoral collaboration and participation, (Sharma et al. 2017, p. 1).

Greater investment in the promotion of mental health and well-being of young people has implications not just on their psychological, emotional and interpersonal relationships (Colizzi et al. 2020), but also on their educational attainment and career prospects (Killackey et al. 2020). By being proactive and strengthening the internal competencies of the individual and the structural support systems, it may be possible to mitigate the need for psychopathological interventions in the future (Dodge, 2020).

While the emphasis on positive mental health has been conceptually well established, the research on effective and sustainable approaches to promote mental health lags behind. This is primarily because most of the approaches have been targeted towards the individual, in this case, the adolescent or emerging adult, rather than including the systemic structures that support their development, such as their family background or their school and university settings. The conflation of the terms, i.e. mental health and mental disorders, has also led to inconsistent evidence, with most strategies being developed to reduce diagnosed or self-reported symptoms of ill-health rather than to promote competencies and adaptive resources. Further heterogeneity of evidence is due to the significant differences in economic, social and political determinants of health across nations (Maselko, 2017). Promisingly, a reformulation of mental health provisions is of interest across the globe, and the importance of socio-cultural and familial context has defined a new era for mental health promotion (Holmes et al. 2018; Killackey et al. 2020).

Socio-ecological and contextual determinants of mental health promotion

Over the last decade, 'resilience' has become a buzzword in the research into mental health promotion. Resilience is defined as a 'dynamic process encompassing positive adaptation within the context of significant adversity' (Luthar et al. 2000, p. 1). This process is 'co-facilitated by individuals and their physical and social ecologies' (Ungar & Theron, 2020, p. 441). The resilience of an individual is proposed to be an interaction between internal factors, such as temperament and emotion regulation skills, and their external context, such as a secure and happy home (Ungar & Theron, 2020). Resilience is said to be an 'ordinary magic' as all young people have the capacity to develop adaptive behaviours and positive mental health when supported by assets and resources within themselves, their family, and their social/professional environment (Masten, 2001). Over the years, the research on resilience and positive mental health has shifted from individual-focused factors to person-social-environmental factors (ahmed Shafi et al. 2020; Sharma et al. 2017) to generate a socio-ecological model of health. Such an approach to mental health promotion emphasises the need for research and practice to be grounded in contextual awareness (Ungar & Theron, 2020).

A qualitative study by Tamburrino et al. (2020) explored the perceptions of youth mental health in disadvantaged adolescents, their parents, their teachers, and professionals (e.g., counsellors, social workers) in Kenya. A range of social, familial and individual factors was identified as core aspects of their mental health. The role of the key support structures, such as the government and parents, social media, positive thinking, and shared responsibility among the youth were identified as responsible for the evasion of mental ill-health and promotion of positive mental health. In a study involving young people across four low- and middle-income countries (Brazil, Kenya, Pakistan, and Turkey), Vostanis et al. (2020) shed light on the context and stressor-dependent variations in resilience strategies. For example, in the face of an external stressor, young people sought interpersonal support and engagement (from family, peers and other elderly members) rather than intrapersonal resources like self-management and emotion-regulation skills. They applied intrapersonal resources such as cognitive reappraisal when faced with situations that evoked a negative effect, e.g., sadness and distress due to adversities in the school or within the family. Such findings demonstrate the importance of a socio-cultural context and support a socio-ecological framework for mental health promotion.

As with the socio-ecological model, social determinants of mental health, i.e., 'the conditions in which people are born, grow, live, work, and age' are integral considerations to effectively support the mental health of young people (WHO, 2008, p. 26). These conditions include dynamic factors such as adverse early life experiences, income inequality, accessibility of mental health provisions and food insecurity as well as relatively stable factors such as racial identity, gender and sexual orientation (Alegría et al. 2019; Shim & Compton, 2018). Furthermore, the meaning and impact of social determinants differ between higher-, middle- and lower-income countries, emphasising the need for cultural appropriateness

Table 4.1 Risk and protective factors across three levels: individual, family and environment

Individual-level risk and protective factors	
Risk factors	*Protective factors*
Low levels of intelligence	Gender
Internalising/externalising behaviours	Self-efficacy
Poor self-regulation	Cognitive skills
Verbal cognitive ability	Self-esteem
Mental health stigma	Positive affect and empathy
Family level risk and protective factors	
Risk factors	*Protective factors*
Parental unemployment	Family support
Parental mental illness	Parental supervision and involvement
Family violence	Positive family relationships
Inadequate care	Proactive parenting
Negative parenting styles	Secure attachment
Environmental risk and protective factors	
Risk factors	*Protective factors*
Low socio-economic status	Peer support
Homelessness	Academic engagement
Community violence and armed conflict	Community cohesion
Lack of educational opportunities	Racial and ethnic identity
Lack of health service provisions	Green and open spaces

Source: Eisenstadt et al. 2021; Gartland et al. 2019; VicHealth, 2015; Woods-Jaeger et al. 2020.

of evidence and strategies (Maselko, 2017). Thus, researchers and practitioners are encouraged to examine resilience and mental health promotion as an interactive process between the young people and their social, economic and cultural context (ahmed Shafi et al. 2020). Table 4.1 lists some of the risk and protective factors that have been identified in the literature. These factors do not function in isolation but present as complex interrelations that can impact the mental health and well-being of young people (Fritz et al. 2018).

Types of interventions for mental health promotion

Interventions targeting the promotion of mental health and well-being amplify the protective resources and assets within the individual and/or their context. The choice of the interventions depends on characteristics of the young people (e.g., gender, age, their geography), whether the whole population or a subgroup of the population is targeted, whether it is theory-based, and/or whether it targets multiple domains, such as the young person, their teachers and their families (Bjerre et al. 2020; Twum-Antwi et al. 2020). This chapter focuses on universal interventions which are aimed at the general population of interest (e.g., university students), regardless of their at-risk status. Furthermore, the chapter elaborates on promotive resource-focused or process-focused interventions which reinforce adaptive systems and/or mobilise resources within the community and the young person to promote positive mental health and well-being (Khanlou & Wray, 2014; Masten & Barnes, 2018).

To provide an overview of the types of interventions available to promote the mental health of young people, the following section briefly introduces the different types of interventions at the levels of the individual, their family and their educational institution.

Individual-level interventions

Individual-level interventions assume that equipping young people with relevant adaptive skills will help them navigate through the challenges in life. These approaches may target social, cognitive and emotional competencies to enhance their self-regulation skills, capacity to develop interpersonal relationships, psychological flexibility and adaptive emotion-regulation strategies (Fusar-Poli et al. 2020; Weissberg et al. 2015).

- **Cognitive-behavioural interventions:** Several individual-level interventions target cognitive and behavioural competencies, such as self-regulation and emotion regulation. Emotion-regulation strategies help individuals to regulate their emotions and modulate their responses to emotion-provoking situations (Li et al. 2020). These strategies, such as cognitive reappraisal and cognitive reframing, aid the maintenance and enhancement of positive affect which can contribute to flexible and creative forms of thoughts (Basson & Rothmann, 2018). Cognitive-behavioural interventions can enhance self-compassion (Inwood & Ferrari, 2018), stress-management skills (Thomas & Zolkoski, 2020), and cognitive flexibility (Pandey et al. 2018) in young people. These interventions can be incorporated into digital avenues such as online resources and personal digital assistants which are increasingly accessible to young people (Bergin et al. 2020). However, for most of these interventions, positive mental health is operationalised as a reduction in symptoms of anxiety and depression and have short-term effectiveness (Dray et al. 2017; Schmidt et al. 2020).
- **Mindfulness-based interventions**: Mindfulness emphasises purposeful and detached observation and attention to thoughts and feelings to enhance awareness towards sensory processes that help to regulate emotions (Agarwal & Dixit, 2017). Mindfulness-based interventions target emotion-regulation capabilities (Brockman et al. 2017), stress-coping skills (Ramasubramanian, 2017), resilience (Roulston et al. 2018), and self-compassion (Bluth et al. 2015). Mindfulness techniques have been incorporated in arts-based interventions, psychosocial interventions and cognitive-behavioural therapies, and these strategies can be incorporated into daily functioning. As with cognitive-behavioural interventions, mindfulness-based interventions often target stress, anxiety and symptoms of depression and demonstrate small but significant positive effects (Dunning et al. 2019).

Illustrative example

'The Mindful Student Study' (Galante et al. 2018).

- **Context:** Cambridge, United Kingdom.
- **Population:** Undergraduate and postgraduate students.
- 309 students were randomised to an eight-week mindfulness course and 307 students were part of the 'mental health support as usual' group.
- **Intervention:** The mindfulness course was intended to optimise resilience and well-being with meditation techniques targeting flexible thoughts, self-discovery, self-compassion and empowerment.
- **Outcomes:** Psychological resilience was operationalised as psychological distress (measured using the Clinical Outcomes in Routine Evaluation Outcome Measure) and mental well-being (measured using the 14-item Warwick-Edinburgh Mental Well-being Scale).
- **Findings:** The mindfulness programme was found to be more effective than the usual provisions for mental health support in reducing psychological distress and building psychological resilience.

- **Arts-based interventions:** Participation in creative activities have been found to enhance self-esteem, social skills, confidence, and resilience in young people (Bungay & Vella-Burrows, 2013). These interventions incorporate aspects of drama, visual arts, dance and music to foster meaningful social interactions, improve peer relations, modulate cognitions and reduce risk behaviours (MacDonald et al. 2020; Zarobe & Bungay, 2017). These can be embedded in the community or educational settings and provide the opportunity for inclusive and accessible social engagement. Arts-based interventions can be aligned with mindfulness programmes which can together improve social and problem-solving skills, and build creative thinking, resilience and self-esteem (Coholic, 2020). While the efficacy of these interventions needs further investigation due to large methodological and contextual variations (Zarobe & Bungay, 2017), these can be provided in conjunction with other health-promoting strategies for a cumulative positive influence on young people (Bungay & Vella-Burrows, 2013).

Additional forms of interventions include psycho-education (O'Connor et al. 2018), companion animal/canine therapies (Purewal et al. 2017), and physical activity-based interventions (Pascoe et al. 2020). Psycho-educational interventions have been identified to be most effective to promote the mental health literacy of young people (Salazar de Pablo et al. 2020). While long-term effects are still to be established, animal-assisted therapies have demonstrated short-term improvements in happiness and stress reduction in young people (Ward-Griffin et al. 2018). Overall, there is a danger of individual-level interventions leading to 'victim-blaming' if young people are unable to adapt and adjust positively (Masten, 2001; Ryan, 1971). This makes embedding these interventions with pragmatic public health and 'whole sector' reforms imperative.

Family-based interventions

For most young people, especially adolescents, considerable development occurs at home with parents. Relationships with parents and family cohesiveness confer significant risk or protection to young people. Supportive parents can ameliorate the effects of environmental stressors on young people, including chronic stressors such as poverty (Lee & Clancy, 2020), and have a cascading positive effect into adulthood (Berzin, 2010; Cluver et al. 2018). Family-based mental health promotion strategies including (and not limited to) parental training programmes, psycho-education and self-monitoring tools can support the development of lasting adaptive emotional, cognitive and behavioural skills in young people and families (Pedersen et al. 2019). Family-based interventions have a positive influence on young people to develop their psychosocial skills and resilience, as well as for parents to develop self-sufficiency and personal agency to support the development of young people (Pedersen et al. 2019; Sanders & Mazzucchelli, 2013). Importantly, in both research and practice, it is vital to recognise that parenting styles and family environments are dynamic systems that are rooted in the socio-economic and cultural context (Twum-Antwi et al. 2020).

Illustrative example

'Parenting for Lifelong Health' (Cluver et al. 2017, 2018).

- **Context:** Eastern Cape province, South Africa
- **Population:** 552 families with adolescents aged 10–18 years old
- **Intervention:** The intervention included activity-based learning, role-plays and home practices with parents and adolescents. The intervention targeted parent and adolescent social support, parent–adolescent communication, non-violent and inconsistent disciplining, and included mindfulness-based exercises.
- **Outcomes:** Primary outcomes included measures of abusive parenting, poor parental supervision, punishment styles, positive parenting, among others. Secondary outcomes included measures of caregiver and adolescent attitudes towards punishment styles, adolescent externalising behaviour, adolescent depression and suicidality, parental stress and parental depression, and social support for caregivers and adolescents. Additional measures were adolescents' exposure to community violence, academic motivation, and alcohol and drug use.
- **Findings:** The parenting programme improved parenting style and supervision, improved family planning and household economic welfare, reduced parents' symptoms of depression and stress and improved social support for both parents and adolescents. There was a reduction in adolescent rule-breaking and aggressive behaviour.

Interventions in educational settings

Educational settings, such as schools and universities, are a source of stability for most young people, with the potential for engaging with stimulating activities to promote social and emotional competencies (Barry et al. 2017; Carey, 2020). Schools and universities may be the only source of support and mental health resources for many

(Weare & Nind, 2011). With increasing participation in education across the globe (KC & Lutz, 2017), Fazel et al. (2014, p.277) propound that delivering mental health-promoting intervention in schools 'democratises access to services.' A mentally healthy educational setting requires a shift away from identification of the deficits of the students, and instead towards the holistic facilitation of positive well-being through all aspects of the educational experience (Baik et al. 2019; Came & Tudor, 2020).

Effective interventions in schools and universities can promote resilience and socio-emotional skills, educational attainment, as well as prevent the occurrence of maladaptive skills and risk behaviours (Fenwick-Smith et al. 2018; O'Reilly et al. 2018). Most school- and university-based interventions have been based on cognitive-behavioural or mindfulness-based approaches to improve psychological and social well-being (Cilar et al. 2020). However, there is a tendency to adopt discrete individual-based interventions rather than embedding sustainable strategies for mental health promotion across all aspects of the students' educational journey (Barry et al. 2017; Nielsen et al. 2015). A whole educational setting-based approach includes review and reform of academic provisions such as the curriculum, assessment strategies, peer-learning opportunities and adoption of inclusive teaching methods (Jones et al. 2020; Woolf et al. 2019). Among other adaptive skills, opportunities to develop stress-management skills, resilience, self-efficacy and a sense of belonging should be embedded across educational, social, welfare and financial support systems for students (Universities UK, 2020).

Illustrative example

'SEHER – A Whole-School Health Promotion Intervention' (Shinde et al. 2017, 2020).

- **Context:** Bihar, India
- **Population:** Secondary school children from 75 state-funded schools (n = 15232, 55 per cent boys, mean age = 14.7 years old)
- **Intervention:** A multi-component intervention, SEHER (Strengthening Evidence base on scHool-based intERventions), emphasised on the role of a positive school climate by developing supportive relationships among all members of the school community. The priority areas were the promotion of social skills, engagement with the school community, participation of students in the school-level decision-making process, access to knowledge about health and risk behaviours, and problem-solving skills. The intervention was either delivered by a counsellor or a teacher.
- **Outcomes:** Primary outcome was the school climate (measured using adapted version of Beyond Blue School Climate Questionnaire). Secondary outcomes were symptoms of depression, experiences of bullying, violence, attitudes towards gender equity, and knowledge of reproductive and sexual health. Behavioural outcomes included questions about current levels of smoking, drinking alcohol, sexual behaviour, consumption of other substances and suicide attempts.
- **Findings:** Teacher-delivered intervention had no effects. Counsellor-delivered intervention led to a positive school climate and a reduction in depression symptoms, bullying and violence. An understanding of the context is important to interpret these findings because there is a strict hierarchy between a teacher and student in India, while a counsellor was possibly perceived as being able to support students confidentially and collaboratively.

Future directions and conclusion

Overall, due to the difficulties in implementing multiple-domain interventions, most mental health-promoting strategies are fragmented and focus primarily on the individual-level characteristics of young people. A recent systematic review by Salazar de Pablo and colleagues (2020) evaluated the efficacy of universal and targeted interventions that aim to promote positive mental health in young people. Of the 276 studies examined, most studies targeted a universal population (61.9 per cent) and focused on promoting social skills followed by self-perception skills. The interventions had a small to medium magnitude of effect for promoting positive mental health. They had no significant impact, however, on improving behaviour, family relationships, and other self-regulatory strategies. Similar findings by Bjerre et al. (2020) highlight the heterogeneity in the magnitude of efficacy for different interventions in different contexts. Additionally, limited information is available regarding gender, socio-economic and ethnic differences (Barry et al. 2017; Brewer et al. 2019).

This chapter has presented an overview of the need for, and characteristics of, mental health promotion strategies for young people based on the extant literature. The key assertions made in this chapter are (1) mental health promotion is the focus on positive skills and assets rather than of the absence of mental disorders, and (2) effective mental health promotion includes a multi-modal approach that embeds protective resources across multiple domains. The chapter challenges the flawed assumption of the global applicability of promotive approaches to promote mental health and well-being in young people without contextual awareness.

To date, the most effective mechanisms underpinning mental health-promoting interventions remain inconclusive. Further evidence towards the sustainability of multi-domain interventions for a whole population group, i.e., universal interventions, is required (Fusar-Poli et al. 2020). However, the short-term benefits of promotive approaches are promising; to improve their effectiveness and sustainability, advancements are necessary. Apart from the need for robust study designs, an investigation into causal mechanisms, and methodological advancements, progress in this field requires:

- co-creation, i.e., the inclusion of the stakeholders (in this case, young people) as active collaborators in the development and design of appropriate programmes; co-creation of intervention strategies validates the lived experiences of young people and acknowledges their role as active agents rather than being subjects for research and practice (Bevan Jones et al. 2020)
- understanding the role of multiple ecologies; along with the socio-cultural context, biological (e.g., brain function) and natural ecology (e.g., nature and blue spaces) also positively impact the mental health and well-being of young people (Britton et al. 2020; Tillmann et al. 2018).
- diversity of evidence; much of the research on mental health promotion has been conducted in higher-income nations and further research in lower- and middle-income countries is anticipated (Vostanis et al. 2020). Additionally, much of the current evidence is from English-speaking countries. Considerable

research remains to be done to understand the mechanisms of social determinants of mental health in lower- and middle-income countries. Care needs to be maintained to apply evidence-based practices from higher-income countries without appropriate contextualisation (Maselko, 2017).

Mental health promotion needs to be considered alongside transformative public policy, social norms and funding, which largely differs across communities and countries (Shim & Compton, 2018). Ultimately, within each context, researchers and practitioners can assist in the promotion of positive mental health and well-being by optimising supportive resources and creating safe and healthy environments to empower young people.

Further reading

Ungar, M., & Theron, L. (2020). Resilience and mental health: How multisystemic processes contribute to positive outcomes. *The Lancet Psychiatry, 7*(5), 441–448. https://doi.org/10.1016/S2215-0366(19)30434-1

Patel, V., Saxena, S., Lund, C., Thornicroft, G., Baingana, F., Bolton, P., … UnÜtzer, Jü. (2018). The Lancet Commission on global mental health and sustainable development. *The Lancet Commissions, 392*(10157), 1553–1598. https://doi.org/10.1016/S0140-6736(18)31612-X

Fusar-Poli, P., Salazar de Pablo, G., De Micheli, A., Nieman, D. H., Correll, C. U., Kessing, L. V., … van Amelsvoort, T. (2020). What is good mental health? A scoping review. *European Neuropsychopharmacology, 31*, 33–46. https://doi.org/10.1016/j.euroneuro.2019.12.105

References

Agarwal, A., & Dixit, V. (2017). The role of meditation on mindful awareness and life satisfaction of adolescents. *Journal of Psychosocial Research, 12*(1), 59.

ahmed Shafi, A., Templeton, S., Middleton, T., Millican, R., Vare, P., Pritchard, R., & Hatley, J. (2020). Towards a dynamic interactive model of resilience (DIMoR) for education and learning contexts. *Emotional and Behavioural Difficulties, 25*(2), 183–198. https://doi.org/10.1080/13632752.2020.1771923

Alegría, M., NeMoyer, A., Falgas, I., Wang, Y., & Alvarez, K. (2019). Social determinants of mental health: Where we are and where we need to go. *Current Psychiatric Reports, 20*(11). https://doi.org/10.1007/s11920-018-0969-9

Baik, C., Larcombe, W., & Brooker, A. (2019). How universities can enhance student mental well-being: The student perspective. *Higher Education Research and Development, 38*(4), 674–687. https://doi.org/10.1080/07294360.2019.1576596

Barry, M. M., Clarke, A. M., & Dowling, K. (2017). Promoting social and emotional well-being in schools. *Health Education, 117*(5), 434–451. https://doi.org/10.1108/HE-11-2016-0057

Basson, M. J., & Rothmann, S. (2018). Flourishing: Positive emotion regulation strategies of pharmacy students. *International Journal of Pharmacy Practice, 26*(5), 458–464. https://doi.org/10.1111/ijpp.12420

Becker, C. M., Glascoff, M. A., & Felts, W. M. (2010). Salutogenesis 30 years later: Where do we go from here? *International Electronic Journal of Health Education, 13*, 25–32.

Bergin, A. D., Vallejos, E. P., Davies, E. B., Daley, D., Ford, T., Harold, G., … Hollis, C. (2020). Preventive digital mental health interventions for children and young people: A review of the design and reporting of research. *Npj Digital Medicine, 3*(1). https://doi.org/10.1038/s41746-020-00339-7

Berzin, S. C. (2010). Vulnerability in the transition to adulthood: Defining risk based on youth profiles. *Children and Youth Services Review, 32*(4), 487–495. https://doi.org/10.1016/j.childyouth.2009.11.001

Bevan Jones, R., Stallard, P., Agha, S. S., Rice, S., Werner-Seidler, A., Stasiak, K., … Merry, S. (2020). Practitioner review: Co-design of digital mental health technologies with children and young people. *Journal of Child Psychology and Psychiatry and Allied Disciplines, 61*(8), 928–940. https://doi.org/10.1111/jcpp.13258

Bjerre, N., Lillefjell, M., Magnus, E., & Anthun, K. S. (2020). Effective interventions targeting the mental health of children and young adults: A scoping review. *Scandinavian Journal of Public Health*, (September 2019), 1–13. https://doi.org/10.1177/1403494820901406

Bluth, K., Roberson, P. N. E., & Gaylord, S. A. (2015). A pilot study of a mindfulness intervention for adolescents and the potential role of self-compassion in reducing stress. *Explore, 11*(4), 292–295. https://doi.org/10.1016/j.explore.2015.04.005

Brewer, M. L., van Kessel, G., Sanderson, B., Naumann, F., Lane, M., Reubenson, A., & Carter, A. (2019). Resilience in higher education students: A scoping review. *Higher Education Research and Development, 38*(6), 1105–1120. https://doi.org/10.1080/07294360.2019.1626810

Britton, E., Kindermann, G., Domegan, C., & Carlin, C. (2020). Blue care: A systematic review of blue space interventions for health and wellbeing. *Health Promotion International, 35*(1), 50–69. https://doi.org/10.1093/heapro/day103

Brockman, R., Ciarrochi, J., Parker, P., & Kashdan, T. (2017). Emotion regulation strategies in daily life: Mindfulness, cognitive reappraisal and emotion suppression. *Cognitive Behaviour Therapy, 46*(2), 91–113. https://doi.org/10.1080/16506073.2016.1218926

Bungay, H., & Vella-Burrows, T. (2013). The effects of participating in creative activities on the health and well-being of children and young people: A rapid review of the literature. *Perspectives in Public Health, 133*(1), 44–52. https://doi.org/10.1177/1757913912466946

Came, H. A., & Tudor, K. (2020). The whole and inclusive university: A critical review of health promoting universities from Aotearoa New Zealand. *Health Promotion International, 35*(1), 102–110. https://doi.org/10.1093/heapro/day091

Carey, S. L. (2020). Promoting positive mental health in adolescent boys: Actions to tackle suicide in Australian secondary schools. *Issues in Educational Research, 30*(2), 452–472. http://www.iier.org.au/iier30/carey-abs.html

Chisholm, B. (1951). *Outline for a study group on World Health and the survival of the human race: Material drawn from articles and speeches.* https://apps.who.int/iris/bitstream/handle/10665/330666/MH.276.51-eng.pdf?sequence=1&isAllowed=y

Cilar, L., Štiglic, G., Kmetec, S., Barr, O., & Pajnkihar, M. (2020). Effectiveness of school-based mental well-being interventions among adolescents: A systematic review. *Journal of Advanced Nursing*, (April), 2023–2045. https://doi.org/10.1111/jan.14408

Cluver, L. D., Lachman, J. M., Ward, C. L., Gardner, F., Peterson, T., Hutchings, J. M., … Redfern, A. A. (2017). Development of a parenting support program to prevent abuse of adolescents in South Africa: Findings from a pilot pre-post study. *Research on Social Work Practice, 27*(7), 758–766. https://doi.org/10.1177/1049731516628647

Cluver, L. D., Meinck, F., Steinert, J. I., Shenderovich, Y., Doubt, J., Romero, R. H., … Gardner, F. (2018). Parenting for lifelong health: A pragmatic cluster randomised controlled trial of a non-commercialised parenting programme for adolescents and their families in South Africa. *BMJ Global Health, 3*(1), 1–15. https://doi.org/10.1136/bmjgh-2017-000539 Creative Commons Attribution (CC BY 4.0) https://creativecommons.org/licenses/by/4.0/

Coholic, D. A. (2020). Promoting resilience in youth through participation in an arts-based mindfulness group program. *Arts-Based Research, Resilience and Well-Being Across the Lifespan*, 63–80. https://doi.org/10.1007/978-3-030-26053-8_5

Colizzi, M., Lasalvia, A., & Ruggeri, M. (2020). Prevention and early intervention in youth mental health: Is it time for a multidisciplinary and trans-diagnostic model for care? *International Journal of Mental Health Systems*, *14*(1), 1–14. https://doi.org/10.1186/s13033-020-00356-9

De Girolamo, G., Dagani, J., Purcell, R., Cocchi, A., & McGorry, P. D. (2012). Age of onset of mental disorders and use of mental health services: Needs, opportunities and obstacles. *Epidemiology and Psychiatric Sciences*, *21*(1), 47–57. https://doi.org/10.1017/S2045796011000746

Dodge, K. A. (2020). Annual Research Review: Universal and targeted strategies for assigning interventions to achieve population impact. *Journal of Child Psychology and Psychiatry and Allied Disciplines*, *61*(3), 255–267. https://doi.org/10.1111/jcpp.13141

Dray, J., Bowman, J., Campbell, E., Freund, M., Wolfenden, L., Hodder, R. K., … Wiggers, J. (2017). Systematic review of universal resilience-focused interventions targeting child and adolescent mental health in the school setting. *Journal of the American Academy of Child and Adolescent Psychiatry*, *56*(10), 813–824. https://doi.org/10.1016/j.jaac.2017.07.780

Dunning, D. L., Griffiths, K., Kuyken, W., Crane, C., Foulkes, L., Parker, J., & Dalgleish, T. (2019). Research Review: The effects of mindfulness-based interventions on cognition and mental health in children and adolescents – a meta-analysis of randomized controlled trials. *Journal of Child Psychology and Psychiatry and Allied Disciplines*, *60*(3), 244–258. https://doi.org/10.1111/jcpp.12980

Eisenstadt, M., Merrick, H., Town, R., Dutta, S., Lally-Francis, A., Garland, L., … Edbrooke-Childs, J. (2021). *A brief review of protective factors for positive mental health among children and young people of colour* (Vol. March). https://www.ons.gov.uk/peoplepopulationandcommunity/birthsdeathsandmarriages/deaths/articles/

Erskine, H. E., Baxter, A. J., Patton, G., Moffitt, T. E., Patel, V., Whiteford, H. A., & Scott, J. G. (2017). The global coverage of prevalence data for mental disorders in children and adolescents. *Epidemiology and Psychiatric Sciences*, *26*(4), 395–402. https://doi.org/10.1017/S2045796015001158

Fazel, M., Hoagwood, K., Stephan, S., & Ford, T. (2014). Mental health interventions in schools 1: Mental health interventions in schools in high-income countries. *The Lancet Psychiatry*, *1*(5), 377–387. https://doi.org/10.1016/S2215-0366(14)70312-8

Fenwick-Smith, A., Dahlberg, E., & Thompson, S. (2018). Systematic review of resilience-enhancing universal primary school-based mental health promotion programs. *BMC Psychology*, *6*(39), 1–17. https://doi.org/10.1186/s40359-018-0242-3

Fledderus, M., Bohlmeijer, E. T., Smit, F., & Westerhof, G. J. (2010). Mental health promotion as a new goal in public mental health care: A randomized controlled trial of an intervention enhancing psychological flexibility. *American Journal of Public Health*, *100*(12), 2372–2378. https://doi.org/10.2105/AJPH.2010.196196

Fritz, J., de Graaff, A. M., Caisley, H., van Harmelen, A. L., & Wilkinson, P. O. (2018). A systematic review of amenable resilience factors that moderate and/or mediate the relationship between childhood adversity and mental health in young people. *Frontiers in Psychiatry*, *9*. https://doi.org/10.3389/fpsyt.2018.00230

Fusar-Poli, P., Salazar de Pablo, G., De Micheli, A., Nieman, D. H., Correll, C. U., Kessing, L. V., … van Amelsvoort, T. (2020). What is good mental health? A scoping review. *European Neuropsychopharmacology*, *31*, 33–46. https://doi.org/10.1016/j.euroneuro.2019.12.105

Galante, J., Dufour, G., Vainre, M., Wagner, A. P., Stochl, J., Benton, A., … Jones, P. B. (2018). A mindfulness-based intervention to increase resilience to stress in university students (the Mindful Student Study): A pragmatic randomised controlled trial. *Lancet Public Health*, *3*, 72–81. https://doi.org/10.1016/S2468-2667(17)30231-1 Creative Commons Attribution (CC BY 4.0) https://creativecommons.org/licenses/by/4.0/

Gartland, D., Riggs, E., Muyeen, S., Giallo, R., Afifi, T. O., Macmillan, H., … Brown, S. J. (2019). What factors are associated with resilient outcomes in children exposed to social adversity?

A systematic review. *BMJ Open, 9*(4), 1–14. https://doi.org/10.1136/bmjopen-2018-024870, This is an open access article distributed in accordance with the Creative Commons Attribution Non Commercial (CC BY-NC 4.0) license, http://creativecommons.org/licenses/by-nc/4.0/.

Holmes, E. A., Ghaderi, A., Harmer, C. J., Ramchandani, P. G., Cuijpers, P., Morrison, A. P., … Craske, M. G. (2018). The Lancet Psychiatry Commission on psychological treatments research in tomorrow's science. *The Lancet Psychiatry Commission, 5*, 237–286. https://doi.org/10.1016/S2215-0366(17)30513-8

Inwood, E., & Ferrari, M. (2018). Mechanisms of change in the relationship between self-compassion, emotion regulation, and mental health: A systematic review. *Applied Psychology: Health and Well-Being, 10*(2), 215–235. https://doi.org/10.1111/aphw.12127

Jones, E., Priestley, M., Brewster, L., Wilbraham, S. J., Hughes, G., & Spanner, L. (2020). Student well-being and assessment in higher education: The balancing act. *Assessment & Evaluation in Higher Education, 46*(3), 438–450. https://doi.org/10.1080/02602938.2020.1782344

Khanlou, N., & Wray, R. (2014). A whole community approach toward child and youth resilience promotion: A review of resilience literature. *International Journal of Mental Health and Addiction, 12*(1), 64–79. https://doi.org/10.1007/s11469-013-9470-1

Killackey, E., Hodges, C., Browne, V., Gow, E., Varnum, P., McGorry, P., & Purcell, R. (2020). *A global framework for youth mental health: Investing in future mental capital for individuals, communities and economies.* http://www3.weforum.org/docs/WEF_Youth_Mental_Health_2020.pdf

Lee, K., & Clancy, B. (2020). Impact of poverty on adolescent drug use: Moderation effects of family support and self-esteem. *Journal of Social Work Practice in the Addictions, 20*(4), 272–291. https://doi.org/10.1080/1533256X.2020.1838860

Li, J., Yao, M., & Liu, H. (2020). From social support to adolescents' subjective well-being: The mediating role of emotion regulation and prosocial behavior and gender difference. *Child Indicators Research, 14*, 77–93. https://doi.org/10.1007/s12187-020-09755-3

Luthar, S. S., Cicchetti, D., & Becker, B. (2000). The construct of resilience: A critical evaluation and guidelines for future work. *Child Development, 100*(2), 130–134. https://doi.org/10.1016/j.pestbp.2011.02.012

MacDonald, A., Baguley, M., Barton, E., & Kerby, M. (2020). How arts-based methods are used to support the resilience and well-being of young people: A review of the literature. In L. McKay (Ed.), *Arts-Based Research, Resilience and Well-Being Across the Lifespan* (Vol. 36, pp. 111–137). Springer.

Maselko, J. (2017). Social epidemiology and global mental health: Expanding the evidence from high-income to low- and middle-income countries. *Current Epidemiology Reports, 4*(2), 166–173. https://doi.org/10.1007/s40471-017-0107-y

Masten, A. S. (2001). Ordinary magic: Resilience processes in development. *American Psychologist, 56*(3), 227–238. https://doi.org/10.1037//0003-066X.56.3.227

Masten, A. S., & Barnes, A. (2018). Resilience in children: Developmental perspectives. *Children, 5*(7), 98. https://doi.org/10.3390/children5070098

Nielsen, L., Meilstrup, C., Nelausen, M. K., Koushede, V., & Holstein, B. E. (2015). Promotion of social and emotional competence: Experiences from a mental health intervention applying a whole school approach. *Health Education, 115*(3/4), 339–356. https://doi.org/10.1108/HE-03-2014-0039

O'Connor, C. A., Dyson, J., Cowdell, F., & Watson, R. (2018). Do universal school-based mental health promotion programmes improve the mental health and emotional wellbeing of young people? A literature review. *Journal of Clinical Nursing, 27*(3–4), e412–e426. https://doi.org/10.1111/jocn.14078

O'Reilly, M., Svirydzenka, N., Adams, S., & Dogra, N. (2018). Review of mental health promotion interventions in schools. *Social Psychiatry and Psychiatric Epidemiology, 53*(7), 647–662. https://doi.org/10.1007/s00127-018-1530-1

Pandey, A., Hale, D., Das, S., Goddings, A. L., Blakemore, S. J., & Viner, R. M. (2018). Effectiveness of universal self-regulation-based interventions in children and adolescents: A systematic review and meta-analysis. *JAMA Pediatrics, 172*(6), 566–575. https://doi.org/10.1001/jamapediatrics.2018.0232

Pascoe, M., Bailey, A. P., Craike, M., Carter, T., Patten, R., Stepto, N., & Parker, A. (2020). Physical activity and exercise in youth mental health promotion: A scoping review. *BMJ Open Sport and Exercise Medicine, 6*(1), 1–11. https://doi.org/10.1136/bmjsem-2019-000677

Pedersen, G. A., Smallegange, E., Coetzee, A., Hartog, K., Turner, J., Jordans, M. J. D., & Brown, F. L. (2019). A systematic review of the evidence for family and parenting interventions in low- and middle-income countries: Child and youth mental health outcomes. *Journal of Child and Family Studies, 28*(8), 2036–2055. https://doi.org/10.1007/s10826-019-01399-4

Polanczyk, G. V., Salum, G. A., Sugaya, L. S., Caye, A., & Rohde, L. A. (2015). Annual research review: A meta-analysis of the worldwide prevalence of mental disorders in children and adolescents. *Journal of Child Psychology and Psychiatry and Allied Disciplines, 56*(3), 345–365. https://doi.org/10.1111/jcpp.12381

Purewal, R., Christley, R., Kordas, K., Joinson, C., Meints, K., Gee, N., & Westgarth, C. (2017). Companion animals and child/adolescent development: A systematic review of the evidence. *International Journal of Environmental Research and Public Health, 14*(3). https://doi.org/10.3390/ijerph14030234

Ramasubramanian, S. (2017). Mindfulness, stress coping and everyday resilience among emerging youth in a university setting: A mixed methods approach. *International Journal of Adolescence and Youth, 22*(3), 308–321. https://doi.org/10.1080/02673843.2016.1175361

Roulston, A., Montgomery, L., Campbell, A., & Davidson, G. (2018). Exploring the impact of mindfulnesss on mental well-being, stress and resilience of undergraduate social work students. *Social Work Education, 37*(2), 157–172. https://doi.org/10.1080/02615479.2017.1388776

Ryan, W. (1971). *Blaming the victim.* Orbach & Chambers.

Salazar de Pablo, G., De Micheli, A., Nieman, D. H., Correll, C. U., Kessing, L. V., Pfennig, A., … Fusar-Poli, P. (2020). Universal and selective interventions to promote good mental health in young people: Systematic review and meta-analysis. *European Neuropsychopharmacology, 41*, 28–39. https://doi.org/10.1016/j.euroneuro.2020.10.007

Samir, K. C., & Lutz, W. (2017). The human core of the shared socioeconomic pathways: Population scenarios by age, sex and level of education for all countries to 2100. *Global Environmental Change, 42*, 181–192. https://doi.org/10.1016/j.gloenvcha.2014.06.004

Sanders, M. R., & Mazzucchelli, T. G. (2013). The promotion of self-regulation through parenting interventions. *Clinical Child and Family Psychology Review, 16*(1), 1–17. https://doi.org/10.1007/s10567-013-0129-z

Schmidt, M., Werbrouck, A., Verhaeghe, N., Putman, K., Simoens, S., & Annemans, L. (2020). Universal mental health interventions for children and adolescents: A systematic review of health economic evaluations. *Applied Health Economics and Health Policy, 18*(2), 155–175. https://doi.org/10.1007/s40258-019-00524-0

Sharma, A., Sharma, S. D., & Sharma, M. (2017). Mental health promotion: A narrative review of emerging trends. *Current Opinion in Psychiatry, 30*(5), 339–345. https://doi.org/10.1097/YCO.0000000000000347

Shim, R. S., & Compton, M. T. (2018). Addressing the social determinants of mental health: If not now, when? If not us, who? *Psychiatric Services, 69*(8), 844–846. https://doi.org/10.1176/appi.ps.201800060

Shinde, S., Pereira, B., Khandeparkar, P., Sharma, A., Patton, G., Ross, D. A., … Patel, V. (2017). The development and pilot testing of a multicomponent health promotion intervention (SEHER) for secondary schools in Bihar, India. *Global Health Action, 10*(1). https://doi.org/10.1080/16549716.2017.1385284 Creative Commons Attribution (CC BY 4.0) https://creativecommons.org/licenses/by/4.0/

Shinde, S., Weiss, H. A., Khandeparkar, P., Pereira, B., Sharma, A., Gupta, R., … Patel, V. (2020). A multicomponent secondary school health promotion intervention and adolescent health: An extension of the SEHER cluster randomised controlled trial in Bihar, India. *PLoS Medicine, 17*(2), 1–17. https://doi.org/10.1371/JOURNAL.PMED.1003021

Tamburrino, I., Getanda, E., O'Reilly, M., & Vostanis, P. (2020). "Everybody's responsibility": Conceptualization of youth mental health in Kenya. *Journal of Child Health Care, 24*(1), 5–18. https://doi.org/10.1177/1367493518814918

Thomas, C., & Zolkoski, S. M. (2020). Preventing stress among undergraduate learners: The importance of emotional intelligence, resilience, and emotion regulation. *Frontiers in Education, 5*(June), 1–8. https://doi.org/10.3389/feduc.2020.00094

Tillmann, S., Tobin, D., Avison, W., & Gilliland, J. (2018). Mental health benefits of interactions with nature in children and teenagers: A systematic review. *Journal of Epidemiology and Community Health, 72*, 958–966. https://doi.org/10.1136/jech-2018-210436

Twum-Antwi, A., Jefferies, P., & Ungar, M. (2020). Promoting child and youth resilience by strengthening home and school environments: A literature review. *International Journal of School and Educational Psychology, 8*(2), 78–89. https://doi.org/10.1080/21683603.2019.1660284

Ungar, M., & Theron, L. (2020). Resilience and mental health: How multisystemic processes contribute to positive outcomes. *The Lancet Psychiatry, 7*(5), 441–448. https://doi.org/10.1016/S2215-0366(19)30434-1

UNICEF. (2016). *State of the world's children: A fair chance for every child.* New York. https://www.unicef.org/reports/state-worlds-children-2016

Universities UK. (2020). *Stepchange: Mentally healthy universities.* https://www.universitiesuk.ac.uk/policy-and-analysis/reports/Documents/2020/uuk-stepchange-mhu.pdf

VicHealth. (2015). *Epidemiological evidence relating to resilience and young people: A literature review.* Melbourne. https://www.vichealth.vic.gov.au/~/media/ResourceCentre/PublicationsandResources/Mental health/Epidemiological evidence relating to resilience and young people. pdf?la=en

Vostanis, P., Haffejee, S., Yazici, H., Hussein, S., Ozdemir, M., Tosun, C., & Maltby, J. (2020). Youth conceptualization of resilience strategies in four low- and middle-income countries. *International Journal of Child, Youth and Family Studies, 11*(1), 91–110. https://doi.org/10.18357/ijcyfs111202019475

Ward-Griffin, E., Klaiber, P., Collins, H. K., Owens, R. L., Coren, S., & Chen, F. S. (2018). Petting away pre-exam stress: The effect of therapy dog sessions on student well-being. *Stress and Health, 34*(3), 468–473. https://doi.org/10.1002/smi.2804

Weare, K., & Nind, M. (2011). Mental health promotion and problem prevention in schools: What does the evidence say? *Health Promotion International, 26*(SUPPL. 1). https://doi.org/10.1093/heapro/dar075

Weissberg, R. P., Durlak, J. A., Domitrovich, C. E., & Gullotta, T. P. (2015). Social and emotional learning: Past, present, and future. In J. A. Durlak, C. E. Domitrovich, R. P. Weissberg, & T. P. Gullotta (Eds.), *Handbook of Social and Emotional Learning: Research and Practice* (pp. 3–19). New York, NY, US: The Guilford Press.

Woods-Jaeger, B., Siedlik, E., Adams, A., Piper, K., O'Connor, P., & Berkley-Patton, J. (2020). Building a contextually-relevant understanding of resilience among African American youth exposed to community violence. *Behavioral Medicine, 46*(3–4), 330–339. https://doi.org/10.1080/08964289.2020.1725865 This is an open access article distributed in accordance with the Creative Commons Attribution Non Commercial (CC BY-NC 4.0) license, http://creativecommons.org/licenses/by-nc/4.0/.

Woolf, S., Zemits, B., Janssen, A., & Knight, S. (2019). Supporting resilience in first year of university: Curriculum, consideration and cooperation. *Journal of Academic Language and Learning, 13*(1), 108–123.

World Health Organization. (2008). *Commission on social determinants of health: Closing the gap in a generation: Health equity through action on the social determinants of health.* Geneva.

World Health Organization. (2018). Mental health: Strengthening our response. February 17, 2021, from https://www.who.int/en/news-room/fact-sheets/detail/mental health-strengthening-our-response

Zarobe, L., & Bungay, H. (2017). The role of arts activities in developing resilience and mental wellbeing in children and young people a rapid review of the literature. *Perspectives in Public Health, 137*(6), 337–347. https://doi.org/10.1177/1757913917712283

Quotation from a young person who participated in Lynn McKeague's (2013) Doctoral Dissertation, University College Dublin:

'Once that label is put on them, once "depression" is put on them [children], "major depression" or "ADHD", or whatever other names they want to give it, well then that's it – they're marked for life, aren't they? It doesn't go away. It's not something you can get rid of. It's not a broken leg that heals and goes away, it's a lifelong tag you have to wear. [...] So not only are you trying to deal with this thing that's wrong with you, you're also thinking that you're in some way defective. And then society doesn't help when you're literally labelled as defective. You know, you're labelled with a disorder, not an illness, a disorder. Implying that other people work this way, and you work that way.'

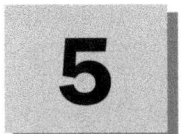

5 Stigma

Lorraine Swords
Trinity College Dublin, Ireland

Eilis Hennessy
University College Dublin, Ireland

Caroline Heary
National University of Ireland, Galway, Ireland

Introduction

'You didn't want to be labelled "bonkers" or "crazy" or "madhouse"[...] so [...] you hide it and the problem just gets worse' ('Sarah').

'Now having a mental illness is my biggest secret because I need to protect myself from the stigma' ('Ely').

'Sarah' and 'Ely' are young adults and former in-patients of a child and adolescent mental health service in Ireland (Byrne and Swords, 2015, pg. 69, 71).

The challenges of living with mental health difficulties are compounded for those affected when they also have to contend with stigma associated with their condition. Stigma is a formidable socially constructed phenomenon that is profoundly discrediting, exerting persistent and pervasive negative effects on the lives it touches. With few exceptions, adolescents experiencing mental disorders are consistently more stigmatised than peers who have physical illness or disability, learning difficulties, or developmental delay (Kaushik et al. 2016). The stigma they experience can exacerbate the symptoms characteristic of their mental health problem and act as another hurdle to disclosing difficulties and seeking treatment, thereby perpetuating the problem and ultimately generating an array of negative psychological and social consequences (Ferrie et al. 2020).

Although the body of research focused on the expression, perception or experience of mental disorder stigma in younger populations is much smaller in comparison to that centred on adult populations, it has been developing steadily over the past twenty years. Recent reviews have emphasised how the unique position of children and young people within society, along with their unique psychological and social needs, can amplify the experience of stigma (DeLuca, 2019; Heary et al. 2017). Therefore, those whose research on stigma focuses on younger age groups have emphasised the need to study how stigma is enacted and experienced in childhood, adolescence and early adulthood, rather than simply translating findings gleaned from older adult groups.

The experience and expression of mental disorder stigma

Many mental disorders first appear in childhood or adolescence and can persist into and throughout adulthood (Kessler et al. 2007; Merikangas et al. 2010). As a developmental period already featuring a surge of physical, psychological, emotional and social changes, the additional burden of a mental disorder and associated stigma in adolescence can impact considerably upon young lives. Self-concept and identity formation, for example, although lifelong processes, are key tasks of adolescence (Erikson, 1968). Cultivating a positive identity can be difficult for a young person when simultaneously dealing with the challenges posed by unchecked symptoms of a mental disorder or stigmatising responses from others. Indeed, because identity development is largely based on membership of social groups, concern about being identified as a member of a devalued group can interfere with healthy identity formation (DeLuca, 2019) and result in less than equal participation in society, including seeking help for mental disorders.

Experiencing stigma during adolescence is also particularly problematic considering the importance young people in this life stage place on peer relationships. Peer acceptance is an important contributor to healthy psychological adjustment during adolescence, while negative peer responses, such as victimisation, are implicated in a range of issues such as anxiety, loneliness and social withdrawal (Brown & Larson, 2009). For adolescents with mental health issues, the peer group can be a source of social support, with some reporting positive experiences when disclosing to close and trusted friends. However, many studies also report young people's concerns about social exclusion. For example, some adolescents in Kranke et al.'s (2010) study stated that they concealed from peers their diagnosis and the use of medication to treat their symptoms in order to avoid embarrassment, being teased, or feeling 'different'. These concerns likely have sound basis, as noted by Wahl and colleagues (2012, p. 654): 'At an age when peer approval and inclusion are especially important and when many serious mental health problems emerge, a student experiencing such problems will not be well served by encounters with classmates with negative and rejecting views'.

The adults in young people's lives can play an important role in modelling positive attitudes and behaviours regarding mental disorders and creating environments conducive to acceptance. Yet, stigmatising responses from parents, teachers and healthcare professionals have been recorded in the literature. Moses (2010), for example, reported how half of the 60 adolescents interviewed in her study said that they were treated in some way differently (e.g. blamed, rejected, avoided) by their family members due to their mental health issues. Over a third of respondents believed that school staff had treated them in negative and demeaning ways (e.g. being underestimated, excluded and feared). The emerging adults interviewed by Byrne and Swords (2015) who had spent time as in-patients in a child and adolescent mental health service spoke about parents and professionals colluding with them to keep their diagnosis and treatment hidden from others, further compounding their sense that their situation was offensive and unacceptable. One young man stated, 'My own parents [...] clench up [...] they're so, the older people are so terrified of what their friends will think or their neighbours. [...] they're embarrassed of it [...] they have [...] an awful lot of regrets like [...] how did it happen to my son?' (p. 69). Such reactions from important people in their social networks only serve to invalidate the young person's illness, induce feelings of shame and embarrassment, lower self-esteem, and self-worth, prompt them to limit their social interactions, and hinder help-seeking and adherence to treatment (Ferrie et al. 2020).

When it comes to exploring the beliefs and attitudes of adolescents towards peers or adults with mental disorders, their capacity to stereotype, react with prejudice, and propose discriminatory behavioural intentions or actual behaviours is apparent (DeLuca, 2019). For example, adolescents have been found to link the symptoms of mental health problems with being 'weird', 'rare' and 'taboo' (MacLean et al. 2013) and generate a range of negative terms such as 'disturbed', 'nuts' and 'psycho' when asked for words or phrases that they associate with someone experiencing such problems (Rose et al. 2007). Prejudicial, affective responses in the form of fear, anger and indifference have also been noted when young people are evaluating others described as having mental health conditions. Responses are particularly negative when individuals are perceived as being in some way responsible for their condition (Corrigan et al. 2005). Conversely, if they are perceived as having little control over the cause of their condition, individuals tend to receive more sympathy and social acceptance (Dolphin & Hennessy, 2016). Prejudicial responses, generated by negative stereotypes, are associated with stigmatising behavioural intentions or actual responses, such as social exclusion. Hanlon and Swords (2020), for example, found that adolescents who believed that symptoms of social anxiety disorder were signs of personal weakness, rather than reflective of a real medical condition, were more likely to exhibit prejudice in the form of more anger and fear, and less pity. These responses then related to greater discrimination as measured by social distance. Further to this, stigmatising responses had a negative relationship with adolescents' willingness to give help to this peer.

Having ascertained that adolescents can exhibit stigmatising responses to individuals with mental disorders, it should be noted that the extent to which the different components of stigma, or aspects of these components, are endorsed vary according to the type of mental disorder. For example, Jorm and Wright (2008) found that individuals with psychosis and depression did not receive significantly different endorsements that they were 'weak' rather than 'sick', but the person with psychosis was considered by young people to be more dangerous and unpredictable than the person with depression. The extent to which stigma is endorsed for different mental disorders also varies according to characteristics of the stigmatiser. Beliefs and attitudes can change through adolescence and into adulthood as young people accumulate life experience and develop cognitively, morally, emotionally and socially. For example, the increasing importance placed on peer group membership, cohesion and social order in adolescence is proposed by O'Driscoll et al. (2012) to explain how older adolescents (15–16 years old) were less accepting and more prejudicial than those younger (10–11 years old) towards peers with ADHD and depression. Later qualitative work by these researchers highlighted how adolescents' expectations that peers with mental disorders may not conform to the norms of friendship are reasons for their rejection (O'Driscoll et al. 2015). Participant gender too may play a role in the expression of stigma. Typically, boys report more negative appraisals of mental disorders and those affected by them than girls (e.g. Dolphin & Hennessy, 2016; O'Driscoll et al. 2012), though this can vary depending on the gender of the peer being evaluated and what mental health condition they present with (e.g. Swords et al. 2011).

Conceptualising and theorising the stigma of mental disorders

Mental disorder stigma is a complex concept that manifests in many ways. Two fundamental manifestations are public stigma and self-stigma.

Public stigma occurs when indicators of an attribute deemed to be undesirable are detected in an individual or group of individuals so that they become set apart in the eyes of society and devalued, demeaned or discriminated against (Corrigan & Watson, 2002). This form of stigma is described as being dependent on inequalities of power, where, for example, groups of higher social standing determine what is undesirable or deviant, fashioning 'in-groups' and 'out-groups', and placing borders between 'us' and 'them' (Corrigan & Kosyluk, 2014). Research has shown that public stigma is not only associated with having a mental health diagnosis, but also seeking professional help for a mental health issue, a sub-type called 'treatment stigma' (Vogel et al. 2017). It is important to note that individuals can be conscious of collectively held stigmatising beliefs without personally endorsing them. Thus, 'perceived public stigma', or stigma awareness, may or may not align with 'personal stigma', or stigma agreement.

Self-stigma occurs when stigmatised individuals become aware of public stigma, agree with it, and begin to apply it to themselves (Corrigan et al. 2011; Vogel et al. 2013). This internalisation can have ramifications for their self-concept, self-esteem and sense of self-efficacy. Adolescents and adults with mental health difficulties have reported how self-stigma induces feelings of shame and encourages secrecy about their condition as they attempt to avoid rejection or other negative reactions. Withdrawing socially or otherwise limiting interactions with others is commonly reported, as is delaying or avoiding seeking help (Clement et al. 2015). In these ways, self-stigma can compound already challenging symptoms leading to poorer long-term outcomes (Corrigan & Watson, 2002).

Given our focus on youth mental health, it is useful to consider the developmental basis of stigma. Very little developmental theory focuses on stigma per se. There are, however, accounts of the emergence of stereotypes and prejudices, with prejudice the more commonly used term to refer to bias towards characteristics such as gender and ethnicity (Phelan et al. 2008), in developmental science research. Knowledge of group differences has been observed in the pre-school years, particularly for very salient characteristics such as gender and race. In addition, the capacity to tune into behavioural differences has been observed from early primary-school years (Hennessy et al. 2008). Bigler and Liben (2007) argue that the developmental origins of prejudice originate in the classification of others into groups on the basis of characteristics that are particularly salient. Once individuals are categorised according to salient attributes, there is potential for negative stereotypes and prejudices to develop. Children may be exposed to the stereotypes that are prevalent in their families and communities and through repeated experience they may come to identify meaningful patterns in terms of how different social groups are treated in their social and cultural contexts. These social experiences coupled with cognitive biases (such as essentialism and in-group preferences) influence the development of stereotypes and prejudices towards social groups. DeLuca (2020) argues that at the stage of adolescence, young people are able to differentiate between their own personally endorsed stigma and their perceptions of public stigma.

Our broader theoretical understanding of the expression and experience of mental health stigma frequently draws on social psychology, sociology and evolutionary perspectives. These theories tend to be generic in nature, with little focus on developmental or lifespan issues. It is beyond the remit of this chapter to review all stigma theories so the following paragraphs will highlight those that are key to our understanding of the origins of stigma, and broader cross-cutting frameworks that seek to guide research and intervention development.

Historically, the seminal work of Goffman (1963) influenced early conceptualisations of stigma within the social sciences. Goffman defined stigma as 'an attribute that is deeply discrediting' which reduces the individual 'from a whole and usual person to a tainted, discounted one' (p. 3). Language, labelling effects and the social construction of disease and disability received much focus within sociological writings (for further information see Jones & Corrigan, 2014; Link et al. 1989). Since then, stigma has been widely researched and considered from a range of different theoretical perspectives.

Cognitive psychological approaches to stigma have prevailed in the literature over time. Social categorisation and self-identification are fundamental cognitive processes underpinning the origins of stigma whereby we tend to spontaneously and automatically allocate ourselves and others to social groups (Stangor et al. 2014). Research has consistently supported the idea that more positive characteristics are ascribed to the groups we are part of, our 'in-groups', than the groups we are not part of, called 'out-groups'. These processes can also result in the tendency to exaggerate the differences between groups and to magnify the similarities within groups (Stangor, 2009). The tendency to view members of out-groups as similar, a phenomenon termed 'out-group homogeneity' (Tajfel, 1969) lays the foundation for the application of stereotypes and exaggerated, overly simplistic ideas about group characteristics.

Many theoretical models focus on the individual (either the stigmatiser or the stigmatised) and the psychological pathways embedded in the stigma process. In contrast, Pescosolido and Martin (2015) argue for a systems approach ranging 'from the individual to the society, and processes, from the molecular to the geographic and historical, that constructs, labels, and translates difference into marks' (p. 101). Two such potential frameworks are the FINIS: A Framework Integrating Normative Influences on Stigma (Pescosolido et al. 2008) and the Health Stigma Discrimination Framework (Stangl et al. 2019). These frameworks are applicable across a range of health conditions, and place greater emphasis on the social, economic, political and cultural forces that structure stigma. While neither of these models focus specifically on youth, the emphasis on social, historical and cultural processes may guide our efforts to understand inter-generational influences that may permeate young people's experiences of mental health stigma, as well as broader structural barriers that young people may face, and the influence of youth culture on youth stigma experiences (or lack thereof).

One of the most commonly applied stigma frameworks is the tripartite social-cognitive model of mental-illness stigma which focuses on cognitive, affective and behavioural components of stigma and highlights how stereotypes may influence our judgements of members of out-groups (e.g. Corrigan, 2004). It proposes that the activation of negative cognitions in the form of stereotypical schemas or beliefs (e.g. this person is dangerous) result in affective, prejudicial reactions (e.g. I am fearful of this person) and discriminatory behaviours (e.g. I will avoid this person). Differences in social power between groups provide an enabling context for negative stereotypes and prejudices to contribute to discriminatory behaviour (Rüsch et al. 2005).

Negative stereotypes can also lead to self-fulfilling prophecies whereby the expectation of 'abnormal' behaviour from individuals with mental disorders may shape future interactions with them. Stereotype threat can influence the beliefs and behaviours of those who are the targets of stigmatisation. For example, Jones and Corrigan (2014) suggest that a student with a diagnosis of schizophrenia who is faced with a negative stereotypical assertion like 'all schizophrenics have cognitive impairments' (p. 14) may experience greater vulnerability if they have a strong identification with their health condition.

Reference to the tripartite conceptualisation of stigma is recurrent in the adult mental health literature and has recently been empirically endorsed with an adolescent sample (Silke et al. 2016). Individual components of this model have also been assessed with children and young people. However, only a few studies have considered all three stigma components and how they interrelate in the same study (e.g. Hanlon & Swords, 2020; McKeague et al. 2015). Such variations in the operationalisation of stigma across studies hampers the synthesis of findings.

The cultural context of stigma

Despite widespread evidence that mental disorders are associated with shame or disgrace in many societies around the world (Thornicroft et al. 2009), we know little about the way in which young people's experiences of stigma vary from culture to culture or how stigma can be compounded by other social identities such as race, gender and sexuality. For example, cultural differences may be manifest in differences between stigma responses in different countries or between different cultural groups within countries. This implies that the findings of research on the antecedents, correlates and/or consequences of stigma, from one country or culture cannot be assumed to apply in another. Although there is very limited research that focuses on comparing cultural, racial or ethnic experiences or expressions of stigma in adolescents and young adults, there is evidence from research with parents of younger children (e.g. Turner et al. 2015) that the implications of parents' concerns about the stigma of mental disorders for their help-seeking intentions differs between ethnic groups in the USA. In this research, Turner et al. (2015) explored parental attitudes, help-seeking intentions and concern about mental health stigma. The authors found that Hispanic Americans who reported more stigma were less likely to report that they would seek treatment for a son or daughter with a suspected mental health problem, whereas this relationship did not hold for the African Americans or European Americans within the study. Differences like these in the relationship between stigma and help-seeking in different cultural groups, for example, could have important implications for developing appropriately targeted mental health services but also for ensuring that anti-stigma messages and interventions are culturally appropriate. Knifton (2012) is critical of the fact that in many countries national campaigns to reduce stigma do not engage with minority groups at all and do not feature members of these groups within the campaign.

Research on the stigma of mental disorders in adolescence and early adulthood has, to date, also failed to adequately investigate the ways in which such stigma may be increased by membership of a marginalised social group (for example, linked to race, ethnicity, gender or sexuality) or having another stigmatised health condition (such as HIV/AIDS). Taylor and Richards (2019) argue that an intersectional approach, which takes account of overlapping forms of marginalisation, is necessary to understand the experiences of some societal groups who may be disproportionately affected by the absence of culturally appropriate services and by structural barriers to diagnosis and treatment. In other words, although the majority of individuals with a serious mental disorder may experience some level of stigma, a young, Black, gay man may have a very different experience from a young, heterosexual, white man even if they both have similar diagnosed mental disorders.

Interventions to combat mental health stigma

In light of the challenges and risks that the existence of mental health stigma creates for young people with diagnosed or suspected mental disorders, it is clearly important to attempt to reduce levels of stigma as early as possible in a young person's life. To this end, multiple school- and college-based anti-stigma interventions have been developed and implemented in the last twenty years, examples of these are outlined below. Interventions that effectively reduce stigma would facilitate the integration of youth with mental disorders with their peer group, thereby promoting and supporting the development of healthy peer relationships and the important learning that results from those relationships (Rubin et al. 2015). Over time effective interventions would reduce the levels of stigma in society and in particular the discrimination experienced by adults with serious mental disorders in areas such as housing and employment (Corrigan et al. 2003). A further potential positive consequence of reducing stigma would be to increase willingness to seek professional help for mental distress because there is evidence that among adolescents, perceptions of stigma are a barrier to seeking professional help (Radez et al. 2020).

The nature of anti-stigma interventions

Despite the need for such interventions, the total number developed, implemented and rigorously evaluated is relatively small and almost all focus on 12–18-year-olds. Most of these interventions are implemented in schools and colleges and are very diverse in their content including, for example, lectures, videos, role play, drama, discussion or some combination of these activities. Although they also vary in their duration, the majority are brief, lasting only a few hours. For example, in Flanigan and Climie's (2020) review, the interventions to reduce stigma associated with schizophrenia lasted anything between two hours and one week but the majority are completed in just one or two short sessions.

Rüsch and colleagues (2005) classify anti-stigma interventions into three broad types. The first type of intervention is 'contact based' meaning that its primary aim is to reduce stigma by providing participants with an opportunity to learn about and engage with an individual who has been diagnosed with a serious mental disorder (for example, see Chisholm et al. 2015; Link et al. 2020). Ideally this is a very carefully managed process of engagement which is comfortable for all involved. For example, in the 'SchoolSpace' intervention (Chisholm et al. 2016) a young person with experience of a mental disorder worked with a class for a morning without mentioning their mental disorder. Once the class had spent some time with the individual, they revealed their diagnosis and engaged in discussion with the members of the class and answered questions about the experience of living with a mental disorder. It is not always possible to arrange personal contact, so some interventions use 'indirect contact' in which a video is shown instead depicting a young person with a diagnosed mental disorder talking about their experience. A review of anti-stigma interventions incorporating video (Janoušková et al. 2017) indicates its potential value, particularly when the video includes both the story of a person who experienced a mental disorder and additional educational information.

The second type of intervention is usually classified as 'education' and the primary aim of such programmes is to increase understanding of mental health and mental disorders (including, for example, how to maintain positive mental health, the nature and duration of mental disorders, treatments, sources of help) and directly address the many myths that surround individuals with diagnosed mental disorders. For example, this might be debunking ideas about dangerousness and providing information on positive outcomes associated with early interventions. Some of these programmes may also include elements of direct or indirect contact as part of the curriculum (e.g. Pinfold et al. 2003; Schulze et al. 2003).

The third type of intervention described by Rusch et al. (2005) is 'protest'. Protest interventions aim to proclaim the injustices that are perpetuated by stigma (Corrigan et al. 2012) and to change public attitudes by drawing attention to their existence. Protest as a mechanism of stigma reduction is much less extensively researched than either contact or education and we are unaware of any account of the use of protest in schools or colleges or in another context with adolescents or emerging adults.

Evaluating anti-stigma interventions

There are now several systematic reviews that synthesise and evaluate the outcomes from anti-stigma interventions with young people (e.g. Flanigan & Climie, 2020; Mellor, 2014; Waqas et al. 2020). Although most note the positive short-term effects typically reported for these interventions, they also note these findings must be interpreted with caution. Reasons for caution include the lack of control/comparison groups, small sample sizes, poor reporting quality and absence of data on behavioural outcomes. Another important limitation in the anti-stigma intervention literature is that so few provide any information regarding the theory of change on which the intervention is based. While it could be argued that many interventions are implicitly based on a model of change whereby knowledge, attitude and behaviour exist along a continuum (Stuart et al. 2012), we are not aware of any studies that have explicitly elaborated on the change mechanisms that they expect. Chen et al. (2018) provide an excellent description of how hypothesised mechanisms of change can be elaborated using a logic model. Although one systematic review (Mehta et al. 2015) has focused on synthesising evidence for long-term (>4 week) reduction in stigma, it did not focus specifically on young people although approximately one third of the studies were conducted in schools or colleges. The authors' conclusions about the long-term positive effects of interventions indicate that they are modest at best, with only a medium-sized effect on knowledge outcomes and a small effect on attitudinal outcomes. Furthermore, the number of studies reporting no significant positive effects was almost equal to the number that reported a significant positive effect.

A further criticism frequently levelled at stigma interventions is that the great majority of these studies have been carried out in high-income countries. Several recent reviews have specifically sought to focus on research carried out in low- and middle-income countries (Hartog et al. 2020; Mehta et al. 2015; Waqas et al. 2020). Unfortunately, each review identified only a very small number of anti-stigma interventions and although most reported some positive effects on mental health understanding, attitudes and/or social distance, the criticism applied to the interventions in high-income countries also apply to these studies. Thus, there remains an urgent need for high-quality evaluations of interventions to reduce mental health stigma in low- and middle-income countries.

In summary, this brief overview of anti-stigma interventions indicates that a growing number of interventions are being implemented in education settings and that many have positive outcomes, at least in the short term. Limitations of the evaluations of these interventions have also been highlighted. Before leaving this topic, it is important to highlight some final points. Having noted that the great majority of interventions are implemented in educational settings, a clear consequence is that young people who are not in secondary or tertiary education are much less likely to be provided with such interventions. Because the proportion of older adolescents and emerging adults enrolled in education varies substantially around the world, this can mean that in some countries a very high proportion of youth may never be educated about mental health or stigma.

Anti-stigma interventions are one important contribution to a wider effort to ensure that young people's mental health is given due attention and that they have access to mental health supports when they need them. Another important element of this effort is the provision of youth-friendly mental health services that are specifically designed to avoid the stigma that has proved such a barrier to help-seeking among young people. These services are typically developed in consultation with young people and retain a strong youth focus in the development and design of the services offered. A recent review by Hetrick et al. (2017) indicates that young people rate the services positively and, without these services, they may not have otherwise sought help. These services are described in more detail in Chapter 13.

Conclusion

Many young people experiencing mental disorders also encounter the additional burden of stigma related to their condition or their attempts to secure treatment for it. The extent of this stigma may vary depending on characteristics of the stigmatisers or the target of their prejudicial responses, but in general is accepted as significant enough to be associated with a range of negative outcomes that cast shadows over young lives.

Stigma is a complex, multifaceted concept. The tripartite model of mental-illness stigma has emerged as one of the predominant theoretical frameworks that helps guide our thinking about the processes involved. Its key cognitive, affective and behavioural components translate, respectively, into stereotypes, prejudice and discrimination. These manifest as public stigma, or the reaction of the public towards stigmatised groups, like those with mental disorders. Young people in these stigmatised groups can internalise this public reaction and self-stigmatise. The consequences of both public stigma and self-stigma for psycho-social well-being are substantial, and young people who experience multiple forms of marginalisation may be disproportionately affected.

Well-designed studies that explore how stigma surrounding mental disorders is expressed and experienced by young people will provide valuable information for intervention efforts aimed at eliminating it. Yet research in this area is still in its infancy. If, as it is proposed, stereotypes, prejudice and discrimination are conceptually distinct components in the stigma process, it is also possible that there are distinct factors that influence or modify each one. Research that fully explores all these avenues is needed if we are to advance to a comprehensive understanding of stigma that can reliably inform effective anti-stigma programmes. At present, it seems that intervention efforts, using a variety of approaches typically within educational settings, are increasing and show potential for positive outcomes. However, more research with systematic evaluation is needed. Appeals to make mental health service provision more youth friendly are also gaining traction. This vision of services that incorporate young people's views into policy, planning and delivery shows promise for their treatment engagement and satisfaction, and ultimately breaking down stigma as a barrier to help-seeking.

Further reading

Martinez, A., & Hinshaw, S. P. (2016). Mental health stigma: Theory, developmental issues, and research priorities. In D. Cicchetti & D. J. Cohen (Eds.), *Developmental psychopathology* (4ᵗʰ ed.) (pp. 997–1039). Hoboken, NJ: Wiley.

Goodwin, J., Saab, M. M., Dillon, C. B., Kilty, C., McCarthy, A., O'Brien, M., & Philpott, L. F. (2021). The use of film-based interventions in adolescent mental health education: A systematic review. *Journal of Psychiatric Research* May (137), 158–172.

References

Bigler, R. S., & Liben, L. S. (2007). Developmental intergroup theory: Explaining and reducing children's social stereotyping and prejudice. *Current directions in psychological science, 16*(3), 162–166.

Brown, B.B., & Larson, J. (2009). Peer relationships in adolescence. In Lerner R.M., & Steinberg, L. (Eds.), *Handbook of adolescent psychology.* (pp. 74–103). John Wiley & Sons.

Byrne, A., & Swords, L. (2015). "Attention seeker", "drama queen": The power of talk in constructing identities for young people with mental health difficulties. *Mental Health Review Journal, 20* (2), 65–78.

Chen, J. (2018). Some people may need it, but not me, not now: Seeking professional help for mental health problems in urban China. *Transcultural Psychiatry, 55*(6), 754–774.

Chisholm, K., Patterson, P., Torgerson, C., Turner, E., Jenkinson, D., & Birchwood, M. (2015). Impact of contact on adolescents' mental health literacy and stigma: The SchoolSpace cluster randomised controlled trial. *BMJ Open* 2016;6:e009435. DOI: 10.1136/bmjopen-2015-009435

Clement, S., Schauman, O., Graham, T., Maggioni, F., Evans-Lacko, S., Bezborodovs, N., ... & Thornicroft, G. (2015). What is the impact of mental health-related stigma on help-seeking? A systematic review of quantitative and qualitative studies. *Psychological Medicine, 45*(1), 11–27.

Corrigan, P. W., Rafacz, J., & Rüsch, N. (2011). Examining a progressive model of self-stigma and its impact on people with serious mental illness. *Psychiatry Research, 189*(3), 339–43.

Corrigan, P. W., & Kosyluk, K. A. (2014). Mental illness stigma: Types, constructs, and vehicles for change. In P. W. Corrigan (Ed.), *The stigma of disease and disability: Understanding causes and overcoming injustices* (pp. 35–56). American Psychological Association. https://doi.org/10.1037/14297-003

Corrigan, P., Markowitz, F. E., Watson, A., Rowan, D., & Kubiak, M. A. (2003). An attribution model of public discrimination towards persons with mental illness. *Journal of Health and Social Behavior*, 162–179.

Corrigan, P. (2004). How stigma interferes with mental health care. *American Psychologist, 59*(7), 614.

Corrigan, P. W., Morris, S. B., Michaels, P. J., Rafacz, J. D., & Rüsch, N. (2012). Challenging the public stigma of mental illness: A meta-analysis of outcome studies. *Psychiatric Services, 63*(10), 963–973. https://doi.org/10.1176/appi.ps.201100529

Corrigan, P. W., & Watson, A. C. (2002). The paradox of self-stigma and mental illness. *Clinical Psychology: Science and Practice, 9*(1), 35–53.

Corrigan, P. W., Lurie, B. D., Goldman, H. H., Slopen, N., Medasani, K., & Phelan, S. (2005). How adolescents perceive the stigma of mental illness and alcohol abuse. *Psychiatric Services, 56*, 544–550. https://doi.org/10.1176/appi.ps.56.5.544, https://doi.org/10.1093/oxfordjournals.schbul.a007096.

DeLuca, J. S. (2020). Conceptualizing adolescent mental illness stigma: Youth stigma development and stigma reduction programs. *Adolescent Research Review*, 5, 153–171. https://doi.org/10.1007/s40894-018-0106-3

Dolphin, L., & Hennessy, E. (2016). Depression stigma among adolescents in Ireland. *Stigma and Health*, 1(3), 185.

Erikson, E. (1968) *Identity, Youth, and crisis*. New York: W. W. Norton.

Ferrie, J., Miller, H., & Hunter, S. C. (2020). Psychosocial outcomes of mental illness stigma in children and adolescents: A mixed-methods systematic review. *Children and Youth Services Review*, 104961.

Flanigan, L. K., & Climie, E. A. (2020). A review of school-based interventions to reduce stigma towards schizophrenia. *Psychiatric Quarterly*, 91, 983–1002 https://doi.org/10.1007/s11126-020-09765-y

Goffman, E. (1963) *Stigma: notes on the management of spoiled identity*. Prentice-Hall.

Hanlon, H. R., & Swords, L. (2020). Adolescent endorsement of the "weak-not-sick" stereotype for generalised anxiety disorder: Associations with prejudice, discrimination, and help-giving intentions toward peers. *International Journal of Environmental Research and Public Health*, 17(15), 5415.

Hartog, K., Hubbard, C. D., Krouwer, A. F., Thornicroft, G., Kohrt, B. A., & Jordans, M. J. (2020). Stigma reduction interventions for children and adolescents in low-and middle-income countries: Systematic review of intervention strategies. *Social Science & Medicine*, 246, 112749. https://doi.org/10.1016/j.socscimed.2019.112749

Heary, C., Hennessy, E., Swords, L., & Corrigan, P. (2017). Stigma towards mental health problems during childhood and adolescence: Theory, research and intervention approaches. *Journal of Child and Family Studies*, 26(11), 2949–2959.

Hennessy, E., Swords, L., & Heary, C. (2008). Children's understanding of psychological problems displayed by their peers: A review of the literature. *Child: Care, Health and Development*, 34(1), 4–9.

Hetrick, S. E., Bailey, A. P., Smith, K. E., Malla, A., Mathias, S., Singh, S. P., ... & McGorry, P. D. (2017). Integrated (one-stop shop) youth health care: Best available evidence and future directions. *Medical Journal of Australia*, 207(S10), S5–S18. DOI: 10.5694/mja17.00694.

Janoušková, M., Tušková, E., Weissová, A., Trančík, P., Pasz, J., Evans-Lacko, S., & Winkler, P. (2017). Can video interventions be used to effectively destigmatize mental illness among young people? A systematic review. *European Psychiatry*, 41(1), 1–9. DOI: 10.1016/j.eurpsy.2016.09.008

Jones, N., & Corrigan, P. W. (2014). Understanding stigma. In P. W. Corrigan (Ed.), *The stigma of disease and disability: Understanding causes and overcoming injustices* (pp. 9–34). American Psychological Association.

Jorm, A. F., & Wright, A. (2008). Influences on young people's stigmatising attitudes towards peers with mental disorders: National survey of young Australians and their parents. *The British Journal of Psychiatry*, 192(2), 144–149.

Kaushik, A., Kostaki, E., & Kyriakopoulos, M. (2016). The stigma of mental illness in children and adolescents: A systematic review. *Psychiatry Research*, 243, 469–494.

Kessler, R. C., Amminger, G. P., Aguilar-Gaxiola, S., Alonso, J., Lee, S., & Ustun, T. B. (2007). Age of onset of mental disorders: a review of recent literature. *Current Opinion in Psychiatry*, 20(4), 359.

Knifton, L. (2012). Understanding and addressing the stigma of mental illness with ethnic minority communities. *Health Sociology Review*, 21(3), 287–298. https://doi.org/10.5172/hesr.2012.21.3.287

Kranke, D., Floersch, J., Townsend, L., & Munson, M. (2010). Stigma experience among adolescents taking psychiatric medication. *Children and Youth Services Review*, 32(4), 496–505.

Link, B. G., Cullen, F. T., Struening, E., Shrout, P. E., & Dohrenwend, B. P. (1989). A modified labeling theory approach to mental disorders: An empirical assessment. *American Sociological Review*, *54*(3), 400–423.

Link, B. G., DuPont-Reyes, M. J., Barkin, K., Villatoro, A. P., Phelan, J. C., & Painter, K. (2020). A school-based intervention for mental illness stigma: A cluster randomized trial. *Pediatrics*, *145*(6). DOI: 10.1542/peds.2019-0780

MacLean, A., Hunt, K., & Sweeting, H. (2013). Symptoms of mental health problems: Children's and adolescents' understandings and implications for gender differences in help seeking. *Children & Society*, *27*(3), 161–173.

McKeague, L., Hennessy, E., O'Driscoll, C., & Heary, C. (2015). Retrospective accounts of self-stigma experienced by young people with attention-deficit/hyperactivity disorder (ADHD) or depression. *Psychiatric Rehabilitation Journal*, *38*(2), 158.

Mellor, C. (2014). School-based interventions targeting stigma of mental illness: Systematic review. *The Psychiatric Bulletin*, *38*(4), 164–171. DOI: 10.1192/pb.bp.112.041723

Merikangas, K. R., He, J. P., Burstein, M., Swanson, S. A., Avenevoli, S., Cui, L., ... & Swendsen, J. (2010). Lifetime prevalence of mental disorders in US adolescents: Results from the National Comorbidity Survey Replication–Adolescent Supplement (NCS-A). *Journal of the American Academy of Child & Adolescent Psychiatry*, *49*(10), 980–989.

Mehta, N., Clement, S., Marcus, E., Stona, A. C., Bezborodovs, N., Evans-Lacko, S., ... & Thornicroft, G. (2015). Evidence for effective interventions to reduce mental health-related stigma and discrimination in the medium and long term: Systematic review. *The British Journal of Psychiatry*, *207*(5), 377–384.

Moses, T. (2010). Being treated differently: Stigma experiences with family, peers, and school staff among adolescents with mental health disorders. *Social Science & Medicine*, *70*(7), 985–993.

O'Driscoll, C., Heary, C., Hennessy, E. & McKeague, L. (2015). Adolescents' explanations for the exclusion of peers with mental health problems: An insight into stigma. *Journal of Adolescent Research*, *30*(6), 710–728.

O'Driscoll, C., Heary, C., Hennessy, E., & McKeague, L. (2012). Explicit and implicit stigma towards peers with mental health problems in childhood and adolescence. *Journal of Child Psychology and Psychiatry*, *53*(10), 1054–1062.

Pescosolido, B. A., & Martin, J. K. (2015). The stigma complex. *Annual Review of Sociology*, *41*, 87–116.

Pescosolido, B. A., Martin, J. K., Lang, A., & Olafsdottir, S. (2008). Rethinking theoretical approaches to stigma: A framework integrating normative influences on stigma (FINIS). *Social Science & Medicine*, *67*(3), 431–440.

Phelan, J. C., Link, B. G., & Dovidio, J. F. (2008). Stigma and prejudice: one animal or two?. *Social Science & Medicine*, *67*(3), 358–367.

Pinfold, V., Toulmin, H., Thornicroft, G., Huxley, P., Farmer, P., & Graham, T. (2003). Reducing psychiatric stigma and discrimination: Evaluation of educational interventions in UK secondary schools. *British Journal of Psychiatry*, *182*, 342–6.

Radez, J., Reardon, T., Creswell, C., Lawrence, P. J., Evdoka-Burton, G., & Waite, P. (2020). Why do children and adolescents (not) seek and access professional help for their mental health problems? A systematic review of quantitative and qualitative studies. *European Child & Adolescent Psychiatry*, 1–29. https://doi.org/10.1007/s00787-019-01469-4.

Rose, D., Thornicroft, G., Pinfold, V., & Kassam, A. (2007). 250 labels used to stigmatise people with mental illness. *BMC Health Services Research*, *7*(1), 97.

Rubin K. H., Bukowski W., & Bowker J. (2015). Children in peer groups. In M. Bornstein & T. Leventhal (Volume Eds.) and R. M. Lerner (Series Ed.). *Handbook of child psychology and developmental science*, *(Vol. 4: Ecological settings and processes, 7th ed.)* (pp. 175–222). New York, NY: Wiley.

Rüsch, N., Angermeyer, M. C., & Corrigan, P. W. (2005). Mental illness stigma: Concepts, consequences, and initiatives to reduce stigma. *European Psychiatry*, *20*(8), 529–539.

Schulze, B., Richter-Werling, M., Matschinger, H., & Angermeyer, M. C. (2003). Crazy? So what! Effects of a school project on students' attitudes towards people with schizophrenia. *Acta Psychiatrica Scandinavica, 107,* 142–50.

Silke, C., Swords, L., & Heary, C. (2016). The development of an empirical model of mental health stigma in adolescents. *Psychiatry Research, 242,* 262–270.

Stangor, C. (2009). The study of stereotyping, prejudice, and discrimination within social psychology: A quick history of theory and research. In T. D. Nelson (Ed.), *Handbook of prejudice, stereotyping, and discrimination.* (pp. 1–22). Psychology Press.

Stangor, C., Jhangiani, R., & Tarry, H. (2014). *Principles of social psychology.* BCcampus.

Stangl, A. L., Earnshaw, V. A., Logie, C. H., van Brakel, W., Simbayi, L. C., Barré, I., & Dovidio, J. F. (2019). The health stigma and discrimination framework: A global, crosscutting framework to inform research, intervention development, and policy on health-related stigmas. *BMC Medicine, 17*(1), 1–13.

Stuart, H., Arboleda-Florez, J., & Sartiorius, N. (2012). Paradigms lost: Fighting stigma and the lessons learned. Oxford University Press.

Swords, L., Heary, C., & Hennessy, E. (2011). Factors associated with acceptance of peers with mental health problems in childhood and adolescence. *Journal of Child Psychology and Psychiatry, 52*(9), 933–941.

Tajfel, H. (1969). Cognitive aspects of prejudice 1. *Journal of Social Issues, 25*(4), 79–97.

Taylor, D., & Richards, D. (2019). Triple jeopardy: Complexities of racism, sexism, and ageism on the experiences of mental health stigma among young Canadian Black Women of Caribbean descent. *Frontiers in Sociology, 4,* 43. DOI: 10.3389/fsoc.2019.00043

Thornicroft, G., Brohan, E., Rose, D., Sartorius, N., Leese, M., & INDIGO Study Group (2009). Global pattern of experienced and anticipated discrimination against people with schizophrenia: A cross-sectional survey. *The Lancet, 373*(9661), 408–415. DOI:10.1016/S0140-6736(08)61817-6

Turner, E. A., Jensen-Doss, A., & Heffer, R. W. (2015). Ethnicity as a moderator of how parents' attitudes and perceived stigma influence intentions to seek child services. *Cultural Diversity and Ethnic Minority Psychology, 21*(4), 613 – 618. http://dx.doi.org/10.1037/cdp0000047

Vogel, D. L., Bitman, R. L., Hammer, J. H., & Wade, N. G. (2013). Is stigma internalized? The longitudinal impact of public stigma on self-stigma. *Journal of Counseling Psychology, 60*(2), 311–316. https://doi.org/10.1037/a0031889

Vogel, D. L., Strass, H. A., Heath, P. J., Al-Darmaki, F. R., Armstrong, P. I., Baptista, M. N., ... & Zlati, A. (2017). Stigma of seeking psychological services: Examining college students across ten countries/regions. *The Counseling Psychologist, 45*(2), 170–192.

Wahl, O., Susin, J., Lax, A., Kaplan, L., & Zatina, D. (2012). Knowledge and attitudes about mental illness: A survey of middle school students. *Psychiatric Services, 63*(7), 649–654.

Waqas, A., Malik, S., Fida, A., Abbas, N., Mian, N., Miryala, S., Amray, A.N, Shah, Z. & Naveed, S. (2020). Interventions to reduce stigma related to mental illnesses in educational institutes: A systematic review. *Psychiatric Quarterly, 91,* 887–903. https://doi.org/10.1007/s11126-020-09751-4

6 Help-seeking

Debra Rickwood
University of Canberra, Australia

Introduction

Help-seeking is a critical focus for youth mental health because of the high need for effective mental healthcare and the many access barriers experienced by young people. Addressing youth mental health problems is not simply a process of a young person developing symptoms and then receiving treatment and support. Symptoms, themselves, do not routinely trigger help-seeking behaviour and there is a large gap between the incidence of mental ill-health and treatment. This gap is greatest for young people in their teen and early adult years, a time when there is the most unmet need for mental healthcare and effective help-seeking is essential. Help-seeking for mental health problems is a complex process affected by many personal, social, and environmental factors, with the impact of these most evident during adolescence and emerging adulthood.

This chapter defines help-seeking and describes the help-seeking process. It explains the importance of seeking help for mental healthcare, by young people in particular. Young people's help-seeking preferences, along with key barriers and facilitators to them seeking help for mental health issues, are presented. Family, peers, schools and technology are highlighted as having special roles for enabling young people's help-seeking. The chapter concludes with a warning that raising help-seeking awareness must be associated with a commensurate increase in the availability and accessibility of youth-appropriate sources of mental healthcare and support.

Help-seeking process

Help-seeking is a term that refers to taking action to obtain information, support and treatment for a health condition. It is pertinent to all health issues, but has assumed special significance for mental healthcare, mainly because of the reluctance of people to reach out to obtain the help they need when experiencing mental ill-health.

Help-seeking is an active, problem-focused, coping strategy. It is a complex behaviour, entailing reaching out to other people and sources of assistance to obtain information, understanding, support, advice and treatment for the symptoms and impacts of mental health problems and disorders. Help can be sought from diverse sources that vary in their relationship to the help-seeker, formal role and level of expertise. The three main types of help-seeking are:

- **Self-help**: sourcing information and advice from books, websites, and media; often facilitated by technology and use of the internet.

- **Informal** help-seeking: from within a person's informal social network, usually family and friends; engaging support through available social connections.
- **Formal** help-seeking: from professionally based relationships including teachers, coaches, youth workers, community workers, clergy and healthcare workers. People in these formal professional roles may or may not have skills in mental healthcare, so it is useful to delineate:
  - **Semi-formal** sources: people in professional roles who are not healthcare workers (teachers, coaches).
  - **Formal** or **professional** sources: professionals with a legitimate role and specific expertise in mental health; generalist and specialist professionals with recognised training in mental healthcare (family doctors, psychologists, counsellors, social workers, psychiatrists).

The basic help-seeking process is presented in Figure 6.1, showing multiple stages involving many decision points. Several similar descriptions have been proposed (Barker, 2007; Srebnik et al. 1996). The process comprises symptom recognition, deciding to seek help, choosing a source of help, and accessing and engaging with that help-source. Seeking help commences with the advent of symptoms, which must be recognised by the person (or others) and appraised as something that requires action. A decision can then be made about the type of action deemed appropriate. To access help, the decision to seek help must be acted on. Importantly, the help-seeking process must be both initiated and then progressed, as effective help-seeking continues beyond the first point of access, requiring engagement with the help-source until the desired outcomes for the help-seeker are attained.

Although Figure 6.1 presents the process as sequential with discrete stages, this is a simplified depiction and non-linear progression, including regression and overlapping steps, and is likely to be the norm. The process is often complicated by multiple decisions, contacts and lengthy delays. It applies for all help-seeking sources: self-help, informal, semi-formal and formal. Pathways for these sources may be unique, sequential or concurrent. Because most research has been cross-sectional – investigating either future intentions to seek help or past help-seeking behaviour with little research applying a prospective longitudinal design – the proposed process has not been well-validated empirically, but still provides a useful conceptualisation.

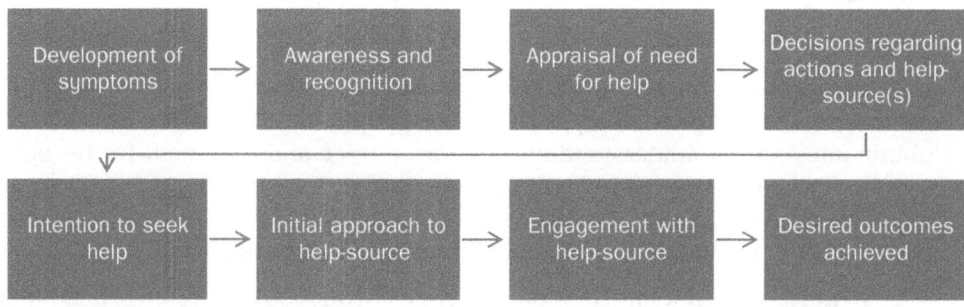

Figure 6.1 Help-seeking process

Help-seeking for mental health problems

Historically, the help-seeking concept originates from the medical sociology literature examining 'illness behaviour' – a term that refers to human health behaviour, describing the ways people monitor their bodies, define and interpret their symptoms, take preventive or remedial action, and utilise the healthcare system (Mechanic, 1962). The study of illness behaviour emerged in response to recognition that people do not consult healthcare professionals whenever they experience symptoms, and the changing nature of illness from acute to chronic and fluctuating conditions (like mental disorders). As far back as the 1970s, it was reported that people consult a doctor for only about 1 in 10 medically significant symptoms they experience (Tuckett, 1976). Complex, multi-level models of health-service use were proposed, acknowledging that illness behaviour involves many factors affecting how people respond to health symptoms and use healthcare.

Many personal, social and environmental factors affect the help-seeking process for both physical and mental health problems, which are increasingly recognised as interdependent. The help-seeking construct is particularly salient for mental health, however, due to our generally poor understanding of mental disorders and the heightened reluctance of people to seek help for symptoms of mental health problems. Without effective early intervention, mental health problems often progress or recur and have an increasingly negative impact on the course of people's lives. Consequently, attaining appropriate mental healthcare in a timely manner is critical for reducing the burden of mental ill-health on individuals, their families and the community. As shown in Chapter 9, young people are at greatest risk, with the prevalence of most mental health problems peaking during this life stage, making addressing the treatment gap more urgent.

Young people's help-seeking patterns

Young people are notably unwilling to seek help for mental health problems, although patterns vary depending on the source of help, type of problem and socio-demographic characteristics. Their help-seeking reluctance is most pronounced for professional help-seeking. This was starkly evident in a large Australian national survey revealing that 30 per cent of young women and only 13 per cent of young men aged 16–24 years old experiencing mental disorder had sought professional help in the past year (Slade et al. 2009). A more recent Australian national survey showed higher rates of health-service use, with 61 per cent of 12–17-year-olds with a mental health problem accessing a health-service provider in the past 12 months, but still substantial unmet need (Lawrence et al. 2015). While service access rates vary widely depending on the sample and method, a large and concerning mental health treatment gap is evident for young people internationally, even in high-income countries with good access to healthcare.

Young people show a marked preference for informal rather than formal help and prefer to talk to people they know and trust about their personal thoughts and feelings (Rickwood et al. 2005). Informal support is often the first step in seeking professional help (Rickwood, Mazzer, et al. 2015). This means that the social supports of family and friends are essential – of themselves and as a conduit to professional help-seeking. Consequently, the help-seeking attitudes, knowledge and behaviours of family and friends have a major impact on young people. It is often only through strong encouragement from informal supports that professional help-seeking takes place.

There are distinct developmental trends and pronounced gender patterns in informal help-seeking. These reflect expected maturation processes, with young people moving from reliance on family to close friends and intimate partners. During early adolescence, help-seeking is mostly from parents, usually mothers. As girls mature, they become more likely to talk to their friends. For boys, this is not the case; they do not disclose to friends and increasingly rely on no one but themselves, although parents remain their main source of help. A shift occurs for young men when they gain an intimate partner, who may then become their key support and help-seeking influence. So, for younger adolescents, parents are the most important source of support; for older adolescents, friends and family are relevant for girls, and boys are increasingly self-reliant; in early adulthood, friends and family are key for young women, and family and partner for young men, although young men are the population group most reticent to seek help at all. Notably, family retains a central role in seeking help among adolescents (Heerde & Hemphill, 2018), meaning that the mental health and help-seeking knowledge and attitudes of parents are crucial (Mizzi et al. 2020).

Beyond family and friends, people in formal positions, but who are not health or mental health experts have an important semi-formal role in the help-seeking context (Mazzer & Rickwood, 2014). Young people often have strong attachments to teachers, coaches, youth workers, clergy – the people with whom they have regular contact through their daily activities related to study, sport, recreation and work. These are the people who are known and trusted and often seen as role models. Such connections are especially important for young people who do not have strong family support, including those experiencing family conflict, in out-of-home care, and who are homeless. Homeless young people receiving support from community-based providers, like youth workers, were more likely to seek professional mental healthcare (Crosby et al. 2018).

In today's 'digital age', self-help enabled by technology increasingly precedes both informal and formal help-seeking. This pathway has expanded rapidly through a plethora of websites and online information about mental health, responding to young people's immersion in the digital world. The internet is fast becoming their primary source of mental health information and support. For example, over one-third of young people diagnosed with psychotic and mood disorders reported using the internet as their main source of mental health information during their pathway to care, including using social media to discuss their symptoms and understand their experiences (Bimbaum et al. 2015). Importantly, help-seeking in the online environment is quite different from other pathways; young people are mostly self-directed online, and this starts at a young age (Rickwood, Mazzer, et al. 2015). Without parental or other adult guidance, direction to credible online sources, moderated social media platforms and guided self-help are critical to the safety and effectiveness of help-seeking in the online environment.

The type of mental health problem strongly influences help-seeking, although the very nature of most of the mental health problems experienced by young people works against them reaching out for help from others (Rickwood, 2021). This includes social withdrawal and hopelessness for depressive disorders; the fear and avoidance that characterise anxiety disorders; the illicit nature of substance use; the shame that often accompanies self-harm and eating disorders; and the social withdrawal, lack of insight and paranoia that may be present in psychosis. Help-negation is a term referring to the opposite of help-seeking; it is the refusal to accept or access available help resources. It was first noted for suicidal ideation, whereby strong suicidal thoughts were associated with actively avoiding seeking help (Rudd et al. 1995). Help-seeking is least likely for more stigmatised and shameful conditions, like self-harm, suicidal ideation, alcohol and other drug use. This was demonstrated in a large national Australian survey where only 11 per cent of respondents aged 16–24 years old with a substance-use problem sought help, compared with 32 per cent with an anxiety disorder, and 49 per cent with an affective disorder (ABS, 2010).

Although help-seeking is an intensely personal and individual process, demographic and socio-cultural characteristics exert strong influences. The effects of age and gender are most researched and best understood. Gender is relevant to many aspects of mental ill-health, including age of onset, type of disorder, trajectory and long-term outcomes, as well as help-seeking. Socio-cultural variations in help-seeking patterns are less well understood as these tend to be specific to cultural and ethnic groups, and often depend upon confounded socio-economic and cultural assimilation factors. Generally, however, in high-income countries, young people from minority backgrounds are less likely to seek help and experience additional barriers to doing so. Considerable research, often from the United States, shows, for example, that help-seeking is substantially less among Asian American (Kim & Zane, 2016), Vietnamese (Guo et al. 2015) and African-American (Planey et al. 2019) young people.

While there are unique circumstances for some cultural groups, particularly young adult refugees (Valibhoy et al. 2017), the factors affecting young people's help-seeking are remarkably similar across population groups. Variations are largely due to some population groups being more exposed to, or more profoundly affected by, the barriers and facilitators. For example, a large Canadian review reported that accessing mental healthcare for Black youth was impacted at multiple levels comprising: systemic (wait times, poor access to practitioners, geographical challenges, financial barriers); practitioner-related (racism and discrimination from providers, inability to provide culturally competent care, lack of organisational support); and personal and community-related barriers (internalised stigma, stigma from community); and that support from family and friends, and good relationships with providers, were facilitators (Fante-Coleman & Jackson-Best, 2020). Many of these are common factors affecting all young people's help-seeking, but their impact is exacerbated for some population groups. (See Chapter 5 for more information on stigma and youth mental health.)

Barriers and facilitators for seeking help

A large body of research has grown about the factors that affect help-seeking for mental health problems. A major systematic review, of both qualitative and quantitative studies of young people's perspectives, identified the main barriers as problems recognising symptoms, a preference for self-reliance, and perceived stigma and embarrassment (Gulliver et al. 2010). Facilitators were less well researched, with evidence for positive past help-seeking experiences and encouragement from the informal social support network. A more recent review of professional help-seeking among adolescents confirmed that the most common barriers were limited mental health knowledge and poor perceptions of help-seeking, followed by stigma, and the therapeutic relationship with providers, including confidentiality and trust (Radez et al. 2020). A fourth theme was structural barriers from the service system itself, which is characterised world-wide by long wait times, inflexible and fragmented service models, administrative and eligibility blocks, high and unknown costs, and complex service pathways (MacDonald et al. 2021). These factors have been recognised for some time – yet, the barriers stubbornly remain and facilitators are still not well understood.

Mental health literacy

Logically, help-seeking should commence with the development of symptoms, but there is generally only a weak association between symptoms and help-seeking, particularly professional help (Zachrisson et al. 2006). Nevertheless, symptom awareness is the first filter in the help-seeking process, and the more distressing, unusual or disruptive the symptoms, the more likely the process will begin. Typically, however, young people will first attempt to ignore, hide or normalise their symptoms, hoping they will go away.

Recognition of symptoms as a mental health problem requires noticing changes in a young person's thoughts, feelings or behaviour, and defining these as a mental health issue. However, because adolescence is characterised by major changes in multiple domains, it can be difficult for young people and their family and friends to differentiate normal developmental changes from indicators of mental ill-health. This is further exacerbated by the high prevalence of mental health problems in adolescence, meaning that many mental health symptoms are regarded as typical of this life stage (e.g. moodiness, sleep problems, irritability, withdrawal from family). Consequently, young people and their social supports tend to minimise the significance of symptoms, attributing them to the teenage years. Symptoms are expected to resolve with time and maturity, and such normalisation inhibits appraising symptoms as requiring action. In contrast, labelling symptoms as outside the emotional norm facilitates the help-seeking process.

Consequently, good mental health literacy is fundamental to help-seeking (see Chapter 7). This is the knowledge and beliefs about mental disorders that aid their recognition, management and prevention (Jorm et al. 1997). In particular, the ability to recognise specific mental disorders facilitates the help-seeking process. Differences in mental health literacy have been shown to account for many demographic variations in help-seeking, including the greater reticence of young males to seek help (Haavik et al. 2019).

Stigma and confidentiality

Another pervasive barrier is the stigma of mental and seeking psychiatric care (see Chapter 5). Stigma has a profound impact for young people because peer group relationships and identity formation are crucial developmental tasks at this life stage (Blakemore, 2019). The primacy of the peer group emerges in early adolescence and peaks in mid to late adolescence, at the same time that mental health problems are rapidly rising. To belong to, and be accepted by, the peer group means conforming to peer group norms. Social belonging is critical for the development of emerging self-identity. The strong stigma associated with mental disorders means that young people are very reluctant to adopt or disclose a mental disorder and fear rejection and discrimination if they do so (Mulfinger et al. 2019). Stigma is greater among ethnic minority groups and boys (DuPont-Reyes et al. 2020), partly accounting for their greater reluctance to seek help.

Stigma around mental health difficulties has been the subject of a large body of research, and a systematic review of 144 studies reported it to be one of the highest ranked barriers to help-seeking, with a small to moderate median association size (Clement et al. 2015). Of the many types of stigma, internalised and treatment stigma were most often related to reduced help-seeking. Self-stigma is when the negative stereotypes of mental health difficulties are internalised and applied to the self; young people then assume that other people, including potential help-sources, will view them in this stigmatised way. Becoming known to be a service user having sought treatment is another major fear. Confidentiality is paramount and will remain so while stigma persists. Ensuring that mental health service use is private, and particularly well-hidden from peers, can be essential for young people. This is especially challenging in small or closed communities, such as schools and rural communities, where risk of exposure is more likely.

Self-reliance and social support

Another key developmental task of adolescence and emerging adulthood is becoming an independent adult, so self-reliance is highly valued. Young people prefer to work out their personal problems themselves, even when highly distressed. A large representative survey of Australian adolescents revealed the most common reason for not seeking professional help was a preference to manage the problem alone, reported by 38 per cent of those aged 13–17 years old (Sawyer et al. 2000). This trend is even more pronounced for young people for whom self-sufficiency assumes greater importance, such as young men (Rice et al. 2017) and marginalised young people (Brown et al. 2016). Extreme self-reliance, which is solving problems entirely on your own all the time, was endorsed by almost 17 per cent of a large sample of New York high-school students, and 29 per cent of those at heightened risk of suicide (Labouliere et al. 2015). Consequently, self-help resources that enable young people to independently manage their mental health problem have a vital function in help-seeking.

It is also essential to engage the other trusted people in a young person's social environment as a key influence (Rickwood, 2017). These are those who know young people well, like family, friends and the trusted adults in young people's daily lives. Such people can notice the signs of mental ill-health, be a first source of support, and encourage and enable access to professional treatment.

Peers require special mention as they can be highly influential in helpful or unhelpful ways. Interestingly, a large Israeli study showed that adolescents are more likely to refer their peers for psychological help than themselves (Raviv et al. 2009). This suggests that young people's friends can be enlisted to assist the process of formal help-seeking. The role of peers and development of peer-support models are a growing focus with much potential. Nevertheless, family, particularly mothers, remain the primary mental health support for most young people.

Past experiences

Unsurprisingly, prior experiences of seeking help have a strong impact on the help-seeking process, including one's own and vicarious experiences. Young people often first seek professional help only once, meaning that initial attempts must be positive and successful to ensure ongoing service engagement and future help-seeking (Rickwood et al. 2015). The help-seeking process does not stop at the initial approach, and longer-term engagement is required for effective mental healthcare. Young people are both unlikely to initiate help-seeking and have high rates of premature drop-out from mental healthcare (Seidler et al. 2020). They typically do not engage with sufficient treatment sessions to attain outcomes. Factors that affect ongoing engagement include young people's participation in service development, parental support and involvement, holistic health clinic approaches, use of technology, engagement with schools, and social marketing (Dunne et al. 2017). A critical facilitator is service providers who are non-judgemental, attentive and show respect for young people; promoting a strong sense of hope and optimism is vital (Dowling & Rickwood, 2016). All help-seeking sources – self-help resources, informal and semi-formal supports, as well as healthcare providers – must be accepting, engaging and hopeful.

Unfortunately, negative help-seeking experiences are common and include not being helped, not feeling listened to and not being taken seriously. Negative perceptions of professional mental healthcare are widespread, including the belief that professional help is not effective. Psychiatric treatment has been perceived as doing more harm than good, particularly psychotropic medication (Zieger et al. 2017). Thinking that 'nothing could help' was the second most endorsed barrier to mental healthcare in a representative Australian national survey (Slade et al. 2009).

Despite a strong focus on primary care and the role of general practice in mental healthcare, adolescents are often reluctant to engage with their GP, particularly for mental health concerns, due to a pervasive lack of trust and fears about confidentiality (Corry & Leavey, 2017). Other common sources of formal help, including teachers, are also often reported by adolescents to be unhelpful (Lubman et al. 2017).

Settings to promote young people's help-seeking

Some settings are particularly well suited to promoting young people's help-seeking. One of the best opportunities is through schools, and the entire school environment, including the curriculum and relationships with school staff and other students, have an impact. Schools can be instrumental in multiple ways to improve mental health literacy, reduce stigma and facilitate help-seeking. Connection to school and relationships is key, as young people often form strong relationships with teachers. A large cross-sectional survey of 31,120 grade 6–12 students in Canada showed that the quality of teacher–student relationships, both inside and outside the classroom, affected whether students sought out and received mental health treatment (Halladay et al. 2020). Teachers can be the first to observe early signs of mental health problems, and act as a gateway to formal care (Mazzer & Rickwood, 2014). School systems need to be appropriately set up, however, with strong pastoral care systems and effective pathways to treatment services (Orlando et al. 2018; Rickwood, 2005).

For older adolescents, the transition period between school and work or further education is high risk, when young people can be disengaged from key support systems and special effort is needed to reach out. The tertiary education sector is increasingly recognised as a critical, but neglected, setting (Orygen, 2017). Further education and training settings, including apprenticeship schemes, are well placed to maintain contact with young people and facilitate mental health literacy and access to service pathways. Peer-support approaches are suited to young adults, and can engage high-risk young people to assist them along the help-seeking pathway, as well as provide a valuable learning experience for peer supporters themselves (Crisp et al. 2020).

The other main setting that provides a key opportunity to engage young people is the online environment. Technology is being harnessed in increasingly novel ways for mental health interventions. E-mental health uses technology to provide mental health information, screening and assessment, peer support, treatment, and monitoring and ongoing support. Research into online services shows they reach unique client groups who may not otherwise seek help or who might wait longer if in-person supports were their only options (Rickwood et al. 2016). Online services lead young people to seek help at an earlier stage of illness and are appealing to young people who have never sought mental health support before. They can also provide immediate help for young people who are highly distressed, including those at risk of self-harm and suicide (Frost & Casey, 2016).

Technology-based services have the potential to address the substantial unmet need for mental healthcare, as in-person services cannot possibly meet demand even in high-income countries. E-mental health can be easily and immediately accessible and remove some of the key barriers to in-person service use, such as cost, geographic accessibility and transport issues, and stigma and confidentiality fears. Online service use can be self-directed and anonymous, upholding young people's self-reliance, while also facilitating strong, supportive social connections.

Technology is not a panacea, however, and a comprehensive review showed that despite the multitude of online services aiming to facilitate help-seeking for young people with mental health problems, only 18 studies had evaluated whether they did so, finding that the majority did not (Kauer et al. 2014). Engagement has been a significant challenge for online interventions, with young people typically engaging only briefly and sporadically. Despite high expectations, the online environment especially struggles to engage and retain adolescent boys (Best et al. 2016). Nevertheless, the review's results showed that young people regularly used these services, would use them again and would recommend them to friends; they found the online services easy to use and satisfactory. If carefully designed to address engagement, satisfaction and efficacy factors (Bakker et al. 2016), there is enormous potential for technology-enhanced help-seeking.

Knowledge gaps and future directions

Despite the large and rapidly growing help-seeking field, there is much yet to learn. The most pressing gap relates to practice – few interventions have been found to improve actual help-seeking behaviour. A comprehensive review of 98 studies (Xu et al. 2018), showed that interventions usually focused on improving predictive factors, like mental health literacy, stigma and motivation, and were generally effective. Interventions to increase formal help-seeking were effective only when delivered to adults with mental health problems, but not for children, adolescents or the general public. Most studies were from high-income countries. Informal help-seeking was particularly hard to change. A rigorous, prospective, randomised control trial of a school-based help-seeking intervention showed that while overall help-seeking was not improved, formal help-seeking did have somewhat greater uptake in the intervention group, although informal help-seeking did not (Lubman et al. 2020). Determining effective interventions to change actual behaviour is challenging, due to the many varied factors that need to be addressed.

Fundamentally, there is no accepted theoretical framework for the help-seeking process. Most studies are atheoretical or purely descriptive. The Theory of Planned Behaviour has sometimes been applied, often in part. It stipulates that attitudes, norms and perceived behavioural control predict behavioural intentions, which then affect behaviour. It incorporates many of the factors that are often investigated. Coping and social support theories have also been occasionally applied, particularly for studies of informal help-seeking (Heerde & Hemphill, 2018), with help-seeking construed as a problem-focused, adaptive, support-seeking form of coping. The help-seeking process aligns strongly with the Transtheoretical Stages of Change Model, corresponding to the precontemplation (lack of awareness), contemplation (recognition of symptoms), preparation (decision intentions), action (seeking help) and maintenance (engagement) stages. This model has rarely been applied, however. An overarching comprehensive conceptual framework, comprising a combination of attitudinal, behaviour change, coping and illness behaviour constructs (such as Andersen's (1995) multi-level behavioural model), is needed to organise the research findings. Without this, the field will remain descriptive and constrained by non-comparable individual studies.

Related to the theory gap, is lack of agreement regarding measurement of help-seeking constructs. The field is marred by confounding of measures of attitudes, orientation, beliefs, facilitating and inhibiting factors, intentions, and behaviours (Rickwood & Thomas, 2012). Of particular concern, past help-seeking behaviour is usually measured, and cross-sectional studies investigate factors associated with *past* behaviour using a predictive approach. Measuring prospective behaviour is complex and dependent on the emergence of a mental health problem. Recent attempts to address this issue have added to the confounding, conceptualising help-seeking as a theoretically undifferentiated, multi-factorial construct (White et al. 2018).

Consequently, empirical validation of the help-seeking process is limited. This is likely to remain the situation until designs are implemented that are prospective, long-term, involve large community samples, and have valid measures. Still, it is unlikely that research will be able to unequivocally demonstrate the help-seeking process with any certainty, as it is such a multi-dimensional, variable, context- and time-bound experience. Nevertheless, a conceptually sound and logically sequenced help-seeking pathway is needed to understand this behaviour – to be able to measure it in replicable ways and investigate the factors that affect different parts of the process.

Very limited research comes from low- and middle-income countries (LMIC); overwhelmingly our understanding derives from high-income, western societies. The treatment gap is much greater in LMIC, where help-seeking is tightly bound by systemic issues related to the health, social and cultural systems in which people live. Young people in many LMIC countries struggle just to survive the impacts of poverty, conflict, climate change and dislocation; health issues, particularly mental health, are neglected. Recent research into the use of technology to overcome some of the systemic barriers in LMIC countries is promising however (Ospina-Pinillos, 2020).

Effective help-seeking behaviour

A final point, critical to emphasise, is that encouraging help-seeking is only appropriate if there are suitable help-seeking options available for young people. If sources of help are not present, not easily accessibles or not able to meet young people's needs, then raising awareness and expectations regarding seeking help may be ineffective and unethical. Importantly, all sources of help are needed to meet demand. This includes self-help options, particularly using innovations in technology and online resources; informal support from family and friends; semi-formal supports, such as teachers; alongside the primary health and mental healthcare systems. Unmet expectations about receiving help could leave young people experiencing mental health problems worse off and less likely to reach out again. It is essential that raised hopes are met by the right response. Along with improving mental health literacy and encouraging young people to seek help, there must be a commensurate focus on ensuring that sources of help are available, accessible and appropriately skilled.

Youth mental health and improving young people's help-seeking are high priorities, and innovations to youth mental health systems are underway in many countries. These acknowledge that young people are disproportionately affected by mental health problems yet face many barriers to seeking help. There are encouraging signs that this focus is leading to substantial improvements, including better mental health literacy, more appropriate service responses and innovative uses of technology, leading to greater likelihood of young people reaching out for help. Such positive trends must be fostered and enhanced. This will be achieved by further efforts to build comprehensive, easily accessible mental health systems that are responsive to young people's needs, supported by good mental health literacy and lack of stigma throughout the entire community.

Further reading

MacDonald, K., Fainman-Adelman, N., Anderson, K.K., & Iyer, S.N. (2018). Pathways to mental health services for young people: A systematic review. *Social Psychiatry and Psychiatric Epidemiology, 53*(10), 1005–1038. https://doi.org/10.1007/s00127-018-1578-y

References

ABS. (2010). Customised report. Australian Bureau of Statistics.

Andersen, R. (1995). Revisiting the behavioral model and access to medical care: Does it matter? *Journal of Health and Social Behavior, 36*(1), 1–10. https://doi.org/10.2307/2137284

Bakker, D., Kazantzis, N., Rickwood, D., & Rickard, N. (2016). Mental health mobile phone apps: Review and evidence-based recommendations for future development. *Journal of Medical Internet Research Mental Health, 3*(1). https://doi.org/10.2196/mhealth.4984

Barker, G. (2007). *Adolescents, social support and help-seeking behaviour: An international literature review and programme consultation with recommendations for action.* World Health Organization.

Best, P., Gil-Rodriguez, E., Manktelow, R., & Taylor, B.J. (2016). Seeking help from everyone and no-one: Conceptualizing the online help-seeking process among adolescent males. *Qualitative Health Research, 26*(8), 1067–1077. https://doi.org/10.1177/1049732316648128

Bimbaum, M.L., Rizvi, A.F., Correll, C.U., & Kane, J. (2015). Role of social media and the Internet in pathways to care for adolescents and young adults with psychotic disorders and nonpsychotic mood disorders. *Early Intervention in Psychiatry, 11*(4), 290–295. https://doi.org/10.1111/eip.12237

Blakemore, S-J. (2019). *Inventing ourselves: The secret life of the teenage brain.* Penguin Random House.

Brown, A., Rice, S., Rickwood, D.J., & Parker, A. (2016). Systematic review of barriers and facilitators to accessing and engaging with mental health care among at-risk young people. *Asia-Pacific Psychiatry, 8*(1), 3–22. https://doi.org/10.1111/appy.12199

Clement, S., Schauman, O., Graham, T., Maggioni, F., Evans-Lacko, S., Bezborodovs, N., Morgan, C., Rüsch, N., Brown, J. S., & Thornicroft, G. (2015). What is the impact of mental health-related stigma on help-seeking? A systematic review of quantitative and qualitative studies. *Psychological Medicine, 45*(1), 11–27. https://doi.org/10.1017/S0033291714000129

Corry, D.A., & Leavey, G. (2017). Adolescent trust and primary care: Help-seeking for emotional and psychological difficulties. *Journal of Adolescence, 54*, 1–8. https://doi.org/https://doi.org/10.1016/j.adolescence.2016.11.003

Crisp, D.A., Rickwood, D.J., Martin, B., & Byrom, N. (2020). Implementing a peer support program for improving university student wellbeing: The experience of program facilitator. *Australian Journal of Education, 64*(2), 113–126. https://doi.org/10.1177/0004944120910498

Crosby, S.D., Hsu, H-T., Jones, K., & Rice, E. (2018). Factors that contribute to help-seeking among homeless, trauma-exposed youth: A social-ecological perspective. *Children and Youth Services Review, 93*, 126–134. https://doi.org/10.1016/j.childyouth.2018.07.015

Dowling, M., & Rickwood, D.J. (2016). Exploring hope and expectations in the youth mental health online counselling environment. *Computers in Human Behavior, 55*, 62–68. https://doi.org/10.1016/j.chb.2015.08.009

Dunne, T., Bishop, L., Avery, S., & Darcy, S. (2017). A review of effective youth engagement strategies for mental health and substance use interventions. *Journal of Adolescent Health, 60*(5), 487–512. https://doi.org/https://doi.org/10.1016/j.jadohealth.2016.11.019

DuPont-Reyes, M.J., Villatoro, A.P., Phelan, J.C., Painter, K., & Link, B.G. (2020). Adolescent views of mental illness stigma: An intersectional lens. *American Journal of Orthopsychiatry, 90*(2), 201–211. https://doi.org/10.1037/ort0000425

Fante-Coleman, T., & Jackson-Best, F. (2020). Barriers and facilitators to accessing mental healthcare in Canada for Black youth: A scoping review. *Adolescent Research Review, 5*(2), 115–136. https://doi.org/10.1007/s40894-020-00133-2

Frost, M., & Casey, L. (2016). Who seeks help online for self-injury? *Archives of Suicide Research, 20*(1), 69–79. https://doi.org/10.1080/13811118.2015.1004470

Gulliver, A., Griffiths, K.M., & Christensen, H. (2010). Perceived barriers and facilitators to mental health help-seeking in young people: A systematic review. *BMC Psychiatry, 10*(1), 1–9. https://doi.org/10.1186/1471-244x-10-113

Guo, S., Nguyen, H., Weiss, B., Ngo, V.K., & Lau, A.S. (2015). Linkages between mental health need and help-seeking behavior among adolescents: Moderating role of ethnicity and cultural values. *Journal of Counseling Psychology, 62*(4), 682–693. https://doi.org/10.1037/cou0000094

Haavik, L., Joa, I., Hatloy, K., Stain, H.J., & Langeveld, J. (2019). Help seeking for mental health problems in an adolescent population: The effect of gender. *Journal of Mental Health, 28*(5), 467–474. https://doi.org/10.1080/09638237.2017.1340630

Halladay, J., Bennett, K., Weist, M., Boyle, M., Manion, I., Campo, M., & Georgiades, K. (2020). Teacher-student relationships and mental health help seeking behaviors among elementary and secondary students in Ontario Canada. *Journal of School Psychology, 81*, 1–10. https://doi.org/10.1016/j.jsp.2020.05.003

Heerde, J.A., & Hemphill, S.A. (2018). Examination of associations between informal help-seeking behavior, social support, and adolescent psychosocial outcomes: A meta-analysis. *Developmental Review, 47*, 44–62. https://doi.org/https://doi.org/10.1016/j.dr.2017.10.001

Jorm, A.F., Korton, A.E., Jacomb, P.A., Christensen, H., Rodgers, B., & Pollitt, P. (1997). "Mental health literacy": A survey of the public's ability to recognise mental disorders and their beliefs about the effectiveness of treatment. *Medical Journal of Australia, 166*, 182–186. https://doi.org/10.5694/j.1326-5377.1997.tb140071.x

Kauer, S.D., Mangan, C., & Sanci, L. (2014). Do online mental health services improve help-seeking for young people? A systematic review. *Journal of Medical Internet Research, 16*(3), e66. https://doi.org/10.2196/jmir.3103

Kim, J.E., & Zane, N. (2016). Help-seeking intentions among Asian American and White American students in psychological distress: Application of the health belief model. *Cultural Diversity and Ethnic Minority Psychology, 22*(3), 311–321. https://doi.org/https://doi.org/10.1037/cdp0000056

Labouliere, C.D., Kleinman, M., & Gould, M.S. (2015). When self-reliance is not safe: Associations between reduced help-seeking and subsequent mental health symptoms in suicidal adolescents. *International Journal of Environmental Research and Public Health, 12*(4), 3741–3755. https://doi.org/10.3390/ijerph120403741

Lawrence, D., Johnson, S., Hafekost, J., Boterhoven De Haan, K., Sawyer, M., Ainley, J., & Zubrick, S.R. (2015). The Mental Health of Children and Adolescents. Report on the Second Australian Child and Adolescent Survey of Mental Health and Wellbeing. Department of Health.

Lubman, D.I., Cheetham, A., Jorm, A.F., Berridge, B.J., Wilson, C., Blee, F., Mckay-Brown, L., Allen, N., & Proimos, J. (2017). Australian adolescents' beliefs and help-seeking intentions towards peers experiencing symptoms of depression and alcohol misuse. *BMC Public Health, 17*(1), 658. https://doi.org/10.1186/s12889-017-4655-3

Lubman, D.I., Cheetham, A., Sandral, E., Wolfe, R., Martin, C., Blee, F., Berridge, B.J., Jorm, A.F., Wilson, C., Allen, N. B., McKay-Brown, L., & Proimos, J. (2020). Twelve-month outcomes of MAKINGtheLINK: A cluster randomized controlled trial of a school-based program to facilitate help-seeking for substance use and mental health problems. *EClinicalMedicine, 18,* 100225. https://doi.org/10.1016/j.eclinm.2019.11.018

MacDonald, K., Ferrari, M., Fainman-Adelman, N., & Iyer, S. N. (2021). Experiences of pathways to mental health services for young people and their carers: A qualitative meta-synthesis review. *Social Psychiatry and Psychiatric Epidemiology, 56*(3), 339–361. https://doi.org/10.1007/s00127-020-01976-9

Mazzer, K.R., & Rickwood, D.J. (2014). Community-based roles promoting youth mental health: Comparing the roles of teachers and coaches in promotion, prevention and early intervention. *International Journal of Mental Health Promotion, 15*(1), 29–42. https://doi.org/10.1080/1462 3730.2013.781870

Mechanic, D. (1962). *Students under stress: A study of the social psychology of adaptation.* Free Press.

Mizzi, A., Honey, A., Scanlan, J.N., & Hancock, N. (2020). Parent strategies to support young people experiencing mental health problems in Australia: What is most helpful? *Health and Social Care in the Community, 28*(6), 2299–2311. https://doi.org/https://doi.org/10.1111/hsc.13051

Mulfinger, N., Rüsch, N., Bayha, P., Müller, S., Böge, I., Sakar, V., & Krumm, S. (2019). Secrecy versus disclosure of mental illness among adolescents: I. The perspective of adolescents with mental illness. *Journal of Mental Health, 28*(3), 296–303. https://doi.org/10.1080/09638237.201 8.1487535

Orlando, C.M., Bradley, W., Collier, T.A., Ulie-Wells, J., Miller, E., & Weist, M.D. (2018). What works in school-based mental health service delivery. In A.W. Leschied, Saklofske, D.H., & Flett, G.L. (Ed.), *Handbook of school-based mental health promotion.* Springer International. https://doi.org/10.1007/978-3-319-89842-1_3

Orygen. (2017). *Under the radar. The mental health of Australian university students.* Orygen, The National Centre of Excellence in Youth Mental Health.

Ospina-Pinillos, L. (2020). Language translation, cultural and contextual adaptation of health information technologies to transform mental health care in low- and middle- income countries: An example of prototypic mental health eClinic for Colombia. University of Sydney. https://hdl.handle.net/2123/21793

Planey, A.M., Smith, S.M., Moore, S., & Walker, T.D. (2019). Barriers and facilitators to mental health help-seeking among African American youth and their families: A systematic review study. *Children and Youth Services Review, 101,* 190–200. https://doi.org/https://doi.org/10.1016/j.childyouth.2019.04.001

Radez, J., Reardon, T., Creswell, C., Lawrence, P.J., Evdoka-Burton, G., & Waite, P. (2020). Why do children and adolescents (not) seek and access professional help for their mental health problems? A systematic review of quantitative and qualitative studies. *European Child and Adolescent Psychiatry, 30,* 183–211. https://doi.org/10.1007/s00787-019-01469-4

Raviv, A., Raviv, A., Vago-Gefen, I., & Fink, A.S. (2009). The personal service gap: Factors affecting adolescents' willingness to seek help. *Journal of Adolescence, 32*(3), 483–499. https://doi.org/10.1016/j.adolescence.2008.07.004

Rice, S., Parker, A., Telford, N., & Rickwood, D.J. (2017). Young men's access to community-based mental health care: Qualitative analysis of barriers and facilitators. *Journal of Mental Health, 27*(1), 59-65. https://doi.org/https://doi.org/10.1080/09638237.2016.1276528

Rickwood, D.J. (2005). Supporting young people at school with high mental health needs. *Australian Journal of Guidance and Counselling, 15*(2), 137–155. https://doi.org/10.1375/ajgc.15.2.137

Rickwood, D.J. (2017). Helping young people get help for mental health problems. In R. Manocha (Ed.), *Growing happy, healthy young minds.* Hachette Australia.

Rickwood, D.J. (2021). Help-seeking in young people. In A.R. Young, P.D. McGorry, & J. Cotter (Eds.), *Youth mental health: Approaches to emerging mental ill-health in young people.* Routledge. https://www.routledge.com/Youth-Mental   health-Approaches-to-Emerging-Mental-Ill-Health-in-Young-People/Yung-McGorry-Cotter/p/book/9780367250645#toc

Rickwood, D.J., Deane, F.P., Wilson, C.J., & Ciarrochi, J. (2005). Young people's help-seeking for mental health problems. *Advances in Mental Health, 4*(Supplement). https://doi.org/10.5172/jamh.4.3.218

Rickwood, D.J., Mazzer, K.R., & Telford, N.R. (2015). Social influences on seeking help from mental health services, in-person and online, during adolescence and young adulthood. *BMC Psychiatry, 15*(40). https://doi.org/https://doi.org/10.1186/s12888-015-0429-6

Rickwood, D.J., Telford, N.R., Mazzer, K.R., Parker, A.G., Tanti, C., & McGorry, P.D. (2015). Services provided to young people through the headspace centres across Australia. *Medical Journal of Australia, 202*(10), 533–536. https://doi.org/10.5694/mja14.01695

Rickwood, D.J., & Thomas, K.A. (2012). Conceptual measurement framework for help-seeking for mental health problems. *Psychology Research and Behavior Management, 5,* 173–183. https://doi.org/10.2147/PRBM.S38707

Rickwood, D J., Webb, M., Kennedy, V., & Telford, N.R. (2016). Who are the young people choosing online mental health support? Findings from the implementation of Australia's national online youth mental health service, eheadspace. *JMIR Mental Health, 3*(3), e40. https://doi.org/10.2196/mental.5988

Rudd, M.D., Joiner, T.E., & Rajab, M.H. (1995). Help negation after acute suicidal crisis. *JMIR Mental Health, 63*(3), 499–503. http://www.sciencedirect.com/science/article/pii/S0022006X02007465

Sawyer, M.G., Arney, F.M., Baghurst, P.A., Clark, J.J., Graetz, B.W., Kosky, R.J., Nurcombe, B., Patton, G.C., Prior, M.R., Raphael, B., Rey, J., Whaites, L.C., & Zubrick, S.R. (2000). The mental health of young people in Australia. Mental Health and Special Programs Branch, Commonwealth Department of Health and Aged Care. http://www.health.gov.au/internet/main/publishing.nsf/content/70DA14F816CC7A8FCA25728800104564/$File/young.pdf

Seidler, Z.E., Rice, S.M., Dhillon, H.M., Cotton, S.M., Telford, N.R., McEachran, J., & Rickwood, D.J. (2020). Patterns of youth mental health service attendance and discontinuation: Population data from Australia's headspace model of care. *Psychiatric Services, 71*(11). https://doi.org/10.1176/appi.ps.202000098

Slade, T., Johnston, A., Teesson, M., Whiteford, H., Burgess, P., Pirkis, J., & Saw, S. (2009). The mental health of Australians 2: Report on the 2007 national survey of mental health and well-being. Department of Health and Ageing.

Srebnik, D., Cauce, A.M., & Baydar, N. (1996). Help-seeking pathways for children and adolescents. *Journal of Emotional and Behavioral Disorders, 4*(4), 210–220. https://doi.org/10.1177/106342669600400402

Tuckett, D. (1976). Becoming a patient. In D. Tuckett (Ed.), *An introduction to medical sociology* (pp. 159–189). Tavistock Publications.

Valibhoy, M.C., Szwarc, J., & Kaplan, I. (2017). Young service users from refugee backgrounds: their perspectives on barriers to accessing Australian mental health services. *International Journal of Human Rights in Healthcare, 10*(1), 68–80. https://doi.org/10.1108/IJHRH-07-2016-0010

White, M.M., Clough, B.A., & Casey, L.M. (2018). What do help-seeking measures assess? Building a conceptualization framework for help-seeking intentions through a systematic review of measure content. *Clinical Psychology Review, 59*, 61–77. https://doi.org/10.1016/j.cpr.2017.11.001

Xu, Z., Huang, F., Kösters, M., Staiger, T., Becker, T., Thornicroft, G., & Rüsch, N. (2018). Effectiveness of interventions to promote help-seeking for mental health problems: Systematic review and meta-analysis. *Psychological Medicine, 48*(16), 2658–2667. https://doi.org/http://dx.doi.org/10.1017/S0033291718001265

Zachrisson, H.D., Rodje, K., & Mykletun, A. (2006). Utilization of health services in relation to mental health problems in adolescents: A population based survey. *BMC Public Health, 6*, 34–37. https://doi.org/10.1186/1471-2458-6-34

Zieger, A., Mungee, A., Schomerus, G., Ta, T., Weyers, A., Böge, K., Dettling, M., Bajbouj, M., von Lersner, U., Angermeyer, M.C., Tandon, A., & Hahn, E. (2017). Attitude toward psychiatrists and psychiatric medication: A survey from five metropolitan cities in India. *Indian Journal of Psychiatry, 59*(3), 341–346. https://doi.org/10.4103/psychiatry.IndianJPsychiatry_190_17

Seen and Heard – a creative piece by young people (18–25 years old), as part of the work of the YOULEAD Research Group, National University of Ireland, Galway, Ireland, and Fregoli Theatre Company, Galway, Ireland in collaboration with SpunOut.ie

'Reaching out for help has been the best thing I've ever done, but also the most difficult. Looking back at my fragile fifteen-year-old self, I wish I could tell her that it would get better and that reaching out was the best thing to do.'

Available at: https://www.youtube.com/watch?v=Wuz-XE8hCao&feature=youtu.be

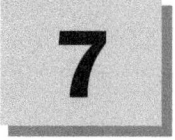

7 Mental health literacy in schools

Yifeng Wei
University of Alberta, Canada

Stan Kutcher
Dalhousie University, Canada

Andrew Baxter
Alberta Health Services, Canada

Wendy Carr
University of British Columbia, Canada

Introduction

The World Health Organization (WHO) (2018) defines mental health as 'a state of well-being in which an individual realizes his or her [their] own abilities, can cope with the normal stresses of life, can work productively and is able to make a contribution to his or her [their] community' (para. 2). The WHO definition of mental health underlines the importance of developing competencies and capacities to support youth (15–24 years old) mental health at both the individual and population level. Youth are at a critical point of their lifetime, a period when most mental disorders manifest, including mood disorders, anxiety disorders, psychoses and substance-use disorders (Merikangas et al. 2010).

The epidemiological fact that common mental disorders in adults first emerge in childhood and adolescence highlights the need for interventions that can create better knowledge and attitudes, and encourage appropriate help-seeking behaviours in this population while they are in school. This can be achieved using a 'pathway through care' approach that links promotion, prevention, early intervention and treatment in a systematic manner. This construct of pathway through care approach was first presented by Hendren et al. (1994) to lay out a comprehensive model to develop and deliver school mental health programming. Ever since, a plethora of interventions addressing promotion, prevention and treatment have been developed and applied to support youth mental health in schools, a context where youth in most countries can be reached conveniently and effectively. While many interventions in these areas have been proposed, implemented and evaluated, interventions are frequently implemented without sufficient evidence of effectiveness to support their full implementation. For example, universal school-based mental health promotion programmes have been applied in many settings, with a focus on improving student social emotional well-being, life skills and resilience. Although some evidence of potential effectiveness for some of these interventions exists, effect sizes range from small to medium, and duration of impact is generally relatively short (O'Connor et al. 2018). Thus, there is a need for further robust studies to guide future practice in this area.

School-based preventive interventions usually refer to 'interventions that occur prior to the onset of a disorder that are intended to prevent or reduce risk for the disorder' (p. 27), and therefore, reduce the incidence of common disorders (US National Research Council, 2009). Many high-income countries have adopted a multitiered approach to include universal (whole population), selective (at-risk populations) and indicated (population with the disorder) interventions in schools. Although there is emerging evidence for such preventive programmes, much of the evidence currently available is relatively weak due to a number of limitations including reliance on small studies, lack of randomisation of available studies, wide variation of outcome measures and difficulty in generalisation to settings outside of where the interventions were applied (Fazel et al. 2014). For example, a recent systematic review and meta-analysis that investigated preventive interventions on depression and anxiety disorders found little evidence of effectiveness of such interventions in both primary and secondary school settings (Caldwell et al. 2019).

Mental health treatments made available through the school setting is another area of interest. Mental health treatments can be delivered through on-site school health centres or by community-partnered school mental health services by staff employed in schools or community-based agencies, including counsellors, social workers and occupational therapists. In some jurisdictions, other providers such as psychologists and psychiatrists are available. On-site mental health treatments usually take place during the school day and are potentially efficient for both youth and their families. Systematic reviews and randomised controlled trials of school-based treatments, such as interpersonal therapy, demonstrated evidence of effectiveness to treat depression and emotional disturbances among children and youth (Mufson et al. 2004; Vernberg et al. 2006). Some studies provide evidence that school-based health centres that include mental health services can provide integrated healthcare (Arenson et al. 2019).

Despite the significant impact of mental disorders on individuals and their families, 40–80 per cent of young people globally do not receive the mental healthcare they need although effective treatments are available (Bruffaerts et al. 2019; Thornicroft, 2007). This may be due to numerous and varied reasons, including the lack of knowledge about mental disorders and their treatments, stigma against mental illness, limited access and other socio-economic or cultural barriers to mental healthcare (Sharp et al. 2006). A systematic review (Gulliver et al. 2010) of perceived barriers and facilitators for mental health help-seeking further indicated that perceived stigma and problems in symptom identification were among the most important barriers to mental health help-seeking. During the past two decades, the field has witnessed rapidly growing interest in mental health literacy as an evidence-based approach to help address child and youth mental health. The mental health literacy approach has been specifically developed to address barriers identified in previous research. And furthermore, it creates the foundation needed to support effective mental health promotion, prevention and treatment (Kutcher et al. 2016), ideally suited to the school setting.

Educators play a key role in effective mental health promotion and prevention. They are very often on the front lines of mental health, being among the first to spot the early signs of mental disorders, particularly in the adolescent years. However, studies have demonstrated concerns about educator competencies to address student mental health (Franklin et al. 2012; Froese-Germain & Riel, 2012). Any school-based mental health intervention must, therefore, consider teacher professional development as a key component in its implementation.

Mental health literacy: definition and constructs

Mental health literacy is defined as 'understanding how to obtain and maintain positive mental health; understanding mental disorders and their treatments; decreasing stigma related to mental disorders; and, enhancing help-seeking efficacy' (Kutcher et al. 2016, p. 155). Mental health literacy originates from health literacy, which evolved from focusing on functional literacy (e.g. reading and writing) to stressing the need for individuals and the general population to develop the knowledge, attitudes and competencies they need to improve their health, better manage their illnesses and advocate for better healthcare (Dewalt et al. 2004). For example, an early definition of health literacy specifies the 'ability to read and comprehend prescription bottles, appointment slips and other essential health-related materials required to successfully function as a patient' (American Medical Association, 1999, p. 552). The WHO advances the notion of health literacy as the 'cognitive and social skills which determine the motivation and ability of individuals to gain access to, understand, and use information in ways which promote and maintain good health' (Nutbeam, 1998, p. 357). Good health literacy is an important factor in determining health and improving healthcare. The WHO has called health literacy 'a stronger predictor of an individual's health status than income, employment status, education level and racial or ethnic group' (WHO, 2013, p. 7). Further, it has the potential to decrease health inequities in populations and enhance the operation of health systems and the development of health policy (WHO, 2013).

Mental health literacy derives from similar foundations to those of health literacy. It was first designed as 'knowledge and beliefs about mental disorders that aid their recognition, management or prevention' (Jorm et al. 1997, p.182) to help individuals understand signs and symptoms of mental disorders (functional literacy). It evolved to more broadly stress the development of lifelong skills for people to better obtain, maintain and sustain their mental health. In this sense, the definition of mental health literacy extends from a limited illness perspective to a holistic approach (Kutcher et al. 2016).

Components of mental health literacy

Knowledge about mental health and its various states

One of the fundamental constructs of mental health literacy is the knowledge and understanding about mental health that identifies the various interrelated states of mental health, including no distress, mental distress (stress), mental health problems and mental disorders/illness. This construct conveys the understanding that almost everyone experiences mental distress daily and may also experience mental health problems at numerous points in their life. Some (about 20 per cent) will also experience a mental disorder. These states are not exclusive of each other: individuals can experience one or more of these states concurrently over different time points of their lives. For example, a person who has a mental disorder can be mentally healthy because of therapeutic interventions and social support. Thus, mental health is not a continuum, in which an individual moves from one state to the other. Rather, mental health is experienced through emotional, behavioural, physical, cognitive and social functions that enable us to think, feel and act in ways that enhance our ability to enjoy life and deal with challenges. For example, we all experience mental distress/stress at some point of our life everyday (e.g. losing keys, being late for school or having an argument with a family member). It is a signal that the brain sends us indicating we need to do something to adapt to the environment. Once we find appropriate strategies to deal with the stress, it will go away and we learn new skills through this process and become more resilient. Developing this understanding in youth enables them to appropriately distinguish between normal distress/stress incurred by everyday life challenges and mental health problems or mental disorders and thus encourages them to seek appropriate sources of help when needed.

Stigma

Mental health literacy includes knowledge, attitudes and skills to fight stigma against mental illness. There are many definitions of stigma; most of these definitions claim that stigma comprises negative attitudes (stereotypes), endorsement of the negative attitudes (prejudice and prejudging) without knowing or understanding, and discriminative behaviours (discrimination) against people with mental illness. For example, Pinto et al. (2012) defined stigma as 'the culmination of negative attitudes and beliefs that motivate the general public to fear, reject, avoid, and enact behaviours of discrimination against people with mental illness' (p. 49). Stigma at the individual, institutional and societal levels creates a significant barrier for people living with mental disorders to access care (Gulliver et al. 2010), and thus adds great burden of illness to the health system. It also impedes people from achieving individual and social success. The inclusion of stigma as a construct of mental health literacy aims to tackle these challenges effectively through early interventions in the school setting and has been demonstrated to be successful in doing so (Hadlaczky et al. 2014; Milin et al. 2016). See Chapter 5 for further discussion of stigma.

Help-seeking efficacy

Help-seeking intentions and behaviours of young people are important for their mental health and, when necessary, for addressing their need for mental health-care. Globally, only 25.3–36.3 per cent of youth with mental disorders seek help from health professionals or families and friends, leading to a greater burden of illness due to the untreated mental disorders (Bruffaerts et al. 2019). Improved knowledge and reduced stigma are considered as facilitators that assist people with mental disorders to seek help (Gulliver et al. 2010; Rickwood et al. 2005; Rusch et al. 2011). Help-seeking efficacy, therefore, is an inextricable component of the mental health literacy conceptual framework. It includes the competencies to know where, when, how and from whom to seek help, and how to take actions when receiving care to help improve the care received. The help-seeking construct is rooted in the theory of planned behaviour, which indicates that attitude, subject norms and perceived behavioural control together shape an individual's behavioural intentions and behaviours (Ajzen, 1991). This theory has informed the current definition of mental health literacy and provides a framework and set of competencies to help young people make more effective health-related decisions and to enhance their ability to seek and benefit from the care they require.

Mental health competencies

Finally, the definition of mental health literacy also includes the knowledge and competencies needed to obtain and maintain mental health (Kutcher et al. 2016; WHO, 2013). This may overlap with more unidimensional mental health promotion interventions, such as social and emotional learning, which may currently be applied in schools and for which evidence is emerging; however, robust evidence of significant and sustained impact has yet to be built, according to the synthesis of systematic reviews (Taylor et al. 2017; Weare & Nind, 2011). Mental health literacy interventions integrate mental and physical health and promote knowledge and competencies in those activities with well demonstrated positive impact. These include, but are not limited to, healthy eating, physical exercise, sleep hygiene, positive relationships and avoidance of dangerous substances. All of these are necessary in promoting both mental health and physical health. Further, young people who are mental health literate can distinguish everyday stress/distress from mental disorders and develop capacity in understanding and using normal everyday distress (the stress response) as a vehicle for learning new skills and adaptive competencies, thus advancing resilience.

School-based mental health literacy interventions

A review of evidence related to the provision of increased levels of mental health treatment in four countries (Jorm et al. 2017) indicated that this did not reduce the prevalence of common mental disorders. The authors hypothesised that this result may be attributed to the lack of sufficient and effective implementation of promotion and prevention activities in both health and education systems. Mental health literacy interventions by trained educators may be an approach to bridge the gap through effective and early identification of youth at risk of mental health problems or disorders and link them to appropriate services, thus reducing the burden on the health system. Further, mental health literacy interventions have been identified as an effective approach to promote youth mental health and increase appropriate use of health services. Therefore, widespread application of such interventions has the potential to support youth to access care they need in a timely and effective way (Bonabi et al. 2016; Rickwood et al. 2005; Rusch et al. 2011).

This evidence is further enhanced in reviews (Hadlaczky et al. 2014; Wei et al. 2013) addressing multiple components (knowledge, attitudes/stigma or help-seeking) of mental health literacy, and in reviews (Schachter et al. 2008;) focusing on stigma reduction strategies. One review (Wei et al. 2013) specifically addressed youth mental health literacy in the secondary school setting, and evaluated knowledge, stigma and help-seeking outcomes. It identified 27 school-based universal programmes, including randomised controlled trials, quasi-experimental studies, and controlled before-and-after studies. All studies claimed that the interventions were effective in promoting knowledge, removing stigma and enhancing help-seeking behaviours. However, the level of evidence of effectiveness of the included interventions was subject to relatively high risk of bias due to the weaknesses of study designs (e.g. lack of randomisation, lack of control of confounders or loss of follow-up data), and authors suggested that future studies focus on applying more robust study designs, such as randomised controlled trials with validated measurement tools.

Examples of school-based mental health literacy interventions

Although research into school-based mental health literacy for youth is still in its infancy, recent studies have started to provide more robust and solid evidence in its application. For example, a Canadian intervention, *Mental Health and High School Curriculum Guide* (the Guide) (Kutcher & Wei, 2017) has been widely applied and researched in different settings in and beyond Canada. The Guide is designed for students aged 13–16 years old to learn mental health literacy in the classroom. It contains six modules with classroom-ready lesson plans including: the stigma of mental illness; understanding mental health and mental illness; information on specific mental illnesses; experiences of mental illness; seeking help and finding support; and the importance of positive mental health. Unlike many other school mental health interventions, the Guide is developed to be taught by classroom teachers who receive training on its delivery, and it doesn't require the fidelity of process; rather, it uses teachers' professional competencies to discharge fidelity of content. This means teachers teach the core content embedded in each module; however, they may decide how the content is delivered using the pedagogical strategies they are familiar with, or adapt the pre-designed classroom activities in each module to meet the unique needs of their students. This approach is consistent with the professional pedagogical approaches that teachers use for classroom teaching globally.

The Guide can be completed in eight to ten hours and can be embedded in different subjects, such as Health, English/Language Arts, Physical Education and others, depending on the school and curriculum requirements. Teachers need to be trained in the use of the Guide, ideally as part of a comprehensive professional development approach that develops teacher mental health literacy. Studies conducted by Wei et al. (2020) show that initial levels of teacher mental health literacy are low. Various approaches with good evidence to develop teacher mental health literacy and support the use of the Guide have been applied. In one, a face-to-face train-the-trainer model has been used wherein each school district establishes a team of core trainers who can then train classroom teachers to apply the Guide in the classroom. Another approach is to provide instructor-guided online training for teachers either in replacement of, or in addition to, face-to-face training (Carr et al. 2017; Wei et al. 2019). This approach can be used in distance learning or extraordinary situations, such as a pandemic. A third approach is for teachers to take a self-directed online professional development course. Currently the course is offered and certified by the University of British Columbia in Canada. Educators taking this course have demonstrated similar positive outcomes in knowledge, attitudes and help-seeking intentions to those who have received face-to-face training in both cohort and controlled studies (Wei et al. 2019).

A substantial body of research has investigated and demonstrated the effectiveness of the Guide. This includes a randomised controlled trial, longitudinal cohort studies and pre- and post-test studies, demonstrating strong evidence of effectiveness in knowledge, stigma and help-seeking outcomes among youth for durations lasting months to one year (Kutcher et al. 2015a; McLuckie et al. 2014; Milin et al. 2016). Educators who received training on the Guide delivery also shared similar results on mental health literacy outcomes (Carr et al. 2017; Wei et al. 2019). It has been adapted, implemented and researched in various international settings, demonstrating similar positive findings on mental health literacy outcomes (Kutcher, Wei, Gilbert et al. 2016; Ravindran et al. 2017).

A companion program, the Go-To Educator Training (GTET) (Wei et al. 2020), is designed to further support educators whom students naturally turn to for help in schools. It focuses on early identification of students at risk of developing mental disorders and linking them with services inside or outside of schools, thus helping them receive appropriate and timely care. The GTET further provides strategies for educators to promote communications among schools, parents/families and services so that related stakeholders build common language and understanding in relation to youth mental health. Research on its impact demonstrated that Canadian teachers improved knowledge about mental health and reduced stigma against mental illness (Wei et al. 2020). One study (Kutcher, Wei, Baxter, Milin & Cawthorpe, 2016) went beyond measuring the core outcomes (knowledge, stigma and help-seeking) to also investigate whether the GTET impacted referrals from schools to mental health services. In this study, students presenting to mental health services from schools were compared on clinical, systemic and demographic variables, based on whether those schools had participated in GTET training or not. Results showed that students presenting to services from trained schools were younger; they were from single-parent families; they were referred more because of adjustment and learning/attention problems; and they had complex social/family issues, thought disturbances and harmful behaviour/thoughts towards others. While they stayed longer in services and had more provisional comorbid diagnoses, they demonstrated positive treatment outcomes at discharge. These outcomes indicate that students from GTET-trained schools were referred with more severe symptoms and were linked earlier with mental health services compared to schools without GTET. This suggests that GTET may improve linkages between education and health sectors.

An additional Canadian school mental health literacy innovation targets both pre-service and in-service teacher professional development (teachmentalhealth. org). A survey of all Canadian teacher education programmes showed limited-to-no pre-service teacher education in mental health literacy (Froese-Germain & Riel, 2012). A collaboration between the Guide developers and four Canadian faculties of Education resulted in a certified university pre-service teacher education course. It is freely available online and can be taken by pre-service teacher candidates or by educators as part of their continuing professional development. It allows participants to build deep understanding about mental health using a modular-based format with practical classroom examples to illustrate each of the mental health literacy constructs, with additional strategies on how to care for their own mental health as educators. It has attracted educators from across the English-speaking world, and research into its impact is ongoing.

An Australian intervention, Mental Health First Aid (MHFA), originally designed for the general public, has also been applied in the secondary and post-secondary settings (Eisenberg & Speer, 2011; Hart et al. 2016). It is a programme providing support to people experiencing a mental health crisis. The programme takes a three-step format to educate the general public: recognising a change in behaviour, responding with a confident conversation, and guiding to appropriate resources and support. Its adapted version for youth, the teen Mental Health First Aid is a three-session classroom-based training programme for students aged 15–18 years old, aiming to improve supportive first-aid behaviours among peers, increase mental health literacy and decrease stigma. Studies on the impact of MHFA among high-school teachers and university/college staff identified increased knowledge, changed beliefs about treatment to be more like those of mental health professionals, reduced stigma and increased self-reported confidence in providing help to students and colleagues (Eisenberg & Speer, 2011; Hart et al. 2016). Similar results were identified among high-school students, including additional positive outcomes addressing students' willingness and comfort-seeking help from appropriate resources (Hart et al. 2016). However, the evidence related to the appropriate identification of youth in need of mental health services has yet to be built for MHFA, although a randomised controlled trial indicated that youth receiving MHFA increased self-reported supportive first-aid intentions towards peers in the short term (Hart et al. 2018).

While school mental health literacy interventions in Canada and Australia have been widely applied and extensively researched in diverse settings, there exist similar interventions elsewhere that address various aspects of mental health literacy among youth. As an example, Mental Health for Everyone in Norway is a three-day universal school intervention for students in Grades 8 to 10 (aged 13–15 years old) (Skre et al. 2013). This programme addresses three themes: (1) self-awareness and identity (well-being, mental health problems and mental disorders) for Grade 8, (2) being different and feeling lonely for Grade 9, (3) and fear of the unknown for Grade 10. The pedagogical approach includes individual tasks, group tasks and plenary sessions, along with illustrative video materials. A non-randomised cluster-controlled study found that students improved recognition of mental disorders and changed prejudiced beliefs about mental health, and there was a shift towards suggesting primary healthcare as a place to seek help

(Skre et al. 2013). In Portugal, *Finding Space for Mental Health* was developed for youth aged 12–14 years old to be delivered in the classroom by mental health professionals. It includes two sessions of 90 minutes that cover topics, including: identification of symptoms and signs of mental disorders; identification of risk factors; promotion of non-stigmatised behaviours, and the social inclusion of people with mental health disorders; identification of help-seeking options; promotion of first-aid skills and self-help strategies for people with mental health problems; and exploration of mental health promoting behaviours. One randomised controlled trial revealed that participants in the experimental group had significantly higher gains compared to the control group in all mental health literacy dimensions, demonstrating the effectiveness of the programme through to follow-up (Campos et al. 2018). In Japan, Grade 8 and 9 teachers apply a curriculum consisting of two 50-minute sessions that explain the signs and symptoms of mental disorders (e.g., depression and schizophrenia), normalise mental disorders, and provide strategies on how youth can help themselves or peers if they are concerned about their mental health. This intervention resulted in significant improvement of youth knowledge and intentions to seek help (Ojio et al. 2015).

There have also been some school-based interventions addressing specific mental disorders that onset during adolescence. An example is the implementation of Adolescent Depression Awareness Program (ADAP) in the United States and other countries (Swartz et al. 2017). ADAP is a didactic curriculum designed to be delivered by Health teachers. It addresses major depression and bipolar disorder, includes evidence-based treatment options, and encourages youth to seek help from a trusted adult. Research findings suggest that ADAP significantly improves youth depression knowledge and facilitates their help-seeking behaviours a few months following ADAP (Beaudry et al. 2019; Swartz et al. 2017). However, an impact of ADAP on stigma reduction was not found (Swartz et al. 2017).

Implications for research and practice

Professional development

In the past five years, there has been significant growth of school mental health literacy interventions delivered by MHL-trained classroom teachers, along with more robust research designs, such as randomised controlled trials providing stronger evidence of effectiveness of these interventions in the school setting. As has been previously noted (Wei et al. 2020), the baseline mental health literacy of teachers is generally poor, so the importance of appropriate professional development to support mental health literacy curriculum implementation – and student outcomes – should not be underestimated. Indeed, one Canadian study showed that a provincial mental health curriculum delivered by teachers who are not MHL-trained actually led to a decrease in student knowledge and an increase in stigma (Milin et al. 2016). Thus, interventions that build capacity within the school system delivered by MHL-trained educators are preferred.

Mental health literacy interventions may also be considered for delivery as targeted interventions for higher-risk youth, for example, by training healthcare providers working with social services or in the juvenile corrections sector to deliver evidence-based mental health literacy interventions. Such programmes do not yet exist, and this may be a future direction for implementation and research. Targeted interventions may also be applied in schools with the facilitation of school mental health professionals to enhance early identification and referral of youth at risk of mental disorders.

Evaluation outcomes

Many mental health literacy interventions have focused on evaluating the core outcomes of knowledge, stigma and help-seeking, and there is a lack of other related outcomes generated from these interventions. For example, some mental health literacy interventions may be able to help youth solve the confusion between everyday life challenges and mental disorders and therefore reduce youth stress levels. Similarly, mental health literacy interventions may also promote youth resilience through successful management of stress and the development of new life skills, thereby enhancing well-being and promoting adaptive competencies. Further, as available evidence on mental health literacy interventions indicates improvement of youth help-seeking efficacy, it is reasonable to hypothesise that such an approach may improve the quality of referrals between schools and health providers and potentially reduce the burden of inappropriate referrals on health systems. Research on these outcomes has started in Canada and Australia. As mentioned earlier in this chapter, a Canadian study demonstrated improved quality of referral for youth admitted to services from MHL-trained schools (Kutcher Wei and Coniglio, 2016). Another example was the investigation of MHFA on its impact on the quality of parent support. This study investigated whether MHFA is able to help parents better identify youth at risk of mental disorders, such as depression and anxiety and provide efficient support for youth to seek professional help. However, researchers did not detect significant changes compared to the control group (Morgan et al. 2019). Advanced research in addressing these outcomes could solidify the impact of a mental health literacy approach in benefiting both education and health systems.

Need for age-appropriate interventions

Mental health literacy interventions must be developmentally appropriate to reflect youth characteristics and needs. In this chapter, we have introduced mental health literacy interventions targeting youth aged 12–18 years old; however, we must be aware that these interventions are not a case of one size fits all. Youth entering post-secondary life may require different interventions specifically designed for this age group and environment. For example, *Transitions: Maximizing Campus Experiences* was created to blend life skills with mental health topics to help youth successfully transition to post-secondary life (Kutcher et al. 2015b). Preliminary research demonstrated improved outcomes of knowledge and stigma and further indicated youth felt more confident about this life change (Hunt et al. 2019; Kutcher et al. 2015b). There have, however, been very few, if any, other similar interventions identified in the literature, and mental health literacy research targeting this age cohort is rare, signifying a significant gap in research and practice. Further, age-appropriate mental health literacy interventions in the elementary/primary-school setting are also scarce. A systematic literature search revealed two interventions (Desocio et al. 2006; Lauria-Horner et al. 2004), but research into these interventions was very preliminary with no further advanced follow-up studies to consolidate and generalise the research findings.

Discussions and conclusion

The concept of mental health literacy first emerged in Australia to educate the public about mental disorders and guide the early identification of people at risk of mental disorders and encourage them to seek appropriate services (Jorm et al. 1997). While it has been widely adapted and adopted in different countries and settings, the concept of mental health literacy and related interventions has also received criticism for using an illness-focused approach due to the inclusion of developing understanding about the signs and symptoms of mental disorders, deeply influenced by Jorm and colleagues' early work in Australia (Mansfield et al. 2020). Critics of mental health literacy suggest a more inclusive model, considering the broader socio-cultural approaches to literacy that go beyond the dichotomy of illness and wellness (Chambers et al. 2015).

Kutcher's model for school mental health literacy has started to address these challenges and criticism through its interpretation of mental health consisting of various states that people may experience concurrently, its integration of help-seeking capacity from appropriate sources in alignment with different mental health states, and its development of self-acquired skills and strategies to achieve good mental health (Kutcher et al. 2016). This model arises from, and is informed by, the wider construct of health literacy (Nutbeam, 1998) and is consistent with the WHO definition (2018, para. 2) of mental health that encourages individuals to develop abilities to cope with everyday life stress, work productively and contribute to the community. To echo the understanding of mental health in various states within this model, measurement of mental health literacy interventions goes beyond evaluating the recognition of mental disorders on which most current mental health literacy interventions focus and addresses numerous other meaningful outcomes such as stress management, resilience, general well-being, help-seeking capacity and stigma reduction.

This chapter has provided a snapshot of mental health literacy concepts, related interventions and implementation work in the context of school settings to support youth transition to early adulthood and enhance their mental health. The adolescent years are a very important development phase in which mental health literacy interventions may have the potential to maximise youth development. Research and practices are evolving rapidly, and evidence of effective interventions is growing. Future focus on strengthening mental health literacy theory through a comprehensive and integrated school mental health model with advanced research studies in different settings and cultural contexts will empower youth with lifelong skills to make informed decisions about their mental health.

Further reading

Jorm, A. F. (2012). Mental health literacy: Empowering the community to take action for better mental health. *American Psychologist, 67*(3), 231–243. https://doi.org/10.1037/a0025957

Kutcher, S., Wei, Y., & Coniglio, C. (2016). Mental health literacy: Past, present, and future. *Canadian Journal of Psychiatry, 61*(3),154–158. DOI: 10.1177/0706743715616609

Milin, R., Kutcher, S., Lewis, S., Walker, S., Wei, Y., Ferrill, N., & Armstrong, M. (2016). Impact of a mental health curriculum on knowledge and stigma among high school students: A randomized controlled trial. *Journal of American Academy of Child and Adolescent Psychiatry, 55*(5), 383–391. DOI: 10.1016/j.jaac.2016.02.018

Weist, M.D., Lever, N.A., Bradshaw, C.P., & Owens, J.S. (2013). *Handbook of school mental health: Research training, practice and policy.* Springer.

References

Ajzen, I. (1991). The theory of planned behavior. *Organizational Behavior and Human Decision Processes, 50*(2): 179–211. DOI:10.1016/0749-5978(91)90020-T

American Medical Association Ad Hoc Committee on Health Literacy. (1999). Report of the scientific council on health literacy. *JAMA,* 281:552–557.

Arenson, M., Hudson, P.J., Lee, N.H., & Lai, B. (2019). The evidence on school-based health centers: A review. *Global Pediatric Health,* 6. DOI: 10.1177/2333794X19828745

Beaudry, M.B., Swartz, K., Miller, L., Scheweizer, B., Glazer, K., & Wilcox, H. (2019). Effectiveness of the Adolescent Depression Awareness Program (ADAP) on depression literacy and mental health treatment. *Journal of School Health, 89*(3), 165–172. DOI:10.1111/josh.12725

Bonabi, H., Müller, M., Ajdacic-Gross, V., Eisele, J., Rodgers, S., Seifritz, E., Rössler, W., & Rüsch, N. (2016). Mental health literacy, attitudes to help-seeking, and perceived need as predictors of mental health service use: A longitudinal study. *Journal of Nervous and Mental Disease, 204*(4), 321–4. DOI: 10.1097/NMD.0000000000000488

Bruffaerts, R., Mortier, P., Auerbach, R.P., Alonso, J., Hermosillo, De la Torre A.E., Cuijpers, P., Demyttenaere, K., Ebert, D.D … Green, J.G. (2019). Lifetime and 12-month treatment for mental disorders and suicidal thoughts and behaviors among first year college students. *International Journal of Methods in Psychiatric Research, 28*(2), 1–15. DOI: 10.1002/mpr.1764

Caldwell, D.M., Davies, S.R., Hetrick, S.E., Palmer, J.C., Caro, P., López-López, J.A.,…Welton, N.J. (2019). School-based interventions to prevent anxiety and depression in children and young people: A systematic review and network meta-analysis. *Lancet Psychiatry, 6*(12). 1011–1020. DOI: 10.1016/S2215-0366(19)30403-1

Campos, L., Dias, P., Duarte, A., Veiga, E., Dias, C.C., & Palha, F. (2018). Is it possible to 'Find Space for Mental Health' in young people? Effectiveness of a school-based mental health literacy promotion program. *International Journal of Environmental Research and Public Health, 15.* 1426. DOI:10.3390/ijerph15071426

Carr, W., Wei, Y., Kutcher, S., & Heffernan, A. (2017). Mental health literacy in pre-service teachers. *Canadian Journal of School Psychology, 33*(4), 314–326. DOI: 10.1177/0829573516688596

Chambers, D., Murphy, F., & Keeley, H.S. (2015). All of us? An exploration of the concept of mental health literacy based on young people's responses to fictional mental health vignettes. *Irish Journal of Psychological Medicine, 32*(1), 129–36. https://doi.org/10.1017/ipm.2014.82

Desocio J., Stember L., & Schrinsky J. (2006). Teaching children about mental health and mental illness: A school nurse health education program. *Journal of School Nursing, 22*(2): 81–86.

Dewalt, D.A., Berkman, N.D., Sheridan, S., et al. (2004). Literacy and health outcomes: a systematic review of the literature. *Journal of General Internal Medicine, 19*(12), 1228–1239.

Eisenberg, D. & Speer N. (2011). Mental Health First Aid for college students: A multi-campus randomized control trial. Final Report for NIMH1RC1MH089757-01.

Fazel, M., Hoagwood, K., Stephan, S., & Ford, T. (2014). Mental health interventions in schools in high-income countries. *Lancet Psychiatry, 1*(5). 377–387. DOI: 10.1016/S2215 0366(14)70312-8.

Froese-Germain, B., & Riel, R. (2012). *Understanding teachers' perspectives on student mental health: Findings from a national survey.* Canadian Teachers Federation.

Franklin, C. G. S., Kim, J. S., Ryan, T. N., Kelly, M. S., & Montgomery, K. L. (2012). Teacher involvement in school mental health interventions: A systematic review. *Children and Youth Services Review, 34*(5), 973–982. DOI: 10.1016/j.childyouth.2012.01.027

Gulliver, A., Griffiths, K.M., & Christensen, H. (2010). Perceived barriers and facilitators to mental health help-seeking in young people: A systematic review. *BMC Psychiatry, 10*, 113.

Hadlaczky, G., Hokby, S., Mkrtchian, A., Carli, V., & Wasserman, D. (2014). Mental health First Aid is an effective public health intervention for improving knowledge, attitudes, and behaviors: A meta-analysis. *International Review of Psychiatry, 26*(4). 467–475. DOI: 10.3109/09540261 .2014.924910.

Hart, L.M., Mason, R.J., Kelly, C.M., Cvetkovski, S., & Jorm, A.F. (2016) 'teen Mental Health First Aid': A description of the program and an initial evaluation. *International Journal of Mental health system, 19*(10). 3. DOI: 10.1186/s13033-016-0034-1

Hart, L.M., Morgan, A.J., Rossetto, R., Kelly, C.M., Mackinnon, A., & Jorm, A.F. (2018). Helping adolescents to better support their peers with a mental health problem: A cluster-randomised crossover trial of teen Mental Health First Aid. *Australian And New Zealand Journal of Psychiatry, 52*(7). 638–651. DOI: 10.1177/0004867417753552

Hendren, R., Birrell Weisen, R., Orley, J.H. & World Health Organization Division of Mental Health. (1994). *Mental health programmes in schools.* World Health Organization. https:// apps.who.int/iris/handle/10665/62308

Hunt, S., Wei, Y., & Kutcher, S. (2019). Addressing mental health literacy in a UK university campus population: Positive replication of a Canadian intervention. *Health Education Journal.* DOI: 10.1177/0017896919826374

Jorm, A.F., Korten, A.E., Jacomb, P.A., Christensen, H., Rodgers, B., & Pollitt, P. (1997). 'Mental health literacy': A survey of the public's ability to recognize mental disorders and their beliefs about the effectiveness of treatment. *The Medical Journal of Australia, 166*(4): 182–6.

Jorm, A.F., Patten, S.B., Brugha, T.S., & Mojtabai, R. (2017). Has increased provision of treatment reduced the prevalence of common mental disorders? Review of the evidence from four countries. *World Psychiatry, 16*(1). 90–99. DOI: 10.1002/wps.20388

Kutcher, S., & Wei, Y. (2017). *Mental health and high school curriculum guide. (Version 3).* https://teenmentalhealth.org/product/mental health-high-school-curriculum/

Kutcher, S., Wei, Y., Baxter, A., Milin, R., & Cawthorpe, D. (2016). School mental health literacy: Early identification & seamless pathways to care. Presentation at the 22nd International Association for Child and Adolescent Psychiatry and Allied Professions World Congress, Calgary, AB: September 18–22.

Kutcher, S., Wei, Y., & Coniglio, C. (2016). Mental health literacy: Past, present, and future. *Canadian Journal of Psychiatry, 61*(3),154–158. DOI: 10.1177/0706743715616609

Kutcher, S., Wei, Y., Gilberds, H., Ubuguyu, O., Njau, T., Brown, A., Sabuni, N., Magimba, A., & Perkins, K. (2016). A school mental health literacy curriculum resource training approach: Effects on Tanzanian teachers' mental health knowledge, stigma and help-seeking efficacy. *International Journal of Mental Health Systems, 10*(1), 50. DOI: 10.1186/s13033-016-0082-6

Kutcher, S., Wei, Y., & Morgan, C. (2015a). Successful application of a Canadian mental health curriculum resource by usual classroom teachers in significantly and sustainably improving student mental health literacy. *Canadian Journal of Psychiatry, 60*(12), 580–586.

Kutcher, S., Wei, Y., & Morgan, C. (2015b). Mental health literacy in post-secondary students. *Health Education Journal, 75*(6). DOI: 10.1177/0017896915610144

Lauria-Horner, B., Kutcher, S., & Brookes, S.J. (2004). The feasibility of a mental health curriculum in elementary school. *Canadian Journal of Psychiatry, 49*(3), 208–211. DOI: 10.1177/070674370404900309

Mansfield, R., Patalay, P., & Humphrey, N. (2020). A systematic literature review of existing conceptualisation and measurement of mental health literacy in adolescent research: Current challenges and inconsistencies. *BMC Public Health, 20.* 607. https://doi.org/10.1186/s12889-020-08734-1

McLuckie, A., Kutcher, S., Wei, Y., & Weaver, C. (2014). Sustained improvements in students' mental health literacy with use of a mental health curriculum in Canadian schools. *BMC Psychiatry, 14*(1), 379. DOI: 10.1186/s12888-014-0379-4.

Merikangas, K. R., Marcy Burstein, M., Swanson, S.A., Avenevoli, S., Cui, L., Benjet, C., Georgiades, K., & Swendsen, J. (2010). Lifetime prevalence of mental disorders in US adolescents: Results from the National Comorbidity Study-Adolescent Supplement (NCS-A). *Journal of the American Academy of Child and Adolescent Psychiatry, 49*(10). 980–989. DOI: 10.1016/j.jaac.2010.05.017

Milin, R., Kutcher, S., Lewis, S., Walker, S., Wei, Y., Ferrill, N., & Armstrong, M. (2016). Impact of a mental health curriculum on knowledge and stigma among high school students: A randomized controlled trial. *Journal of American Academy of Child and Adolescent Psychiatry, 55*(5), 383–391. DOI: 10.1016/j.jaac.2016.02.018.

Morgan, A.J., Fischer, J.A., Hart, L.M., Kelly, C.M., Kitchener, B.A., Reavley, N.J.,… Jorm, A.F. (2019). Does Mental Health First Aid training improve the mental health of aid recipients? The training for parents of teenagers randomised controlled trial. *BMC Psychiatry, 19*(99). https://doi.org/10.1186/s12888-019-2085-8

Mufson, L., Dorta, K.P., Wickramaratne, P., Nomura, Y., Olfson, M., & Weissman, M.M. (2004). A randomized effectiveness trial of interpersonal psychotherapy for depressed adolescents. *Archives of General Psychiatry, 61.* 577–84.

Nutbeam, D. (1998) Health promotion glossary. *Health Promotion International, 13,* 349–364.

O'Connor, C.A., Dyson, J., Cowdell, F., & Watson, R. (2018). Do universal school-based mental health promotion programmes improve the mental health and emotional well-being of young people? A literature review. *Journal of Clinical Nursing, 27*(3–4). e412–e426. DOI: 10.1111/jocn.14078.

Ojio, Y., Yonehara, H., Taneichi, S., Yamasaki, S., Ando, S., Togo, F., Nishida, A., & Sasaki, T. (2015). Effects of school-based mental health literacy education for secondary school students to be delivered by school teachers: A preliminary study. *Psychiatry and Clinical Neurosciences, 69,* 572–579.

Pinto, M.D., Hickman, R., Logsdon, M.C., & Burant, C. (2012). Psychometric evaluation of the Revised Attribution Questionnaire (r-AQ) to measure mental illness stigma in adolescents. *Journal of Nursing Measurement, 20*(1), 47–58. https://doi.org/10.1891/1061-3749.20.1.47

Ravindran, A., Herrera, A., da Silva, T., Henderson, J., Castrillo, M., & Kutcher, S. (2017). Evaluating the benefits of a youth mental health curriculum for students in Nicaragua: A parallel-group, controlled pilot investigation. *Global Mental Health, 5* (e4), 1–12. DOI: 10.1017/gmh.2017.27

Rickwood, D., Deane, F.P., Wilson, C.J., & Ciarrochi, J.V. (2005). Young people's help-seeking for mental health problems. *Australian e-Journal for the Advancement of Mental Health, 4*(3), 1–34.

Rusch, N., Evans-Lacko, S., Henderson, C., Flach, C., & Thornicroft, G. (2011). Public knowledge and attitudes as predictors of help-seeking and disclosure in mental illness. *Psychiatric Services, 62*(6), 675–8.

Schachter, H.M., Girardi, A., Ly, M., Lacroix, D., Lumb, A.B., van Berkom, J., & Gill, R. (2008). Effects of school-based interventions on mental health stigmatization: A systematic review. *Child and Adolescent Psychiatry and Mental Health, 2*(1), 18. DOI: 10.1186/1753-2000-2-18.

Sharp, W., Hargrove, D.S., Johnson, L., & Deal, W.P. (2006). Mental health education: An evaluation of a classroom-based strategy to modify help-seeking for mental health problems. *Journal of College Student Development, 47*(4), 419–438.

Skre, I., Friborg, O., Breivik, C., Johnsen, L.I., Arnesen, Y., & Wang, C. (2013). A school intervention for mental health literacy in adolescents: Effects of a non-randomized cluster-controlled trial. *BMC Public Health, 13*, 873. DOI: 10.1186/1471-2458-13-873.

Swartz, K., Musci, R.J., Beaudry, M.B., Heley, K., Miller, L., Alfes, C.,... Wilcox, H.C. (2017). School-based curriculum to improve depression literacy among US secondary school students: A randomized effectiveness trial. *American Journal of Public Health, 107*, 1970–1976. DOI:10.2105/AJPH.2017.304088

Taylor, R.D., Oberle, E., Durlak, J.A., & Weissberg, R.P. (2017). Promoting positive youth development through school-based social and emotional learning interventions: A meta-analysis of follow-up effects. *Child Development, 88* (4), 1156–1171. https://doi.org/10.1111/cdev.12864

Thornicroft, G. (2007). Most people with mental illness are not treated. *The Lancet, 370*(9590), 807–808.

US National Research Council, Institute of Medicine. (2009). *Preventing mental, emotional, and behavioral disorders among young people: Progress and possibilities*. National Academies Press, Washington, DC.

Vernberg, E.M., Roberts, M.C., Randall, C.J., Biggs, B.K., Nyre, J.E., & Jacobs, A.K. (2006). Intensive mental health services for children with serious emotional disturbances through a school-based, community-oriented program. *Clinical Child Psychology And Psychiatry, 11*, 417–30.

Weare, K., & Nind, M. (2011). Mental health promotion and problem prevention in schools: What does the evidence say? *Health Promotion International,* Suppl 1: i29–69. DOI:10.1093/heapro/dar075.

Wei, Y., Carr, W., Kutcher, S., & Alaffe, R. (2019). Mental health literacy development: Application of online and in-person professional development for preservice teachers to address knowledge, stigma, and help-seeking intentions. *Canadian Journal of Behavioral Science / Revue canadienne des sciences du comportement, 52*(2), 107–114. DOI:10.1037/cbs0000164.

Wei, Y., Hayden, J.A., Kutcher, S., Zygmunt, A., & McGrath, P. (2013). The effectiveness of school mental health literacy programs to address knowledge, attitudes and help-seeking among youth. *Early Intervention Psychiatry, 7*(2), 109–121.

Wei, Y., Kutcher, S., & Baxter, A. (2020). The program evaluation of 'go-to educator' training on educator's knowledge about and stigma towards mental illness in six Canadian provinces. *Early Intervention in Psychiatry.* DOI: 10.1111/eip.13037.

World Health Organization (WHO). (2013). The solid facts: health literacy. World Health Organization. http://www.euro.who.int/__data/assets/pdf_file/0008/190655/e96854.pdf

World Health Organization. (2018). Mental health: strengthening our response. https://www.who.int/news-room/fact-sheets/detail/mental health-strengthening-our-response

8 Youth mental health in low- and middle-income countries: A Kenyan case study

David M. Ndetei
University of Nairobi, Kenya

Victoria Mutiso
Africa Mental Health Research and Training Foundation (AMHRTF), Kenya

Christine Musyimi
Africa Mental Health Research and Training Foundation (AMHRTF), Kenya

Introduction: Setting the context

The focus of this chapter is on youth mental health in Kenya, a country that falls into the 'Low- and Middle-Income Country' (LMIC) classification based on gross national income per capita using data published by the World Bank (Hamadeh et al. 2021). The socio-demographic patterns of young people in LMICs are very different from high-income countries (HICs). Of particular relevance to discussion in this chapter is the fact that almost 90 per cent of the world's children and adolescents live in LMICs, where they form up to 50 per cent of the population of these countries (Kieling et al. 2011). With mental health problems affecting 10–20 per cent of children and adolescents world-wide (Kieling et al. 2011) it is clear that LMICs have significant needs in relation to providing mental health support to their youngest citizens.

The Lancet Commission on Global Mental Health (Patel et al. 2018) notes that around the world, there is underinvestment in mental health services when compared to physical health services and the consequence of this is stark for LMICs because they have a higher proportion of young people in their population and fewer economic resources. For example, Patel (2007) notes that the median number of psychiatrists in high-income countries (HICs) is 200 times greater than that in low-income countries and the disparity in availability of a mental health workforce is clearly illustrated in Figure 8.1. Furthermore, Patel et al. (2018) notes that in many LMICs mental health services are concentrated in in-patient psychiatric hospitals rather than in local community health settings, making them less accessible to the majority of young people. When adolescents and emerging adults do not receive timely and effective treatment for mental health difficulties this leaves them at greater risk of a range of negative long-term outcomes (Gibb et al. 2010).

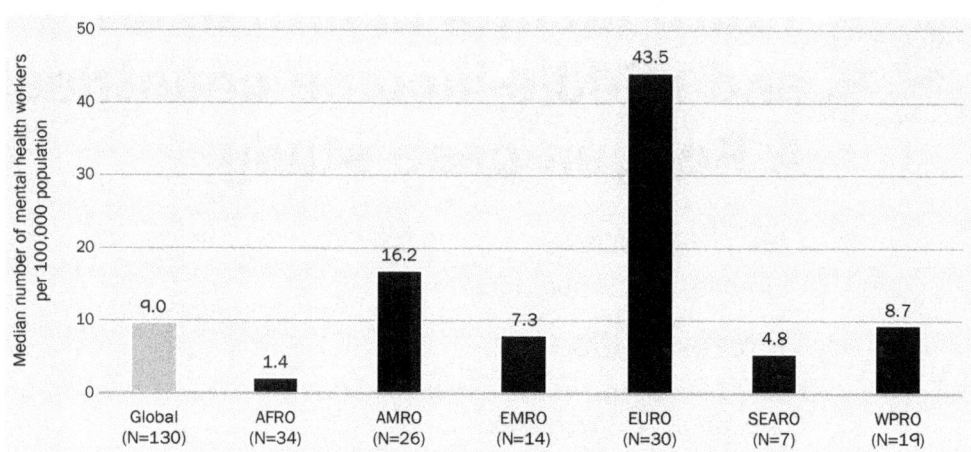

Figure 8.1 Mental health workforce per 100,000 population, by WHO region

Table 8.1 Kenyan population percent ages for ages 10–24 based on 2019 national population census

Age group	National
10–14	6,346,072 (13%)
15–19	5,285 (11%)
20–24	4,447,674 (10%)
Total (10–24)	16,079,603 (34%)

Source: 2019 National Population Census [Kenya National Bureau of Statistics (KNBS)], 2019.

In response to the urgent need to provide support to young people with mental health difficulties, many LMICs have implemented innovative interventions delivered by less specialised health workers (Healy et al. 2018; Patel et al. 2018). This approach to the delivery of mental health interventions (sometimes called task-sharing) can help to overcome the extreme shortage of highly trained mental health specialists in LMICS and thereby increase young people's access to support (Healy et al. 2018).

This chapter describes the situation in Kenya as a case study of the experiences of LMICs in sub-Saharan Africa outlining some of the challenges faced as well as innovative solutions that have been implemented. Located on the East African coast, Kenya has a total area of 580,370 km² and a population currently estimated at 52.6 million; it is classified as a lower-middle-income country (World Bank Group, 2021a). A large proportion of the Kenyan population (c. 70 per cent) live in rural areas (World Bank, 2021b). Due to reported reductions in mortality rates and its relatively high birth rate, the Kenyan population has been continuously increasing in recent years (World Bank Group, 2019). While life expectancy in Kenya is slowly increasing, it is relatively low in global terms, sitting at approximately 66 years old (World Bank Group, 2021a). Table 8.1 summarises Kenyan population data and age distribution. Going by this, Kenyan young people (aged 10–24 years old) make up 34 per cent of the total population.

With such a large proportion of young people, who are the future and posterity of the country, these statistics highlight the importance of investing in good mental health. Early investment in an attempt to cultivate resilient mental health will put these young people on a trajectory to achieve their full potential, be productive members of the society, contribute to the economic well-being of the country and reduce the burden of disease. This strategy was clearly articulated in the October 2011 Lancet series on Global Mental Health (Kieling et al. 2011). The Lancet paper made an urgent call for innovative approaches to address mental health issues in school-aged children and adolescents in LMICs in order to promote mental well-being, support positive cognitive development and break the vicious cycle of mental disorders continuing through adulthood.

The challenge in Kenya is how to achieve the recommendations of the Lancet series, given the socio-cultural and economic context of LMICs. Young people in Kenya live in an environment where there is a dearth of resources, and in particular a dearth of resources for mental health. For example, WHO (2015) data dramatically illustrates the differences in professional mental health supports between HIC and LMIC: the median number of mental health workers per 100,000 population is 43.5 in the European region; 16.2 in the Americas and 1.4 in Africa. Yet the epidemiological evidence demonstrates that mental disorders have similar prevalence in both HICs and LMICs (Mutiso, Musyimi, Tomita et al. 2018). These young people require access to the same kinds of services as those in HICs. Development of such services is time sensitive, thus the young people of Kenya cannot wait until the country catches up with the copious resources of HICs. While making efforts to improve resources, LMICs must be innovative with the resources that they already have. This will be the theme of this chapter.

The Lancet series (Kieling et al. 2011) recommended early and integrated interventions to prevent child and adolescent mental disorders in LMICs using the following 10 possibilities:

1. Establishing the extent of the problem and the perceived need for an intervention within the community.
2. Choosing and designing an intervention that targets risk factors and protective factors for child and adolescent mental health in that setting.
3. Promoting ownership of the intervention by the community, for example, by inclusion of key stakeholders in the design or choice of the intervention.
4. Promoting intervention buy-in by all stakeholders before implementation (e.g. teacher support).
5. Using evidence-based interventions with in-built cultural flexibility (e.g. using interventions that build on existing practices and strengths).
6. Assessing the feasibility and acceptability of the intervention for staff within the setting before implementation (e.g. are sufficient resources and time available?).
7. Ensuring the intervention is acceptable and is perceived as relevant by participants to promote engagement, (e.g. assess the extent to which the intervention fits in with prevailing attitudes, beliefs and current practices).

8. Piloting and assessing the intervention in the new settings, and using the data to inform any modifications to the interventions before scaling up.
9. Integrating interventions into existing services and using existing staff to promote sustainability (e.g. integrating interventions into school settings and healthcare services).
10. Providing intervention with systematic training and providing ongoing monitoring and support for staff. Patel et al. (2009) and Chibanda et al. (2011) have argued that in order to avoid rejection or simply being ignored by stakeholders, integration of a new service into an existing service should be carried out in such a way that it is not seen as intrusive and/or competitive with other priorities. This must be considered when developing youth mental health services.

Over the last 20 years or so, even before the Lancet series, Africa Mental Health Research and Training Foundation (AMHRTF) has taken this path. AMHRTF is a non-governmental organisation based in Kenya which is dedicated to research on mental and neurological health and substance use. AMHRTF's mission is to generate evidence for policy and best practice in the provision of affordable, appropriate, and accessible mental health service, while promoting positive mental health and behaviour. We shall share our experiences in the following areas: (1) our research in epidemiological data on school mental health in Kenya and how Kenya compares to global trends; (2) stigma among children and adolescents towards people with mental disorders; (3) mental health and ego-resilience in children and adolescents; (4) challenges associated with youth-focused mental health interventions in LMIC. It is in this last area where innovations are most needed and where we have developed hypothetical models. Our innovative approach has involved a multi-stakeholder dialogue on mental health in children and young adolescents, including the child/adolescent themselves, their teachers, school counsellors, peer counsellors, parents, community health opinion leaders, and service providers operating within the community (who were also trained with skills to manage mental health issues in school-going children and adolescents). We called the innovation 'The Kenya Integrated Intervention Model for Dialogue and Screening to Promote Children's Mental Well-being (KIDS)' (Mutiso, Musyimi, Musau, et al. 2018). It revolves around the World Health Organization's (WHO) Mental Health Gap Action Programme Intervention Guide (mhGAP-IG; WHO, 2016), and the process of consultation and intervention development is described later in this chapter.

Kenyan epidemiological data on school mental health

In early studies, Ndetei et al. (2008) found a 12.9 per cent prevalence of significant clinical symptoms of anxiety in Kenyan schools. Other school-based studies by the same team found associations between alcohol, cannabis and khat (a psychostimulant herb) use and behavioural problems, emotional problems and poor academic performance (Ndetei et al. 2009); a high prevalence of PTSD (50.5 per cent) (Ndetei, Ongecha-Owuor, Khasakhala, Mutiso et al. 2007); a high prevalence of high-school bullying ranging between 63.2 per cent and 81.8 per cent (Ndetei, Ongecha-Owour, Khasakhala, Syanda et al. 2007) and high levels of psychopathology in adolescents exposed to post-election violence in Kenya (Harder et al. 2011). In more recent studies, we have documented the prevalence and correlates of mental disorders among upper primary school young adolescents (11–13 years old). We adapted and administered the Youth Self Report (YSR, Achenbach, 1991) instrument to 2267 young adolescents drawn from 23 randomly selected schools. The YSR is a multipurpose scale which covers a broad range of behavioural and emotional symptoms. We estimated the prevalence of DSM-IV mental disorders and used logistic regression analyses to examine the socio-demographic factors associated with each disorder. We found the following: the prevalence of any mental disorder among Kenyan young adolescents was 37.7 per cent. Somatic complaints were the most prevalent, followed by affective disorders and conduct disorder. Presence of one or more comorbid mental disorders was seen among 18.2 per cent of young adolescents. Male gender, living in a peri-urban rather than rural area, having divorced or separated parents, and having an employed mother were associated with an increased likelihood of having most of the mental disorders examined, whereas increasing age was associated with a reduced likelihood (Ndetei, Mutiso, Musyimi et al. 2016). In summary, a high prevalence of mental disorders was evident among young adolescents in Kenyan schools, therefore highlighting the need for early detection and initiation of interventions so that these disorders do not interfere with young adolescent's psychological, social and educational development.

Suicide in youth is of great concern, particularly since the advent of COVID-19. We will therefore examine further the trends on suicide in youth, not only in Kenya but globally. On a global scale, suicide is the third leading cause of death among adolescents between 15–19 years old, and the second leading cause of death among emerging adults between 19–29 years old (WHO, 2019). About 79 per cent of global suicide occurs in LMICs (WHO, 2019). More than 90 per cent of suicides in youth result from depression and other mental disorders, often in combination with substance-use disorders (WHO, 2019). These mental disorders are complicated by multiple competing social and family dynamics, such as life events, disciplinary issues such as family or school rules, social isolation, loss of friends and family members, violence, physical and sexual abuse, bullying, lack of support for non-binary gender identity, chronic pain and illness, and media pressures. For many, suicide also is related to availability of means to attempt and or complete suicide, such as poison (Stanford Children's Health, 2021; WHO, 2019). Broader cultural and structural factors also complicate young people's experiences, such as stigma, religious beliefs, explanatory models for suicidal ideas and behaviours, poverty, and lack of appropriate mental health services. In the Kenyan context, although we have good indications on the overall prevalence of suicidal behaviour, there is no integrated information available on how all these variables interact to determine the final trajectory to suicidal behaviour, and how they inform evidence-based strategies to minimise risk for suicide in Kenyan youth. Unlike HICs, Kenya and other LMICs have an acute shortage of specialists in mental healthcare (WHO, 2017).

As part of an ongoing study in Kenya, we have collected data on 9,742 high-school, college, and university undergraduate students in one of the largest institution-based studies on suicide conducted in LMICs (Ndetei et al. 2022).

Focusing on suicidal ideation, we found a 22.6 per cent prevalence of suicidal ideas, the most common being 'thinking of specific ways of taking their life' (19.3 per cent) and least being 'wanting to be dead' (10.7 per cent). Major depression was a risk factor in 20 per cent of participants, psychosis in 8.7 per cent, and stress in 26 per cent. Several indicators of financial insecurity within families were also associated with suicidal ideas. This work underscores how economic indicators at family level (Deaton, 2005; Harttgen & Vollmer, 2013) especially in rural areas (Morris et al. 2000) is regarded as a better measure of the actual status of households than gross domestic product per capita, i.e. the need to focus on the family. Although our study was a cross-sectional one and purely institution-al-based, our pre-COVID-19 pandemic data provide a baseline for comparison of the potential impact of COVID-19 on youth. Our previous school-based work demonstrated similar suicide prevalence with emphasis on suicidal ideas (Culbreth et al. 2018; Ndetei et al. 2022).

In the same study, we looked at the prevalence of substance abuse. We found high prevalence of alcohol abuse, khat, tobacco and cannabis, sedatives, heroin and cocaine. However, more importantly and related to our paper, there was a statistically significant association between various types of substance abuse and psychiatric disorders.

Stigma towards people with mental disorders

It is a well-established fact that stigma towards mental disorders is a major barrier to seeking mental healthcare among adults world-wide, and specific to LMICs (Clement et al. 2015; Schnyder et al. 2017). But what about in children and adolescents? In our literature review, we found that research surrounding stigmatising attitudes towards people with mental disorders by children and adolescents in developing countries was lacking (Ndetei, Mutiso, Maraj et al. 2016). To fill this gap, we carried out a study that aimed to examine socio-demographic factors associated with the endorsement of such stigmatising attitudes among Kenyan school goers. We conducted a cross-sectional survey on 4585 primary-school children and young adolescents (6–13 years old) in the Eastern Province of Kenya. We examined relationships between the endorsement of stigmatising attitudes and age, gender, district, religion, being in the class appropriate for one's age, and parental employment status. We found that stigma scores decreased with increasing age, boys displayed higher stigma scores compared to girls and pupils from the rural district had higher average stigma scores compared to those from the peri-urban district. We concluded that stigmatising attitudes towards people who have a mental disorder are prevalent among primary- school children and young adolescents in Kenya. Thus, anti-stigma interventions are needed, and our findings highlight particular subgroups that should be targeted (Ndetei, Mutiso, Maraj et al. 2016).

Mental health and ego-resilience

Ego-resilience, or trait resilience, has been defined as the 'capacity to adapt one's behaviour to various situational contexts' (Philippe et al. 2011, p. 585).

Ego-resilience incorporates inborn traits and therefore is specific to the individual. Ego-resilience in childhood and early adolescence is linked to positive mental health outcomes but varies across cultures. We hypothesised that ego-resilience traits would be found in Kenyan primary-school children and young adolescents, and we aimed to explore such traits. Specifically, we aimed to: (1) demonstrate ego-resilience in Kenya; (2) determine associated socio-demographic and psychological factors in a non-clinical population of primary-school children and young adolescents; (3) contribute to the global database with Kenyan data; and (4) lay the grounds to inform future and more focused studies in Kenya. We used a socio-demographic questionnaire, the Ego-Resilience Scale (ER-89; Block & Kremen, 1996) and the Youth Self Report Scale (YSR) (Achenbach, 1991). Multivariate analyses showed that the only independent predictors of ego-resilience were female gender and peri-urban region. We did not find any association between ego-resilience and YSR (Achenbach, 1991) scores in this non-clinical population study (Ndetei et al. 2019), but further studies are needed to explain this finding. We are currently following this theme with ongoing studies on building resilience in young people in the context of their families.

Challenges associated with youth-focused mental health interventions in LMIC

Traditionally, youth mental health interventions have focused mainly on institutional approaches, be it based in schools, colleges, universities or youth groups. Our research team has conducted a wide range of such studies in Kenya in the past (Culbreth et al. 2018; Ndetei et al. 2019; Ndetei, Mutiso, Maraj et al. 2016) and we continue to carry out similar projects (Osborn et al. 2021). These approaches are favourable because they are easy to implement. However, they have one major limitation: they do not take into account the total social context of young people's lives, the social drivers of mental health and/or access to services within the community. The total environment in which young people live, and how these environments influence the final pathway to mental disorder or well-being has been ignored. Biological, psychological, social, cultural and economic influences should be considered. In order to understand the total context that determines mental health in children, adolescents and young adults, we recommend the Research Domain Criteria (RDoC) approach (Insel et al. 2010). The RDoC project is an effort to develop a precision-medicine approach for research on mental disorders, which combines contemporary knowledge about domains of human cognitive functioning, clinical neuroscience and genetics, while recognising the importance of development, environmental exposures, and the evolution of psychopathology (Garvey et al. 2016; NIMH, 2010). In response to this, we have developed a hypothetical model that takes into account the various possible drivers of suicide, most of which cannot be addressed through institutional approaches or youth groups. This biopsycho-social model recognises the role of factors intrinsic to the adolescent while regarding family factors as pivotal and also acknowledges the importance of community, peer and institutional factors in determining suicide risk.

We maintain that the family is the key institution for supporting adolescent mental health, not schools, colleges or universities. The family not only forms the most important driver of mental health in children, but is the major decision maker on what to do with a child with a mental disorder. The family is responsible for whether or not the child goes for treatment and, if so, where they go for treatment, depending on family resources and cultural beliefs. Indeed, Patel et al.'s paper in *The Lancet* (2018) notes that the more collectivistic culture in most LMICs gives the family more prominence in decision-making related to mental health than in HICs.

This approach facilitates follow-up regardless of which institution the child attends or will attend. Because African culture and practice are characterised by strong connections between young people and their families, this also facilitates formation of cohorts for long-term follow-up of the effectiveness of interventions. This is more so in rural areas where the majority of families live and where the families have permanent addresses. Thus, this model not only takes into account the total context of young people's lives but also has in-built sustainability. There-fore, one must consider the mental health of the family when considering youth mental health, along with the multiple determinants of mental health in each of the environments. No two families are identical, and therefore each family has to be treated as unique. This cannot be achieved using school mental health models. Taking the family approach is a better investment to ensure positive outcomes for young people as nuclear and extended family arrangements are still the norm in the Kenyan rural population. This approach is feasible given that community health workers (CHW), who are the backbone of most community-based non-mental health issues, could easily incorporate mental health in their activities.

CHWs (also known as community health volunteers) are normally high-school graduates who come from the same communities they serve (Chankova et al. 2009; Dovlo, 2004). They are identified by the communities in consultation with the Ministry of Health. Because the communities are involved in their identification, CHWs occupy positions of great trust in the communities. They undergo training by the Kenyan Ministry of Health on community health education on various types of health issues and disorders including school mental health (Jenkins et al. 2010). They are compensated on mutually agreed arrangements between them-selves, the communities and the Ministry of Health. These CHWs, unlike any other category of health workers, visit every home on a routine basis and know all members of the family. Cumulatively, this has the potential to reach all young people in a particular community. We have made some progress on this as will be discussed under examples of good practice. However, we are far from the finish line, and further development and implementation is still required.

Novel interventions in youth mental health

In Kenya, we have several examples of good practice in the development and implementation of youth mental health interventions, three of which have been evaluated in terms of their feasibility and efficacy. These include: (1) training of life skills to reduce negative mental health symptoms and enhance mental well-being in primary-school-age young adolescents (Ndetei et al. 2018); (2) developing a school mental health service, to promote mental well-being (Mutiso et al. 2018a); (3) a comparison of Shamiri Layperson-Provided Intervention vs Study Skills Control Intervention for depression and anxiety symptoms in adolescents (Osborn et al. 2021). Each of these is considered in turn below. The Shamiri Institute (https://www.shamiri.institute/about-us) is a youth-led organisation that aims at improving the mental health and well-being of Africa's young population. They develop and disseminate evidence-based interventions for young people in sub-Saharan Africa. They believe that young people thrive by improving their mental health, academic grades and social relationships.

(1) Life-skills training: There is significant evidence that training in life skills for primary-school-age children and adolescents improves their physical and mental health status (Burkey et al. 2015; Sancassiani et al. 2015). Life-skills training can also improve academic performance (Lipman et al. 2011; Maynard et al. 2011). However, over 90 per cent of the studies on school-based psychosocial interventions have been conducted in high-income countries (HICs) (Calear et al. 2016; Coombe et al. 2015) whereas less than 10 per cent were conducted in LMICs (Baker-Henningham, 2014; Fazel et al. 2014). In particular, we did not have any such studies reported from Kenya, despite the fact that Kenya has a curriculum and a policy for life-skills training in schools (Kenya Institute of Curriculum Development; KICD, 2008). This development, Life Skills Education (LSE), set out to provide children and adolescents with psychosocial competencies which would enable them to deal effectively and efficiently with the challenges they face in daily life, through developing adaptive and positive behaviours (KICD, 2008). This programme has not been implemented across Kenya due to the lack of local evidence for its efficacy (Waiganjo & Mwangi, 2018). We therefore aimed to determine the efficacy and effectiveness of the life-skill training curriculum for primary schools, which was adapted from the WHO Life Skills recommendation and validated by the Ministry of Education (MoE), Kenya (Kenya Institute of Education, 2002). We randomly selected 23 schools from two randomly selected sub-counties representing urban/peri-urban and rural contexts in Kenya (Ndetei et al. 2018). We collected baseline socio-demographic characteristics, and administered a locally validated YSR (Achenbach, 1991) for 11–18-year-olds at baseline and nine months post-intervention. The students completed the questionnaire in the presence of trained research assistants and in the absence of their teachers. We hired teachers, not from the same schools who had been trained in the MoE curriculum, to administer training for adolescents in upper primary schools immediately after the baseline. The training was spread over eight hours to suit the convenience of the individual schools.

Within the 23 schools taking part in the study (Ndetei et al. 2018), a total of 2044 adolescents met the criteria for YSR and completed all the socio-demographic information. We were able to follow 530 urban and 545 rural adolescents for nine months and who also fully completed all the items on YSR giving a follow-up of 1075 students i.e. a 51.9 per cent follow-up rate. Because of late age entry to school, the age range was wider than would be expected for these schools (11–18 years old) with a mean age of 12.5 years and standard deviation of 1.3. We found significant positive improvements in internalising and externalising YSR symptoms and syndromes in both urban and rural areas. The improvement was over 40 per cent and therefore unlikely to be attributed to placebo effect or natural recovery without intervention. However, attention problems worsened – more in rural sites and particularly in girls. We therefore concluded that life-skills training is efficacious in improving mental health in school-going adolescents in the Kenyan context. However, it is not effective in attention problems which seem to be cognitive in nature (Ndetei et al. 2018).

(2) Developing a school mental health service to promote mental well-being (Mutiso, Musyimi, Musau et al. 2018). School mental health programmes have been successfully piloted in HICs (Wyn et al. 2000, Chapter 4 of this book). We aimed to pilot a school mental health programme in a Kenyan socio-cultural context for the first time. Our approach has been described in detail in two easily available references (Mutiso et al. 2020; Mutiso, Musyimi, Musau et al. 2018)). We also provided a diagrammatic summary of the Theory of Change (ToC) that we developed (Mutiso, Musyimi, Musau et al. 2018) that enables schools to determine what aspects of mental health they wish to target within their school. This ToC starts from what is expected and communally agreed by the stakeholders on what outcomes they want. Then they work backwards to track the path from the beginning to the desired outcomes. Stakeholders then collectively identify the barriers in the pathway depending on the local socio-cultural context. They also collectively identify the potential solutions to known barriers and agree on how to mitigate and negotiate resolutions on any unexpected barriers. This dialogue also addresses the issue of socio-culturally available enablers along the pathway and how to facilitate those enablers.

It is to be noted that ToC takes place as the first step in the development of school-based programmes. In the process of developing ToC and the actual implementation of the school mental health programme, we encountered several challenges and learned several lessons that could be useful to others in developing their own school mental health programme in LMICs. Based on our experience we concluded that different stakeholders can come together to decide together how they want the programme developed. This promotes collective ownership of the process from beginning to end, including ownership of the emerging policy and practice recommendations and feasible seamless transition from programme to policy and practice using readily available community resources. The engagement with stakeholders and focus on the use of existing community resources ensures that the solution is sustainable. This process not only builds social capital for the community to manage mental health problems for the children and adolescents, but also promotes social connectedness in the community around mental health in children and young adolescents beyond the school environment (Mutiso, Musyimi, Musau et al. 2018).

(3) A comparison of Shamiri Layperson-Provided Intervention vs Study Skills Control Intervention for Depression and Anxiety Symptoms in Adolescents Trial (Osborn et al. 2021). This study set out to determine whether scalable psychological interventions that invoke simple psychological principles rather than explicit references to psychopathology, alleviate depression and anxiety symptoms in Kenyan adolescents. We used a randomised clinical trial study design of 413 high school students in Kenya aged 13–18 years old. We employed a four-week layperson-delivered group intervention that teaches growth mindset, gratitude and value affirmation. The layperson was an older student from the same school who had finished high school and not yet joined tertiary training. This student was trained on how to administer the intervention to students still in that school (details are in the recommended reading at the end of this chapter). We found that this type of intervention appeared to significantly reduce depression and anxiety symptoms in symptomatic adolescents compared with the control group, although both groups showed symptom reductions over a period of seven months. This could be a cost-effective intervention delivered by laypeople. However, further studies are needed.

Conclusions

In this chapter we have chosen to use our experience of research on youth mental health in Kenya to illustrate the kinds of challenges faced by LMIC countries in Africa. Kenya's demographic distribution is very different from that of most HICs with many more young people and a much greater proportion of the population living in rural areas. Mental health resources are much scarcer than they are in HICs and so innovative and sustainable solutions are needed to support young people who experience mental health difficulties.

The research we presented clearly demonstrates that mental health problems are widespread among young people in Kenya and that these problems are associated with a range of socio-demographic factors such as family structure and limited availability of resources. A further challenge for young people in Kenya is the high rate of suicide and the existence of stigma towards people with mental disorders that makes help-seeking less likely. Our research clearly indicates that anti-stigma interventions are needed.

We propose that CHWs, who work closely with families in providing a wide range of healthcare supports, are sufficiently trusted by communities and families to be well positioned to take on a significant role in supporting young people's mental health. We have also begun to gather evidence on school-based interventions designed to teach life skills and promote children and adolescents' well-being.

The team at AMHRTF has come to appreciate that youth mental health in LMICs is not a concern limited to researchers and practitioners based in LMICs. It is indeed a global health issue which AMHRTF has received funding for by agencies in HICs, but has also collaborated and published together with researchers from HICs. This is of mutual benefit. Locally, we build capacity for research on evidence-based interventions. Because of the nature of the community approach, we build community capital and also promote social connectedness at community level around youth mental health which extends to other community activities. To our satisfaction we have noticed that our colleagues from HICs come with an open and ardent attitude, with interest in understanding differences and similarities between HICs and LMICs, and what may underpin such contextual variation. This process contributes to the global database and is true to the concept of global mental health. AMHRTF invites collaborations.

Further reading

Mutiso V., Musyimi C., Musau A., Nandoya E., McKenzie K., Ndetei D. Pilot towards developing a school mental health service: Experiences and lessons learnt in implementing Kenya Integrated intervention model for Dialogue and Screening to promote children's mental well-being (KIDS). *Early Intervention in Psychiatry. 2018, 1-7.* DOI: 10.1111/eip.12543

Mutiso V., Musyimi C. W., Mokua C., Andeso P., Malinda S., Ndetei D. (2021) Setting Up School Mental Health Program. In: Okpaku S.O. (Eds.) *Innovations in Global Mental Health.* Springer, Cham. https://doi.org/10.1007/978-3-319-70134-9_81-1

Osborn, T. L., Venturo-Conerly, K. E., Arango, S., Roe, E., Rodriguez, M., Alemu, R. G., Gan J., Wasil A. R., Otieno B. H., Rusch T., Ndetei D. M., Wasanga C., Schleider J. L., & Weisz, J. R. (2021). Effect of Shamiri layperson-provided intervention vs study skills control intervention for depression and anxiety symptoms in adolescents in Kenya: a randomized clinical trial. *JAMA Psychiatry, 78*(8), 829–837. DOI:10.1001/jamapsychiatry.2021.1129

References

Achenbach, T. M. (1991) Manual for the Youth Self-report and 1991 Profile. University of Vermont, Department of Psychiatry.

Baker-Henningham, H. (2014). The role of early childhood education programmes in the promotion of child and adolescent mental health in low-and middle-income countries. *International Journal of Epidemiology, 43*(2), 407–433.

Block, J., & Kremen, A. M. (1996). IQ and ego-resiliency: conceptual and empirical connections and separateness. *Journal of Personality and Social Psychology, 70*(2), 349.

Burkey, M. D., Hosein, M., Purgato, M., Adi, A., Morton, I., Kohrt, B. A., & Tol, W. A. (2015). Psychosocial interventions for disruptive behavioural problems in children living in low-and middle-income countries: Study protocol of a systematic review. *BMJ Open, 5*(5).

Calear, A. L., Christensen, H., Freeman, A., Fenton, K., Grant, J. B., Van Spijker, B., & Donker, T. (2016). A systematic review of psychosocial suicide prevention interventions for youth. *European Child & Adolescent Psychiatry, 25*(5), 467–482.

Chankova, S., Muchiri, S., & Kombe, G. (2009). Health workforce attrition in the public sector in Kenya: A look at the reasons. *Human Resources for Health, 7*(1), 1–8.

Chibanda, D., Mesu, P., Kajawu, L., Cowan, F., Araya, R., & Abas, M. A. (2011). Problem-solving therapy for depression and common mental disorders in Zimbabwe: Piloting a task-shifting primary mental healthcare intervention in a population with a high prevalence of people living with HIV. *BMC Public Health, 11*(1), 1–10.

Clement, S., Schauman, O., Graham, T., Maggioni, F., Evans-Lacko, S., Bezborodovs, N., ... & Thornicroft, G. (2015). What is the impact of mental health-related stigma on help-seeking? A systematic review of quantitative and qualitative studies. *Psychological Medicine, 45*(1), 11–27.

Coombe, J., Mackenzie, L., Munro, R., Hazell, T., Perkins, D., & Reddy, P. (2015). Teacher-mediated interventions to support child mental health following a disaster: A systematic review. *PLoS Currents, 7.*

Culbreth, R., Swahn, M. H., Ndetei, D., Ametewee, L., & Kasirye, R. (2018). Suicidal ideation among youth living in the slums of Kampala, Uganda. *International Journal of Environmental Research and Public Health, 15*(2), 298.

Deaton, A. (2005). Measuring poverty in a growing world (or measuring growth in a poor world). *Review of Economics and Statistics, 87*(1), 1–19.

Dovlo, D. (2004). Using mid-level cadres as substitutes for internationally mobile health professionals in Africa. A desk review. Human resources for health, 2(1), 1–12.

Fazel, M., Patel, V., Thomas, S., & Tol, W. (2014). Mental health interventions in schools in low-income and middle-income countries. *The Lancet Psychiatry, 1*(5), 388–398.

Garvey, M., Avenevoli, S., & Anderson, K. (2016). The national institute of mental health research domain criteria and clinical research in child and adolescent psychiatry. *Journal of the American Academy of Child & Adolescent Psychiatry, 55*(2), 93–98.

Gibb, S. J., Fergusson, D. M., & Horwood, L. J. (2010). Burden of psychiatric disorder in young adulthood and life outcomes at age 30. *The British Journal of Psychiatry, 197*(2), 122–127.

Hamadeh, N., Van Romaey, C., & Metreau, E. (2021). New World Bank country classifications by income level: 2021–2022. https://blogs.worldbank.org/opendata/new-world-bank-country-classifications-income-level-2021-2022

Harder, V. S., Mutiso, V. N., Khasakhala, L. I., Burke, H. M., & Ndetei, D. M. (2011). Postelection violence, posttraumatic stress, and comorbidity of behavioral and emotional problems among Kenyan youth. *Comprehensive Psychiatry, 52*(6), e7–e7.

Harttgen, K., & Vollmer, S. (2013). Using an asset index to simulate household income. *Economics Letters, 121*(2), 257–262.

Healy, E. A., Kaiser, B. N., & Puffer, E. S. (2018). Family-based youth mental health interventions delivered by nonspecialist providers in low-and middle-income countries: A systematic review. *Families, Systems, & Health, 36*(2), 182.

Insel, T., Cuthbert, B., Garvey, M., Heinssen, R., Pine, D. S., Quinn, K., ... & Wang, P. (2010). Research domain criteria (RDoC): Toward a new classification framework for research on mental disorders. *American Journal of Psychiatry 167*, 748–751

Jenkins, R., Kiima, D., Okonji, M., Njenga, F., Kingora, J., & Lock, S. (2010). Integration of mental health into primary care and community health working in Kenya: Context, rationale, coverage and sustainability. *Mental Health in Family Medicine, 7*(1), 37.

Kenya Institute of Curriculum Development Education (2006). *Proposal for funding on up scaling mainstreaming of Life Skills Education into school Curriculum.* Kenya Institute of Curriculum Development, Nairobi, Kenya. https://kicd.ac.ke/

Kenya Institute of Education (2002). Life skills education for behavior change. Facilitator's handbook. Kenya Institute of Education.

Kenya National Bureau of Statistics (KNBS) (2019). *2019 Kenya Population and Houseing Census Volume III: Distribution of Population by Age and Sex.* KNBS.

Kieling, C., Baker-Henningham, H., Belfer, M., Conti, G., Ertem, I., Omigbodun, O., ... Rahman, A. (2011). Child and adolescent mental health world-wide: evidence for action. *The Lancet, 378*(9801), 1515–1525.

Lipman, E. L., Kenny, M., Brennan, E., O'Grady, S., & Augimeri, L. (2011). Helping boys at-risk of criminal activity: Qualitative results of a multi-component intervention. *BMC Public Health, 11*(1), 1–11.

Maynard, A. S., Monk, J. D., & Booker, K. W. (2011). Building empathy through identification and expression of emotions: A review of interactive tools for children with social deficits. *Journal of Creativity in Mental Health, 6*(2), 166–175.

Morris, S. S., Carletto, C., Hoddinott, J., & Christiaensen, L. J. M. (2000). Validity of rapid estimates of household wealth and income for health surveys in rural Africa. *Journal of Epidemiology & Community Health, 54*(5), 381–387.

Mutiso, V., Musyimi, C. W., Mokua, C., Andeso, P., Malinda, S., & Ndetei, D. (2020). Setting Up School Mental Health Program BT – Innovations in Global Mental Health. In S. O. Okpaku (Ed.) (pp. 1–12). Springer International Publishing. http://doi.org/10.1007/978-3-319-70134-9_81-1

Mutiso, V. N., Musyimi, C. W., Musau, A. M., Nandoya, E. S., Mckenzie, K., & Ndetei, D. M. (2018). Pilot towards developing a school mental health service: Experiences and lessons learnt in implementing Kenya Integrated intervention model for Dialogue and Sreening to promote children's mental well-being (KIDS). *Early Intervention in Psychiatry, 12*(5), 972–978.

Mutiso, V. N., Musyimi, C. W., Tomita, A., Loeffen, L., Burns, J. K., & Ndetei, D. M. (2018). Epidemiological patterns of mental disorders and stigma in a community household survey in urban slum and rural settings in Kenya. *International Journal of Social Psychiatry, 64*(2). http://doi.org/10.1177/0020764017748180

National Institute of Mental Health (NIMH). (2010). *Definitions of the RDoC Domains and Constructs.* https://www.nimh.nih.gov/research/research-funded-by-nimh/rdoc/definitions-of-the-rdoc-domains-and-constructs

Ndetei, D., Khasakhala, L., Nyabola, L., Ongecha-Owuor, F., Seedat, S., Mutiso, V., ... Odhiambo, G. (2008). The prevalence of anxiety and depression symptoms and syndromes in Kenyan children and adolescents. *Journal of Child & Adolescent Mental Health, 20*(1), 33–51.

Ndetei, D. M., Khasakhala, L. I., Mutiso, V., Ongecha-Owuor, F. A., & Kokonya, D. A. (2009). Psychosocial and health aspects of drug use by students in public secondary schools in Nairobi, Kenya. *Substance Abuse, 30*(1), 61–68.

Ndetei, D. M., Mutiso, V., Gitonga, I., Agudile, E., Tele, A., Birech, L., ... McKenzie, K. (2018). World Health Organization life-skills training is efficacious in reducing youth self-report scores in primary school going children in Kenya. *Early Intervention in Psychiatry, 13*(5), 1146–1154.

Ndetei, D. M., Mutiso, V., Maraj, A., Anderson, K. K., Musyimi, C., & McKenzie, K. (2016). Stigmatizing attitudes toward mental illness among primary school children in Kenya. *Social Psychiatry and Psychiatric Epidemiology, 51*(1), 73–80. http://doi.org/10.1007/s00127-015-1090-6

Ndetei, D. M., Mutiso, V., Maraj, A., Anderson, K. K., Musyimi, C., Musau, A., ... McKenzie, K. (2019). Towards understanding the relationship between psychosocial factors and ego resilience among primary school children in a Kenyan setting: A pilot feasibility study. *Community Mental Health Journal, 55*(6), 1038–1046.

Ndetei, D. M., Mutiso, V., Musyimi, C., Mokaya, A. G., Anderson, K. K., McKenzie, K., & Musau, A. (2016). The prevalence of mental disorders among upper primary school children in Kenya. *Social Psychiatry and Psychiatric Epidemiology, 51*(1), 63–71. http://doi.org/10.1007/s00127-015-1132-0

Ndetei, D. M., Mutiso, V. N., Weisz, J. R., Okoth, C. A., Musyimi, C., Muia, E. N., Osborn, T. L., Sourander, A., Wasserman, D. & Mamah, D. (2022). Socio-demographic, economic and mental health problems were risk factors for suicidal ideation among Kenyan students aged 15 plus. *Journal of affective disorders, 302*, 74–82. doi.org/10.1016/j.jad.2022.01.055.

Ndetei, D. M., Ongecha-Owour, F. A, Khasakhala, L., Syanda, J., Mutiso, V., Othieno, C. J., ... Kokonya, D. a. (2007). Bullying in public secondary schools in Nairobi, Kenya. *Journal of Child and Adolescent Mental Health, 19*(1), 45–55. http://doi.org/10.2989/17280580709486634

Ndetei, D. M., Ongecha-Owuor, F. A., Khasakhala, L., Mutiso, V., Odhiambo, G., & Kokonya, D. A. (2007). Traumatic experiences of Kenyan secondary school students. *Journal of Child & Adolescent Mental Health, 19*(2), 147–155.

Osborn, T. L., Venturo-Conerly, K. E., Arango, S., Roe, E., Rodriguez, M., Alemu, R. G., Gan, J., Wasil, A. R., Otieno, B. H., Rusch, T., Ndetei, D. M., Wasanga, C., Schleider, J. L., & Weisz, J. R. (2021). Effect of Shamiri layperson-provided intervention vs study skills control intervention for depression and anxiety symptoms in adolescents in Kenya: a randomized clinical trial. *JAMA Psychiatry, 78*(8), 829–837. DOI:10.1001/jamapsychiatry.2021.1129

Patel, V. (2007). Mental health in low-and middle-income countries. *British Medical Bulletin, 81*(1), 81–96.

Patel, V., Goel, D. S., & Desai, R. (2009). Scaling up services for mental and neurological disorders in low-resource settings. *International Health, 1*(1), 37–44.

Patel, V., Saxena, S., Lund, C., Thornicroft, G., Baingana, F., Bolton, P., ... & UnÜtzer, J. (2018). The Lancet Commission on global mental health and sustainable development. *The Lancet, 392*(10157), 1553–1598.

Philippe, F. L., Laventure, S., Beaulieu-Pelletier, G., Lecours, S., & Lekes, N. (2011). Ego-resiliency as a mediator between childhood trauma and psychological symptoms. *Journal of Social and Clinical Psychology, 30*(6), 583–598.

Sancassiani, F., Pintus, E., Holte, A., Paulus, P., Moro, M. F., Cossu, G., … Lindert, J. (2015). Enhancing the emotional and social skills of the youth to promote their well-being and positive development: a systematic review of universal school-based randomized controlled trials. *Clinical Practice and Epidemiology in Mental Health: CP & EMH, 11*(Suppl 1 M2), 21.

Schnyder, N., Panczak, R., Groth, N., & Schultze-Lutter, F. (2017). Association between mental health-related stigma and active help-seeking: systematic review and meta-analysis. *The British Journal of Psychiatry, 210*(4), 261–268.

Stanford Children's Health. (2021). Teen Suicide.

Waiganjo, M. M. & Mwangi, M. W. (2018). Relevance of life skills education in preparing Kenyan youth for national development. *Journal of African Studies in Educational Management and Leadership, 10*, 85–103. http://kaeam.or.ke/articles/v10/Paper6.pdf

World Bank Group. (2021). World Bank Country and Lending Groups.

World Bank. (2021a). Data for lower middle income, Kenya. https://data.worldbank.org/?locations=XN-KE. Accessed October 5, 2021.

World Bank. (2021b). Rural Population, Kenya. https://data.worldbank.org/indicator/SP.RUR.TOTL.ZS?locations=KE Accessed October 5, 2021.

World Health Organization (WHO). (2015). *Mental Health Atlas 2014.*

World Health Organization (WHO). (2017). *Mental Health Atlas 2017.*

World Health Organization (WHO). (2019). WHO Suicide data.

Wyn, J., Cahill, H., Holdsworth, R., & Rowling, L. C. S. (2000). MindMatters, a whole-school approach promoting mental health and well-being. *Australian and New Zealand Journal of Psychiatry, 34*(4), 594–601.

World Health Organization. (2016). *mhGAP intervention guide for mental, neurological and substance use disorders in non-specialized health settings: Mental health Gap Action Programme (mhGAP).* World Health Organization.

Seen and Heard – a creative piece by young people (18–25 years old), as part of the work of the YOULEAD Research Group, National University of Ireland, Galway and Fregoli Theatre Company in collaboration with SpunOut.ie:

Confused, overwhelmed, at sea
Lost
How do I navigate this system?
How can I find myself?

Available at: https://www.youtube.com/watch?v=Wuz-XE8hCao&feature=youtu.be

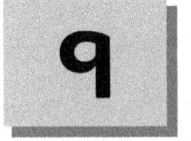

Epidemiology of mental health difficulties in young people

Emma Howard
University College Dublin, Ireland

Barbara Dooley
University College Dublin, Ireland

Introduction

At present, around a quarter of the global population comprises young people aged between 10–24 years old, which is the greatest proportion of this cohort in history (Abidi, 2017; World Health Organization [WHO], 2009). Mental health problems are the leading cause of disability and poor-life outcomes for young people, contributing 45 per cent of the overall burden of disease (Killackey et al. 2020) and young people demonstrate the highest incidence, prevalence, and burden of mental ill-health (Mei et al. 2020). Furthermore, 75 per cent of mental health problems and disorders emerge before 25 years old, which go on to persist into adulthood (Kessler et al. 2007). Mental health problems can also affect mortality; while suicide and self-harm are not mental health problems themselves, they are linked with mental distress and mental disorders. Although self-harm is not necessarily linked with suicide, it can increase the risk of suicide (Mental Health Foundation, 2016). Suicide is the second most common cause of death globally for young people aged 15–29 years old, after road injury, and of the estimated 800,000 people who die by suicide annually, the majority are young people (Killackey et al. 2020). The top two mental health problems are depression followed by anxiety (Global Burden of Disease Study 2013 Collaborators, 2015). It is important to have robust data across studies, across countries and geographic regions for this age group in order to help us understand the societal impact and the need for service provision. Another important issue to consider in assessing the societal burden of mental problems, such as anxiety, depression and suicidal behaviour is whether there is evidence of increasing prevalence in recent years (Twenge et al. 2019).

Thus, the aim of this chapter is to present data selected from studies reporting prevalence on the following: depression, anxiety and suicidal behaviour. These studies have been drawn from high-, middle- and low-income countries and include commonly used self-report measures. We report on studies that illustrate the prevalence of mental health problems globally but this chapter is not a systematic review of all published studies.

Comparing anxiety and depression across studies is difficult for the following reasons: studies use a plethora of different measures, the timeframe often differs (e.g. one week or one month) and the measures reported often have not been validated psychometrically for the population of interest. However, taking a systematic approach, while acknowledging these methodological issues, does add value to our understanding of mental health problems in young people. The data presented in this chapter, reporting on routinely used self-report measures, relate to common mental health problems and therefore should be considered within that context and not as diagnosed mental disorders.

The chapter begins with a broad overview of results concerning the estimated prevalence of anxiety and depression in adolescents and young adults. This is followed by data on suicidal behaviours. The final part of the chapter captures data on anxiety and depression during the COVID-19 pandemic. Mental health is complex, therefore each section reports on relevant risk and protective factors, including coping strategies. The chapter closes with a discussion of interpretations and implications of the reported findings. All sources of the data are provided so that the source can be checked independently to research the findings in more depth.

Methods

A systematic approach was taken to finding papers using three databases (PsychInfo via Proquest, CINAHL, and MEDLINE via Proquest) in order to understand the prevalence of anxiety, depression and suicidal behaviour in youth aged 10–24 years old. The inclusion criteria were: (1) papers published in English; (2) the sample size was large >600; (3) age-range of 10–24 years old; (4) mental health data were collected through self-report; and (5) the study focused on general mental health difficulties (i.e. not formal diagnosis) in the general population of interest (e.g. not specific samples such as rape victims or post a natural disaster). Where studies included populations (or data) outside of the inclusion criteria (e.g. aged 15–29 years old), studies were included if data could be extracted for the relevant population. For studies related to self-harm and suicidal thoughts and behaviour (STB), and to allow for ease of comparisons, there was an additional inclusion criterion that the prevalence must relate to a one-year period prior to data collection. Studies were then selected in order to draw from world-wide locations to ensure inclusion from high-, low-, and middle-income countries. The World Bank (http://data.worldbank.org/about/country-and-lending-groups) classifies countries into four categories: low, low-middle, middle-upper, and upper-income countries. For the purposes of this chapter, three classifications are used: low- (LIC), middle- (MIC) and high-income (HIC) countries. MIC combines low-middle and middle-upper-income categories from the World Bank, in line with previously published papers (Li, You et al. 2021).

Mental health problems

While two aims of this chapter are to provide the prevalence of mental health problems and to reflect on the change in the prevalence over time, comparisons are made difficult by the methodology used, for example the wide variety of measures used, whether the measure is self-report or clinician rate, or the sampling method (e.g. convenience, clustering, stratified etc.). For example, Cheung et al. (2017) investigated the prevalence of adolescent health-related behaviours in two similar regions in the Netherlands using two different data collection methods. In Twente, 9,360 young people were recruited to a mandatory sample, and in IJsselland, 1,952 young people were recruited to a voluntary sample. These regions were considered to be comparable. However, they found that the respondents in the voluntary sample were less likely to report risky behaviour and were more likely to have better mental health status and to be female (61.3 per cent vs 51.5 per cent). To help counteract the problem of oversampling groups, studies may use weighting of participants.

To study how different depression measures classify respondents, Dardas et al. (2019) collected depression data using both the Center for Epidemiologic Studies-Depression scale (CES-D) and the Beck Depression Inventory-II (BDI-II) from a sample of 13–17-year-old adolescents living in Jordan. Using the recommended cut-off[2] of 20 for both measures, the prevalence of depression was 49 per cent for CES-D and 35 per cent for the BDI-II. However, when they adjusted for an alternative recommended cut-off of 24 for the CES-D, they found the prevalence to be 38 per cent. For both CES-D cut-off levels, the difference with the BDI-II remains statistically significant, that is they were more likely to be classified as depressed using the CES-D. Measures used globally to examine mental health include: Beck's Depression Inventory (BDI); Brief Symptom Inventory (BSI); Center for Epidemiologic Studies Depression (CES-D); Depression, Anxiety, and Stress Scales (DASS); Generalised Anxiety Disorder (GAD); General Health Questionnaire (GHQ); Hospital Anxiety and Depression Scale (HADS); Kessler Psychological Distress Scale (K-6); Short Mood and Feelings Questionnaire (SMFQ); Strengths and Difficulties Questionnaire Total (SDQ); Patient Health Questionnaire (PHQ); Psychological Strain Scales (PSS), and; Warwick-Edinburgh Mental Well-being Scale (WEMWBS).

Table 9.1 shows that mental health problems peak during late adolescence (Ferro et al. 2015; Pitchforth et al. 2019; Twenge et al. 2019), are higher in low- and middle-income countries (LMICs), have been increasing over time (Collishaw et al. 2010; Twenge et al. 2019) or remain steady (Pitchforth et al. 2019), and generally females have higher prevalence than males.

Studies show us that there are many risk factors associated with mental health problems including having a chronic health problem (Dardas et al. 2018), learning difficulty (Dardas et al. 2018), hopelessness (Nabunya et al. 2020), lower socio-economic status (Ferro et al. 2015), poorer interpersonal relations (Ferro et al. 2015), having lower self-esteem (Ferro et al. 2015), being dissatisfied with the university culture (Hossain et al. 2019), low and high daily meal intake frequency (Hossain et al. 2019), physical inactivity (Hossain et al. 2019), and sedentary behaviour (Vancampfort et al. 2018). On the other hand, Collishaw et al. (2010) found that over time in the United Kingdom changes in family structure (intact/non-intact families) and ethnicity did not account for the changing trends seen in symptoms of depression and anxiety.

---

[2] A value or criterion that is held to mark the lowest point at which a certain status or category is attained, e.g. depression (APA dictionary)

Family is repeatedly seen as a protective factor for young people's mental health. Studies have found that positive family climate (Klasen et al. 2015), favourable family characteristics (Ferro et al. 2015) or good family relationships (Nabunya et al. 2020) are linked with better mental health in young people. Hickey et al. (2017) found that the strength of the relationship between perceived family support and depressive symptoms is linked to coping, in particular problem solving/planned and seeking social support. Other protective factors include having future goals and aspirations (Almroth et al. 2018), being able to talk about personal problems (Fernandes et al. 2013), and social support generally (Nabunya et al. 2020). Dardas et al. (2018: 6) comment that the most successful documented preventative strategies 'involve (1) identifying at-risk cohorts, such as offspring of depressed parents or adolescents with subsyndromal depression; (2) examining the mechanisms by which risk is imposed; (3) augmenting protective factors; and (4) and utilising expert clinicians to deliver treatments when needed'.

Self-harm and suicidal thoughts and behaviours

The prevalence ranges for self-harm and STB are detailed in Table 9.2 and, as you will observe, quite a lot of variation is reported. For example: self-harm (5.8 per cent in Ireland to 11.1 per cent in England), suicidal ideation (0.7 per cent in Myanmar to 25.7 per cent in Australia), suicidal planning (5.2 per cent in Australia to 19.3 per cent in Africa) and suicidal attempt (<1 per cent in Hanoi to 60.7 per cent in Samoa). In every study, females were more likely to engage in STB than males; this holds for calculated pooled prevalence in all world regions but not in every country (Page et al. 2013). Also, the prevalence was higher in late adolescence rather than early adolescence (Li, You et al. 2021; Zubrick et al. 2016). In addition, there is variation across time. Between 1991–2009, for female students (Lowry et al. 2014), the prevalence of suicide ideation decreased (from 37.2 per cent to 17.4 per cent), before subsequently increasing during 2009–11 to 19.3 per cent. Comparatively, for male students (Lowry et al. 2014), the prevalence of suicide ideation decreased during 1991–2007 (from 20.8 per cent to 10.3 per cent) and then increased during 2007–11 to 12.5 per cent. Between 2001–17 (Price and Khubchandani, 2019), the rates of suicidal planning and attempt have been increasing for females (percentage change are +45.4 per cent and +27.6 per cent respectively) and decreasing for males (percentage change are –13.3 per cent and –10.7 per cent respectively).

Self-harm and STB should be considered in the context of mental health as loneliness (Li, You et al. 2021), anxiety (Li, Zhang et al. 2021), depression (Oh et al. 2021) and mental health disorders (Zubrick et al. 2016) are all strongly associated with STB. Bullying has repeatedly been identified as a risk factor for suicide. Koyanagi et al. (2019) observed this risk in 47 out of 48 LMICs (except Afghanistan). They investigated the relationship between different types of bullying and suicide attempts and found those who were bullied for (in descending order), religion, race, nationality and colour had the highest odds of suicide attempts. Physical bullying, sexual bullying, exclusion, being bullied due to physical appearance, and number of days being bullied were also strongly associated with

Table 9.1 Summary of mental health problem studies

Study	Relevant MH Measures and Cutoff	Prevalence	Study Design	Location	Sample
Almroth et al. (2018)	CES-DC (Swedish version; cutoff of 30) SDQ (cutoff of 18)	CES-DC: 12.1%[*1]; male 3.8%[*]; female 19.7%[*] SDQ: 10.9%[*]; male 7.6%[*]; female 13.9%[*]	KUPOL longitudinal study (baseline data)	Sweden[HIC]	Size: 3,343 Female: 52.2% Age: 13 years
Collishaw et al. (2010)	Malaise Inventory psychological subscale (15 item) GHQ-12	Depressed mood: male (1986 6.6%; 2006 6.6%); female (1986 10.5%; 2006 11.9%) General worries: male (1986 8.3%; 2006 12.8%); female (1986 16.4%; 2006 28.4%) Difficulty coping: male (1986 4.1%; 2006 6.1%); female (1986 5.3%; 2006 8.4%) Worn out/under strain: male (1986 3.6%; 2006 8.6%); female (1986 6.6%; 2006 11.0%) Note: Prevalence for other individual symptoms of depression or anxiety available	Follow-up of the 1970 British Cohort Study (data from 1986) Health Surveys for England 2002/2003 (data from 2006) Response rate: 1986 46%; 2006 51%	England[HIC]	Size: 5,243 Female: – Age: 16–17 years
Dardas et al. (2018)	BDI-II (Arabic version); minimal 0–13; mild 14–19; moderate 10–28; severe 29+)	Depression: minimal 47%; mild 18%; moderate 19%; severe 15%	Cross-sectional school survey Stratified random sampling with strata being country regions Sample size calculated: 1,045 Response rate: 93%	Jordan[MIC]	Size: 2,349 Female: 59% Age: 12–17 years

(continued)

Table 9.1 (continued)

Study	Relevant MH Measures and Cutoff	Prevalence	Study Design	Location	Sample
Fatiregun & Kumapayi et al. (2014)	PHQ-9 (mild 5–9; moderate 10–14; moderately severe 15–19; severe 20+)	Depression: none 44%; mild 34.7%; moderate 16.1%; moderately severe 4.6%; severe 0.5%; overall 21.2%; 10–13 years 20.6%; 14–16 years 20.1%; 17–19 years 28.0%	Cross-sectional Stratified cluster sampling procedure based on public and private schools Sample size calculated: 1,367	Nigeria[MIC]	Size: 1,713 Female: 55.3% Age: 10–19 years
Fernandes et al. (2013)	GHQ-12 (cutoff of 5)	Common mental disorders: 7.9%; female 8.3%; male 7.4%; 16–18 years 7.1%; 19–21 years 7.4%; 22–24 years 9.7%;	Baseline data from an RCT	India[MIC] (Goa)	Size: 3,649 Female: 51% Age: 16–24 years
Ferro et al. (2015)	CES-D (12-item version) Three distinct trajectories of depressive symptoms: Minimal (55%; CES-D<6); Subclinical (39%; CES-D = 9–13); Clinical (6%; CES-D>18)	Depression: Minimal Group: 12–13 years M = 4.0; 14–15 years M = 4.0; 16–17 years M = 5.2; 18–19 years M = 5.3; 20–21 years M = 5.3; 22–23 years M = 5.3 Subclinical Group: 12–13 years M = 9.3; 14–15 years M = 11.3; 16–17 years M = 12.6; 18–19 years M = 12.5; 20–21 years M = 11.5; 22–23 years M = 10.7 Clinical Group: 12–13 years M = 18.6; 14–15 years M = 22.0; 16–17 years M = 24.8; 18–19 years M = 24.7; 20–21 years M = 23.5; 22–23 years M = 21.3	National Longitudinal Survey of Children and Youth (1994–2009)	Canada[HIC]	Size: 2,825 Female: 49% Age: 12–23 years

Study	Relevant MH Measures and Cutoff	Prevalence	Study Design	Location	Sample
Hickey et al. (2017)	DASS-21 (depression scale: normal 0–9; mild 10–13; moderate 14–20; severe 21–27; very severe 28–42)	Depression: normal 69.9%; mild 10.8%; moderate 11.3%; severe 3.7%; very severe 4.3%	My World Survey-Second Level (MWS-SL) Student response rate: 45%	Republic of Ireland[HIC]	Size: 6,085 Female: 51% Age: 12–19 years
Hossain et al. (2019)	PHQ-9 (normal 0–4; mild 5–9; moderate 10–14; moderately severe 15–19; severely severe 20+) GAD-7 (minimal 0–4; mild 5–9; moderate 10–14; severe 15+)	Depression: Normal: baseline 48.4%; follow-up 25.9% Mild: baseline 25.9%; follow-up 27.3% Moderate: baseline 14.8%; follow-up 25.0% Moderately severe: baseline 7.6%; follow-up 15.8% Severely severe: baseline 3.2%; follow-up 6.0% Anxiety Minimal: baseline 65.2%; follow-up 38.1% Mild: baseline 20.4%; follow-up 28.5% Moderate: baseline 10.7%; follow-up 22.1% Severe: baseline 3.7%; follow-up 11.3%	Stratified random sampling with strata being different faculties Fifteen-month follow-up	Bangladesh[MIC] (Dhaka)	Size: 1,140 (baseline); 897 (follow-up) Female: 42% Age: 18–22 years

(continued)

Table 9.1 (continued)

Study	Relevant MH Measures and Cutoff	Prevalence	Study Design	Location	Sample
Liu et al. (2019)	CES–D Youth Self-Report (YSR) depression scales (16 items)	Scores >90th percentile on both scales were used as cutoff points to define clinically relevant depressive symptoms	Shandong Adolescent Behaviour and Health Cohort study (2015) Longitudinal study Cross-sectional design	China[MIC] (Shandong province)	Size: 11,831 Female: 49% Age: M = 15.0 SD = 1.5
Klasen et al. (2015)	CES–DC (German version; cutoff of 16)	Depression: baseline 17%; 1-year follow-up 15%; 2-year follow-up 14%	BELLA study: mental health module of the German National Health Interview and Examination Survey for children and adolescents (KIGGS)	Germany[HIC]	Size: 1,643 Female: 50.6% Age: 11–17 years
Nabunya et al. (2020)	BDI (minimal 0–9; mild 10–18; moderate 19–29; severe 30+)	Depression: Overall: minimal 22.1%; mild 31.8%; moderate 29.7%; severe 16.4% 14–15 years: minimal 22.7%; mild 34.7%; moderate 27.2%; severe 15.5% 16–17 years: minimal 21.4%; mild 28.0%; moderate 33.0%; severe 17.5%	Baseline data from the Suubi4Her study longitudinal randomized clinical trial (2017–2022)	Uganda[LIC]	Size: 1,260 Female: 100% Age: 14–17 years

Study	Relevant MH Measures and Cutoff	Prevalence	Study Design	Location	Sample
Pitchforth et al. (2019)	WEMWBS GHQ (cutoff of >3)	Scotland 13–15 years GHQ: average 9.4% (2003 8.2%; 2008 10.0%; ...; 2012 6.4%; 2013 11.9%; 2014 11.6%; female average 11.91%; male average 6.97%) WEMWBS: average M = 51.1 (2012 M = 51.6; 2013 M = 51.1; 2014 M = 50.6; female M = 50.0; male M = 52.1) Scotland 16–24 years GHQ: average 16.0% (2003 14.0%; 2008 17.0%; ...; 2012 15.5%; 2013 18.3%; 2014 18.9%; female average 19.2%; male average 11.9%) WEMWBS: average M = 49.7 (2008 M = 50.0; 2009 M = 50.0; ...; 2013 M = 49.5; 2014 M = 49.1; female M = 49.1; male M = 50.5) England 13–15 years GHQ: average 10.6% (1995 9.8%; 1997 11.0%; ...; 2009 10.4%; 2010 11.5%; 2012 11.1%; 2014 10.7%; female average 13.9%; male average 7.3%)	Health Survey for England (18 surveys between 1995–2014), Scottish Health Survey (eight surveys 2003–2014) and Welsh Health Survey (eight surveys 2007–2014) Retrospective secondary data analysis Repeated (mostly annual) surveys	England[HIC], Scotland[HIC] and Wales[HIC]	Size: – Female: – Age: 13–24 years

(continued)

Table 9.1 (continued)

Study	Relevant MH Measures and Cutoff	Prevalence	Study Design	Location	Sample
Pitchforth et al. (2019)	WEMWBS GHQ (cutoff of >3)	England 16–24 years GHQ: average 15.4% (1995 16.9%; 1997 17.5%; 1998 16.2%; …; 2010 14.8%; 2012 16.2%; 2014 15.7%; female average 19.2%; male average 10.9%) WEMWBS: average M = 51.3 (2010 M = 50.8; 2011 M = 51.8; 2012 M = 52.2; 2013 M = 51.3; 2014 M = 50.5; female M = 50.7; male M = 52.0) Data available by gender, and for mental disorders, general health and SDQE/SDQ			
Shevlin et al. (2013)	GHQ (cutoff of >3) UCLA Loneliness Scale (cutoff of 42–which is one SD higher than sample mean)	Loneliness: 15.6% Psychiatric morbidity: 28.4%	Young Life and Times Survey 2011 The survey sampling frame was the Northern Ireland Child Benefit Register Response rate: 37%	Northern Ireland[HIC]	Size: 1,434 Female: 55% Age: 16 years
Somrongthong et al. (2013)	CES-D (cutoff of 22)	Depression: 34.9%; female 40.4%; male 27.6%; 12–13 years 37.4%; 14–17 years 34.8%; 18–22 years 33.1%	Random sampling of clusters to select sub-communities Systematic random sampling to identify households	Thailand[MIC] (Bangkok, Klong Toey Slum Community)	Size: 871 Female: 57.2% Age: 12–22 years

Study	Relevant MH Measures and Cutoff	Prevalence	Study Design	Location	Sample
			Simple random sampling of individuals within a household		
Twenge et al. (2019)	K-6 (cutoff of 13)	Psychological Distress: 18–19 years (2008 9.0%; 2009 8.5%; 2010 8.9%; 2011 9.2%; 2012 9.4%; 2013 9.6%; 2014 11.0%; 2015 12.3%; 2016 13.1%; 2017 15.0%; Percentage Change 67%) 20–21 years (2008 8.1%; 2009 8.5%; 2010 9.0%; 2011 7.1%; 2012 8.6%; 2013 8.7%; 2014 9.8%; 2015 10.7%; 2016 12.6%; 2017 14.4%; Percentage Change 78%) 22–23 years (2008 7.0%; 2009 7.6%; 2010 7.2%; 2011 7.1%; 2012 7.5%; 2013 8.0%; 2014 8.3%; 2015 9.1%; 2016 9.8%; 2017 12.0%; Percentage Change 72%)	National Survey on Drug Use and Health (2008–2017) Weighted average response rate: 65.2%	USA[HIC]	Size: – Female: – Age: 18–23 years
Vancampfort et al. (2018)	One yes/no question	Depression[**2]: 28.6% (range Myanmar 14.7% – Zambia 51.5%)	Global School-Based Student Health Survey (2003–2008) Two-stage probability sampling design First stage by schools Second stage by class	LMICs (30 countries)	Size: 67,077 Female: 50.6% Age: 12–15 years

[1*] indicates that the figure has been calculated using data provided in the published study.
[2**] indicates that the figure is available per country.

prevalence of suicide attempts. Oh et al. (2021 p. 558) highlight that 'according to the interpersonal theory of suicide, people experiencing multiple types of abuse may become desensitized to emotional and physical pain (increased distress toler-ance) and acquire irreversible increased capability for suicidal ideation and behaviour'.

Other risk factors for self-harm and STB for young people include: being non-heterosexual (Oh et al. 2021); poorer family financial situation (Zubrick et al. 2016); family history of suicide (Blum et al. 2011); identifying as certain races/ethnicities (Oh et al. 2021); migration status (Blum et al. 2011); poor family func-tioning (Zubrick et al. 2016); single-parent household (Zubrick et al. 2016); and substance use (Blum et al. 2011). Not all of these factors are associated with all STBs; Oh et al. (2021) for example found that race/ethnicity is associated with suicidal ideation but not suicidal planning when accounting for other co-variates. Protective factors for self-harm and STB include both mother and father support (Blum et al. 2011) or family support (Li, You et al. 2021), being religious (Oh et al. 2021), and having close friends (Li, You et al. 2021). Blum et al. (2011) found that 56.4 per cent of young people believe they would talk to their peers if they felt suicidal. However, 32.4 per cent of males and 25.6 per cent of females believe they would talk to no-one, pointing towards the need to support young people to reach out and seek help. On a more positive note, having a supportive figure or a confi-dant helps to lower the risk of self-harm and STB.

COVID-19 pandemic

COVID-19 has impacted the mental health of nations world-wide and rather than being viewed as an outlier event for mental health, it must be viewed as a signifi-cant event which could occur again. Mirroring the variations reported earlier in the chapter, the prevalence of depression (see Table 9.3) ranged from 7.7 per cent (China) to 64.8 per cent (Egypt), and anxiety ranged from 6.7 per cent (China) to 51.6 per cent (Egypt). Considering the adolescent cohort, Zhou et al. (2020b) noted higher depression prevalence in those not participating in distance learning (54.0 per cent vs 38.4 per cent).

Of interest in these studies, are the specific risk and protective factors and cop-ing strategies related to COVID-19 which could be generalised to any future pan-demic situations. For example, in addition to previously identified risk factors, Al Omari et al. (2020) found that pandemic-related risk factors included being exposed to an infected person with COVID-19 (depression and anxiety), being quarantined for 14 days (depression), using the internet after the COVID-19 pandemic was declared (depression, anxiety and stress), being at risk of infection with COVID-19 (depression, anxiety and stress), and having a relative diagnosed with COVID-19 (stress). Similarly, other specific risk factors for depression include exposure risk to COVID-19 (Cao et al. 2021), less face-to-face communication with family members (Li, Zhang et al. 2021), leaving home and going outside (Li, Zhang et al. 2021), paren-tal restrictions on screen and study time (Li, Zhang et al. 2021), and being concerned about COVID-19 (Zhou, Yuan et al. 2020). Most of the Chinese studies also consid-ered living in Hubei province or Wuhan, the source of the COVID-19 outbreak, as a potential risk factor. Zhou, Zhang et al. (2020) found being from Hubei province had an odds ratio of 1.64 and 1.58 for anxiety and depression respectively.

Table 9.2 Summary of self-harm and STB studies

Study	Measure	Prevalence (12 month)	Study Design	Location	Sample
Blum et al. (2012)	Yes/no questions	Suicidal ideation: 8.4%; Hanoi 2.3%; Shanghai 8.1%; Taipei 17.0% Suicidal attempt: 2.5%; Hanoi <1%; Shanghai 1.3%; Taipei 6.9%	Levels of Change in Adolescent Sexual Behaviour in Three Asian Cities study Multistage sampling	Vietnam[MIC] (Hanoi city) China[MIC] (Shanghai) Taiwan[MIC] (Taipei)	Size**: 17,109 Female**: 49% Age: 15–24 years
Kidger et al. (2012)	Yes/no question followed by questions on how, why, how many times etc.	Self-harm: 11.1%*; female 15.0%*; male 5.4%*	Avon Longitudinal Study of Parents and Children (ALSPAC) birth cohort	England[HIC]	Size: 4,810 Female: 58.9% Age: 16–17 years
Koyanagi et al. (2019)	How many times	Suicide attempts**: 10.7%; female 11.2%; male 10.0% Suicide attempt by region: Africa (11.1–28.8%; pooled 18.5%*); Americas (7.8–22.3%; pooled 14.8%*); Eastern Mediterranean (12.5–15.8%; pooled 13.6%*); South-East Asia (3.9–14%; pooled 7.9%*); Western Pacific (5.9–60.7%; pooled 13.7%*)	Global School-Based Student Health Survey (2009–2015) Two-stage cluster design First stage by schools Second stage by class Response rate**: 60–97%	48 countries: Africa (9); Americas (17); Eastern Mediterranean (6); South-East Asia (5); Western Pacific (11) High-income counties (9); Middle-income countries (33); Low-income countries (6)	Size**: 134,229 Female**: 48.9% Age: 12–15 years
Li et al. (2021)	Yes/no questions and homy many times	Suicidal ideation**: 14.5% (female: 16.1%; male 12.5%; 12–13 years 13.6%; 14–15 years 15.1%) Suicidal planning**: 14.6% (female: 16.0%; male 13.3%; 12–13 years 13.4%; 14–15 years 15.1%) Suicide attempt**: 12.7% (female: 13.7%; male 11.3; 12–13 years 12.3%; 14–15 years 12.6%)	Global School-Based Student Health Survey (2009–2015) Two-stage cluster design First stage by schools Second stage by class Average response rate**: 98.1%	46 LMICs: Americas (16); Africa (8); Eastern Mediterranean (6); South-East Asia (5); Western Pacific (11)	Size**: 130,488 Female**: 51.9% Age: 12–15 years

(continued)

Table 9.2 (continued)

Study	Measure	Prevalence (12 month)	Study Design	Location	Sample
		Suicidal ideation, planning, and attempt respectively by region: Africa (16.7%, 19.3%, 17.0%); Americas (16.0%, 14.4%, 12.9%); Eastern Mediterranean (14.8%, 13.9%, 11.9%); South-East Asia (8.2%, 10.5%, 7.4%); Western Pacific (16.5%, 17.1%, 15.8%)			
Lowry et al. (2014)	Yes/no questions followed by how many times	Suicide ideation: female (1991 37.2%; 2009 17.4%; 2011 19.3%); male (1991 20.8%; 2007 10.3%; 2011 12.5%) 2011: Suicidal planning: female 15.0%; male. 10.8% Suicide attempt: female 9.8%; male 5.8%	Youth Risk Behaviour Surveys conducted biennially during (1991–2011) Three-stage probability sampling methodology Response rate: 60–71%	USA[HIC]	Size: Range 10,904–16,410 Female: - Age: Grade 9-12 students
McMahon et al. (2014)	Participants reporting self-harm were asked to describe the self-harm conducted	Self-harm: 5.8%*; female 8.9%; male 2.4%	Child and Adolescent Self-Harm in Europe (CASE) study School response rate: 72.2*	Republic of Ireland[HIC]	Size: 3,631 Female: 52% Age: 15–17 years

Study	Measure	Prevalence (12 month)	Study Design	Location	Sample
Mortier et al. (2018)	Columbia - Suicide Severity and time course of STBs	Suicidal ideation: 17.2% Suicidal planning: 8.8% Suicide attempt: 1.0% Suicidal ideation by country: Australia 25.7%; Belgium 7.0%; Germany 18.8%; Mexico 9.8%; Northern Ireland 18.5%; South Africa 24.3%; Spain 14.7%; USA 18.8%	Cross national data Response rate: 45.5%	Nineteen colleges and universities Eight countries (Australia[HIC], Belgium[HIC], Germany[HIC], Mexico[MIC], Northern Ireland[HIC], South Africa[MIC], Spain[HIC], USA[HIC])	Size**: 13,984 Female: 54.4% Age: First-year students
O'Connor et al. (2014)	Yes/no self-harm questions followed by providing a description	Self-harm: 6%; female 9.3%; male 2.9% Self-harm thoughts without doing so: 12.7%; female 18.0%; male 7.8%	Northern Ireland Lifestyle and Coping Survey Cross-sectional study School response rate: 40%*	Northern Ireland[HIC]	Size: 3,596 Female: 47.6% Age: M = 15 (SD = 0.7)
Oh et al. (2021)	Yes/no questions	Suicidal ideation: 12.6% Suicidal planning: 5.7% Suicide attempt: 1.3%	Healthy Minds Study 2019 Cross-sectional survey Response rate: 16%	USA[HIC]	Size: 62,171 Female: 66.0%; Male: 31.9%; Transgender: 2.1% Age: 18+ years White: 65.1%
Page et al. (2013)	Yes/no questions	Suicidal ideation**: 15.3% Suicidal ideation by region: Africa (11.6–31.1%; pooled 22.1%*); Americas (10.2–23.2%; pooled 17.4%*); Asia (0.7–16.8%; pooled 12.1%*); Middle East/Europe (7.2–19.8%; 12.9%**)	Global School-Based Student Health Survey (2003-2010) Two-stage cluster design (with weighting) First stage by schools Second stage by class	38 countries: Africa (7); Americas (17); Asia (6); Middle East/Europe (8);	Size: 127,694* Female: - Age: 13–15 years

(continued)

Table 9.2 (continued)

Study	Measure	Prevalence (12 month)	Study Design	Location	Sample
Price & Khubchandani (2019)	Yes/no questions and how many times	Suicidal ideation: 2001 (male: 9.2% female: 17.2%); 2003 (male: 10.3% female: 14.7%); 2005 (male: 7.0% female: 17.1%); 2007 (male: 8.5% female: 18.0%); 2009 (male: 7.8% female: 18.1%); 2011 (male: 9.0% female: 17.4%); 2013 (male: 10.2% female: 18.6%); 2015 (male: 6.6% female: 22.4%) 2017 (male: 9.0% female: 17.4%) Suicidal Planning: 2001 (male: 7.5% female: 13.0%); 2003 (male: 8.4% female: 12.4%); 2005 (male: 5.5% female: 13.5%); 2007 (male: 7.1% female: 12.0%); 2009 (male: 6.2% female: 13.3%); 2011 (male: 8.4% female: 13.9%); 2013 (male: 7.7% female: 13.1%); 2015 (male: 10.6% female: 17.3%); 2017 (male: 6.5% female: 18.9%); Percentage Change (male: - 13.3% female: 45.4%)	Youth Risk Behaviour Surveys (2001–2017)	USA[HIC]	Size: 26,197* (range: 1,768–3,590) Female: - Age: Grade 9–12 students African-American: 100%

Study	Measure	Prevalence (12 month)	Study Design	Location	Sample
		Suicide attempt: 2001 (male: 7.5% female: 9.8%); 2003 (male: 7.7% female: 9.0%); 2005 (male: 5.2% female: 9.8%); 2007 (male: 5.5% female: 9.9%); 2009 (male: 5.4% female: 10.4%); 2011 (male: 7.7% female: 8.8%); 2013 (male: 6.8% female: 10.7%); 2015 (male: 7.2% female: 10.2%); 2017 (male: 6.7% female: 12.5%); Percentage Change (male: -10.7% female: 27.6%)			
Zubrick et al. (2016)	Yes/no questions and how many times and whether the suicide attempt resulted in medical treatment etc.	Suicidal ideation: 12–17 years 7.5%; 16–17 years 11.2%; 12–15 years 5.6% Suicidal planning: 12–17 years 5.2%; 16-17 years 7.8%; 12–15 years 3.8% Suicide attempt: 12–17 years 2.4%; 16–17 years 3.8%; 12–15 years 1.7%	Second Australian Child and Adolescent Survey of Mental Health and Wellbeing (2013–2014)	Australia[HIC]	Size: 2,653 Female: - Age: 12–17 years

*Indicates that the figure has been calculated using data provided in the published study. **Indicates that the figure is available per country

Zhou, Zhang et al. (2020) found that protective factors against anxiety and depression specifically during COVID-19 included an awareness of COVID-19 (COVID-19 knowledge, prevention and control measures, and projections of COVID-19 trend). They conducted their survey in March 2020 when many countries world-wide were entering lockdown, when there was limited knowledge of COVID-19 generally, and adolescents were required to undertake distance learning. Considering coping strategies, Cho et al. (2021) found that 41.2 per cent of their sample was taking at least one substance as a coping strategy to deal with the pandemic situation; many of whom had a history of emotional issues. Cauberghe et al. (2021) investigated three coping strategies for handling anxiety and depression during the COVID-19 lockdown: active coping, social relation coping and humorous coping. They found that 'social media can be used as a constructive coping strategy for adolescents to deal with anxious feelings during the COVID-19 quarantine' (p. 1). This is particularly relevant for individuals feeling lonely and isolated during lockdown.

Overall, these studies indicate that in the event of future pandemics, mental health issues may be improved by providing accurate information and considering coping strategies that allow for communication between family and friends.

Discussion and conclusion

It is evident from what we have reported in this chapter that prevalence rates for anxiety, depression and STB vary widely. Extracted data found that: mental health problems peak during late adolescence; they are higher in LMICs; that overall, they have been increasing over time; and that generally females have higher prevalence rates than males. Rates for depression and anxiety vary considerably across studies often co-varying with the measure used to establish the prevalence rates. Various risk factors have been linked to mental distress including, but not limited to, low self-esteem, sedentary behaviour, poor interpersonal relations, hopelessness and lower socio-economic status. Protective factors linked to lower levels of mental health problems include good family relationships, being able to talk about personal problems, future goals and aspirations, and appropriate coping strategies (e.g. problem solving/planned coping, seeking social support).

Prevalence data for STB also varied; self-harm (5.8 per cent to 11.1 per cent), suicidal ideation (0.7 per cent to 25.7 per cent), suicidal planning (5.2 per cent to 19.3 per cent) and suicidal attempt (<1 per cent to 60.7 per cent). What is consistent is that (1) females were more likely to engage in STBs than males, which holds true in all world regions, and (2) later adolescence has higher rates than early adolescence. Risk factors associated with STBs include bullying, identifying as non-heterosexual, migration and poor family functioning. Data collected during the pandemic again revealed a wide prevalence range for depression ranging from 7.7 per cent (China) to 64.8 per cent (Egypt), and anxiety ranging from 6.7 per cent (China) to 51.6 per cent (Egypt). In addition to previously identified risk factors, additional pandemic related-risk factors included being exposed to an infected person with COVID-19, being quarantined for 14 days, being at risk of infection with COVID-19, and having a relative diagnosed with COVID-19.

Table 9.3 Summary of COVID-19 studies

Study	Relevant Measures and Cutoff Scores	Prevalence	Location	Sample
Al Omari et al. (2020)	DASS-21 (Arabic version; calculations using depression subscale cutoff of 10, anxiety subscale cutoff of 8, stress subscale cutoff of 15)	Anxiety**: 40.5%* (Saudi Arabia 33.1%* - Egypt 51.6%*) Depression**: 57%* (Saudi Arabia 47.9%* - Egypt 64.8%*) Stress: 38.1%*	Egypt[MIC], Iraq[MIC], Jordan[MIC], Oman[HIC], Saudi Arabia[HIC], United Arab Emirates[HIC]	Size**: 1,057 Female: 71.5% Age: 15-24 years
Cao et al. (2021)	PHQ-9 (cutoff of 5) GAD-7 (cutoff of 5)	Anxiety: 23.7% Depression: 37.9%	Chin[MIC] (Shaanxi, Shandong, Henan, Fujian, and Liaoning provinces)	Size: 11,180 Female: 49.9% Age: 12-18 years
Cauberghe et al. (2021)	CES-D (3 items for happiness) GAD-7 RULS-6	Anxiety: female M = 2.1 SD = 0.8; male M = 1.7 SD = 0.6 Happiness: female M = 2.8 SD = 0.7; male M = 3.2 SD = 0.7 Loneliness: female M = 2.9 SD = 0.8; male M = 2.6 SD 0.8	Belgium[HIC]	Size: 2,165 Female: 66.6% Age: 13-19 years
Chen et al. (2020)	PHQ-9 (cutoff of 10)	Depression: 7.7% Suicidal ideation for past two weeks: 7.2%	China[MIC] (Guangdong province)	Size: 323,489 Female: 59.7% Age: college students
Cho et al. (2021)	Revised Children's Anxiety and Depression Scale - Generalized Anxiety Disorder scale	Generalized anxiety: M = 1.2 SD = 0.8 ranged = 0-3	USA[HIC] (California, Los Angeles)	Size: 2,120 Female: 61.2% Age: M = 21.2 SD = 0.4

(continued)

Table 9.3 (continued)

Study	Relevant Measures and Cutoff Scores	Prevalence	Location	Sample
Dewa et al. (2021)	PHQ-9 Coronavirus Impact Scale (CIS) Poor mental health status is defined as PHQ-9 score >= 15 and/or self-harm present and/or CIS scores indicate persistent worries/severe stress-related symptoms	Poor mental health: 30.3% Self-harm: 10.8%	United Kingdom[HIC]	Size: 796 Female: 78.9% Age: 16–24 years
Li, You et al. (2021)	HADS (Chinese translated version; cutoff subscale score of >7)	Anxiety: 21.6%; female 21.7%; male 21.5% Depression: 24.6%; female 23.5%; male 25.8%	China[MIC] (Wuhan)	Size: 7,890 Female: 52.1% Age: 12–18
Liu et al. (2021)	PHQ-9 (cutoff of 10) GAD-7 (cutoff of 10)	Anxiety: 6.7% Depression: 13.8%	China[MIC] (Shandong province)	Size: 3,836 Female: - Age: Middle and high school
Pierce et al. (2020)	GHQ-12 (cutoff of 4)	Mental distress: 2014/15 19.8%; 2015/16 19.6%; 2016/17 19.7%; 2017/18 23.5%; 2018/19 24.5%; April 2020 36.7%	United Kingdom[HIC]	Size: 1,543 Female: - Age: 16–24 years
Zhou, Zhang et al. (2020)	PHQ-9 (cutoff of 5) GAD-7 (Chinese version; cutoff of 5)	Anxiety: 37.4%; female 38.4%; male 36.2%; rural 40.4%; urban 32.5% Depression: 43.7%; female 45.5%; male 41.7%; rural 47.5%; urban 37.7% Combination: 31.3%	China[MIC]	Size: 8,079 Female: 53.5% Age: 12–18 years
Zhou, Yuan et al. (2020)	CES-D (Chinese version; cutoff of 16)	Depression: 39.5%; 11-14 years 30.8%; 15–18 years 46.3%; distance learning 38.4%; not participating in distant learning 54.0%	China[MIC]	Size: 4,085 Female: 100% Age: 11–18 years

*Indicates that the figure has been calculated using data provided in the published study. **Indicates that the figure is available per country

From a methodological perspective, it is important to consider how and what was measured to understand whether or not the observed differences are due to real or methodological differences. While we are able to compare self-harm and STB prevalence rates globally, given that the method to record suicidal ideation was stable across studies, identifying the prevalence of aspects of general mental health is more complex. This is a recognised problem. Issues that confound the data include: the measure used (e.g. BDI-II, CES-D); the timeframe used in the measure (e.g. in the past week vs the last month); the number of items in the measure; the establishment of cut-off scores; classification based on a dichotomy (e.g. depressed/not depressed) or scale (normal, mild, moderate, severe, very severe). For many large-scale studies, for example the Global School-based Student Health Survey, depression and anxiety were measured using one item rather than a validated measure, again a limitation. A potential explanation for this approach is that this lowers the number of questions for participants, reducing the burden to participants and encouraging participants to complete the survey.

To facilitate comparisons, some funders have tried to solve one of these methodological problems through recommending the use of specific measures for inclusion in the study of mental health. For example, the Wellcome Trust recommends that anxiety and depression studies include one or more of the following: PHQ, GAD, Revised Child Anxiety and Depression Scale and the World Health Organization Disability Assessment Schedule (WHODAS). The drawback of this is that these measures may not account for all conditions and measurement invariance across key demographic variables, such as gender, age, ethnicity, and geographic location. However, such a systematic approach would enhance our understanding of the mental health problems of young people.

Despite the inherent limitations outlined, data are necessary in contributing to our understanding of the mental health problems of young people within a global context to identify where resources should be targeted in terms of prevention, early intervention and treatment using a youth-focused model of service delivery.

Further reading

Dooley, B., & Fitzgerald, A. (2013). Methodology on the My World Survey (MWS): A unique window into the world of adolescents in Ireland. *Early Intervention in Psychiatry*, 7(1), 12–22. https://doi.org/10.1111/j.1751-7893.2012.00386.x

Solmi, M., Radua, J., Olivola, M., Croce, E., Soardo, L., de Pablo, G. S., Shin, J. I., Kirkbride, J. B., Jones, P., Kim., J. H., Kim, J. Y., Carvalho, A. F., Seeman, M. V., Correll, C. U., & Fusar-Poli, P. (2021). Age at onset of mental disorders world-wide: Large-scale meta-analysis of 192 epidemiological studies. *Molecular Psychiatry*. https://doi.org/10.1038/s41380-021-01161-7

References

Abidi, S. (2017). Paving the way to change for youth at the gap between child and adolescent and adult mental health services. *Canadian Journal of Psychiatry*, 62(6), 388–392. https://doi.org/10.1177/0706743717694166

Al Omari, O., Al Sabei, S., Al Rawajfah, O., Abu Sharour, L., Aljohani, K., Alomari, K., Shkman, L., Al Dameery, K., Saifan, A., Al Zubidi, B., Anwar, S., & Alhalaiqa, F. (2020). Prevalence and predictors of depression, anxiety, and stress among youth at the time of COVID-19: An online cross-sectional multicountry study. *Depression Research and Treatment, 2020.* https://doi.org/10.1155/2020/8887727

Almroth, M. C., László, K. D., Kosidou, K., & Galanti, M. R. (2018). Association between adolescents' academic aspirations and expectations and mental health: A one-year follow-up study. *European Journal of Public Health, 28*(3), 504–50. https://doi.org/10.1093/eurpub/cky025

Blum, R., Sudhinaraset, M., & Emerson, M. R. (2012). Youth at risk: Suicidal thoughts and attempts in Vietnam, China, and Taiwan. *The Journal of Adolescent Health, 50*(3 Suppl), S37–S44. https://doi.org/10.1016/j.jadohealth.2011.12.006

Cao, Y., Huang, L., Si, T., Qun Wang, N., Qu, M., & Yang Zhang, X. (2021). The role of only-child status in the psychological impact of COVID-19 on mental health of Chinese adolescents. *Journal of Affective Disorders, 282,* 316–321. https://doi.org/10.1016/j.jad.2020.12.113.

Cauberghe, V., Van Wesenbeeck, I., De Jans, S., Hudders, L., & Ponnet, K. (2021). How adolescents use social media to cope with feelings of loneliness and anxiety during COVID-19 lockdown. *Cyberpsychology, Behavior, and Social Networking, 24*(4), 250–257. https://doi.org/10.1089/cyber.2020.0478

Chen, R-n., Liang, S-w., Peng, Y., Li, X-g., Chen, J-b., Tang, S-y., & Zhao, J-b. (2020). Mental health status and change in living rhythms among college students in China during the COVID-19 pandemic: A large-scale survey. *Journal of Psychosomatic Research, 137.* https://doi.org/10.1016/j.jpsychores.2020.110219

Cheung, K. L., ten Klooster, P. M., Smit, C. de Vries, H., & Pieterse, M. E. (2017). The impact of non-response bias due to sampling in public health studies: A comparison of voluntary versus mandatory recruitment in a Dutch national survey on adolescent health. *BMC Public Health, 17.* https://doi.org/10.1186/s12889-017-4189-8

Cho, J., Bello, M. S., Christie, N. C., Monterosso, J. R., & Leventhal, A. M. (2021). Adolescent emotional disorder symptoms and transdiagnostic vulnerabilities as predictors of young adult substance use during the COVID-19 pandemic: Mediation by substance-related coping behaviors. *Cognitive Behavior Therapy, 50*(4), 276–294. https://doi.org/10.1080/16506073.2021.1882552

Collishaw, S., Maughan, B., Natarajan, L., & Pickles, A. (2010). Trends in adolescent emotional problems in England: A comparison of two national cohorts twenty years apart. *Journal of Child Psychology and Psychiatry, 51,* 885–894. https://doi.org/10.1111/j.1469-7610.2010.02252.x

Dardas, L. A., Silva, S. G., Smoski, M. J., Noonan, D., & Simmons, L. A. (2018). The prevalence of depressive symptoms among Arab adolescents: Findings from Jordan. *Public Health Nursing, 35*(2), 100–108. https://doi.org/10.1111/phn.12363

Dardas, L. A., Shoqirat, N., Xu, H., Al-Khayat, A., Bani Ata, S., Shawashreh, A., & Simmons, L. A. (2019). Comparison of the performance of the Beck Depression Inventory-II and the Center for Epidemiologic Studies-Depression Scale in Arab adolescents. *Public Health Nursing, 36*(4), 564–574. https://doi.org/10.1111/phn.12618

Dewa, L.H., Crandell, C., Choong, E., Jaques, J., Bottle, A., Kilkenny, C., Lawrence-Jones, A., Di Simplicio, M., Nicholls, D., & Aylin P. (2021). CCopeY: A mixed-methods coproduced study on the mental health status and coping strategies of young people during COVID-19 UK lockdown. *Journal of Adolescent Health, 68*(4), 666–675. http://dx.doi.org/10.1016/j.jadohealth.2021.01.009

Fatiregun, A. A., & Kumapayi, T. E. (2014). Prevalence and correlates of depressive symptoms among in-school adolescents in a rural district in southwest Nigeria. *Journal of Adolescence, 37*(2), 197–203. https://doi.org/10.1016/j.adolescence.2013.12.003

Fernandes, A. C., Hayes, R. D., & Patel, V. (2013). Abuse and other correlates of common mental disorders in youth: A cross-sectional study in Goa, India. *Social Psychiatry and Psychiatric Epidemiology, 48*(4), 515–523. https://doi.org/10.1007/s00127-012-0614-6

Ferro, M. A. Gorter, J. W., & Boyle, M. H. (2015). Trajectories of depressive symptoms in Canadian emerging adults. *American Journal of Public Health, 105,* 2322–2327, https://doi.org/10.2105/AJPH.2015.302817

Global Burden of Disease Study 2013 Collaborators. (2015). Global, regional, and national incidence, prevalence, and years lived with disability for 301 acute and chronic diseases and injuries in 188 countries, 1990–2013: A systematic analysis for the Global Burden of Disease study. *The Lancet, 386*(9995), 743–800, https://doi.org/10.1016/S0140-6736(15)60692-4

Hickey, E., Fitzgerald, A., & Dooley, B. (2017). The relationship between perceived family support and depressive symptoms in adolescence: What is the moderating role of coping strategies and gender? *Community Mental Health Journal, 53*, 474–481. https://doi.org/10.1007/s10597-017-0087-x

Hossain, S., Anjum, A., Uddin, E., Rahman, A., & Hossain, F. (2019). Impacts of socio-cultural environment and lifestyle factors on the psychological health of university students in Bangladesh: A longitudinal study. *Journal of Affective Disorders, 256*, 393–403. https://doi.org/10.1016/j.jad.2019.06.001

Kessler, R. C., Amminger, G. P., Aguilar-Gaxiola, S., Alonso, J., Lee, S., & Üstün, T. B. (2007). Age of onset of mental disorders: A review of recent literature. *Current Opinion in Psychiatry, 20*, 359–364. https://doi.org/10.1097/YCO.0b013e32816ebc8c

Kidger, J., Heron, J., Lewis, G., Evans, J., & Gunnell, D. (2012). Adolescent self-harm and suicidal thoughts in the ALSPAC cohort: A self-report survey in England. *BMC Psychiatry, 12*(69), 1–12. https://doi.org/10.1186/1471-244X-12-69

Killackey, E., Hodges, C., Browne, V., Gow, E., Varnum, P., McGorry, P., & Purcell, R. (2020). A Global Framework for Youth Mental Health: Investing in Future Mental Capital for Individuals, Communities and Economies. Geneva: World Economic Forum.

Klasen, F., Otto, C., Kriston, L. Patalay, P., Schlack, R., Ravens-Sieberer, U., & The BELLA study group. (2015). Risk and protective factors for the development of depressive symptoms in children and adolescents: Results of the longitudinal BELLA study. *European Child & Adolescent Psychiatry, 24*, 695–703. https://doi.org/10.1007/s00787-014-0637-5

Koyanagi, A., Oh, H., Carvalho, A.F., Smith, L., Haro, J. M., Vancampfort, D., Stubbs, B., & DeVylder, J. E. (2019). Bullying victimization and suicide attempt among adolescents aged 12–15 years from 48 countries. *Journal of the American Academy of Child & Adolescent Psychiatry, 58*(9). https://doi.org/10.1016/j.jaac.2018.10.018

Li, W., Zhang, Y., Wang, J., Ozaki, A., Wang, Q., Chen, Y., & Jiang, Q. (2021). Association of home quarantine and mental health among teenagers in Wuhan, China, during the COVID-19 pandemic. *JAMA Pediatrics, 175*(3), 313–316. https://doi.org/10.1001/jamapediatrics.2020.5499

Li, L., You, D., Ruan, T., Xu, S., Mi, D., Cai, T., & Han, L. (2021). The prevalence of suicidal behaviors and their mental risk factors among young adolescents in 46 low- and middle-income countries. *Journal of Affective Disorders, 281*, 847–855. https://doi.org/10.1016/j.jad.2020.11.050

Liu, J., Liu, C. X., Wu, T., Liu, B-P., Jia, C-X., & Liu, X. (2019). Prolonged mobile phone use is associated with depressive symptoms in Chinese adolescents. *Journal of Affective Disorders, 259*, 128–134. https://doi.org/10.1016/j.jad.2019.08.017

Liu, Y., Yue, S., Hu, X., Zhu, J., Wu, Z., Wang, J., & Wu, Y. (2021). Associations between feelings/behaviors during COVID-19 pandemic lockdown and depression/anxiety after lockdown in a sample of Chinese children and adolescents. *Journal of Affective Disorders, 284*, 98–103. https://doi.org/10.1016/j.jad.2021.02.001

Lowry, R., Crosby, A. E., Brener, N. D., & Kann, L. (2014). Suicidal thoughts and attempts among U.S. high school students: Trends and associated health-risk behaviors, 1991–2011. *The Journal of Adolescent Health, 54*(1), 100–108. https://doi.org/10.1016/j.jadohealth.2013.07.024

McMahon, E. M., Keeley, H., Cannon, M., Arensman, E., Perry, I. J., Clarke, M., Chambers, D., & Corcoran, P. (2014). The iceberg of suicide and self-harm in Irish adolescents: A population-based study. *Social Psychiatry and Psychiatric Epidemiology, 49*(12), 1929–1935. https://doi.org/10.1007/s00127-014-0907-z

Mei C., Killackey E., Chanen A., & McGorry P. D. (2020). Early intervention and youth mental health: Synergistic paradigms to transform mental health outcomes. In S. Okpaku (Ed.)

Innovations in global mental health. Springer. https://doi.org/10.1007/978-3-319-70134-9_ 77-1

Mental Health Foundation. (2016). Fundamental Facts About Mental Health 2016. Mental Health Foundation.

Mortier, P., Auerbach, R. P., Alonso, J., Bantjes, J., Benjet, C., Cuijpers, P., Ebert, D. D., Green, J. G., Hasking, P., Nock, M. K., O'Neill, S., Pinder-Amaker, S., Sampson, N. A., Vilagut, G., Zaslavsky, A. M., Bruffaerts, R., Kessler, R. C., & WHO WMH-ICS Collaborators. (2018). Suicidal thoughts and behaviors among first-year college students: Results From the WMH-ICS Project. *Journal of the American Academy of Child and Adolescent Psychiatry, 57*(4), 263–273. e1. https://doi.org/10.1016/j.jaac.2018.01.018

Nabunya, P., Damulira, C., Byansi, W. Muwanga, J., Bahar, O. S., Namuwonge, F., Ighofose, E., Brathwaite, R., Tumwesige, W., & Ssewamala, F. M. (2020). Prevalence and correlates of depressive symptoms among high school adolescent girls in southern Uganda. *BMC Public Health, 20.* https://doi.org/10.1186/s12889-020-09937-2

O'Connor, R. C., Rasmussen, S., & Hawton, K. (2014). Adolescent self-harm: A school-based study in Northern Ireland. *Journal of Affective Disorders, 159,* 46–52. https://doi.org/10.1016/j. jad.2014.02.015

Oh, H. Y., Marinovich, C., Jay, S., Zhou, S., & Kim, J. H. J. (2021). Abuse and suicide risk among college students in the United States: Findings from the 2019 Healthy Minds Study. *Journal of Affective Disorders, 282,* 554–560, https://doi.org/10.1016/j.jad.2020.12.140

Page, R. M., Saumweber, J., Hall, P. C., Crookston, B. T., & West, J. H. (2013). Multi-country, cross-national comparison of youth suicide ideation: Findings from Global School-based Health Surveys. *School Psychology International, 34*(5), 540–555. https://doi.org/10.1177/ 0143034312469152

Pierce, M., Hope, H., Ford, T., Hatch, S., Hotopf, M., John, A., Kontopantelis, E., Webb, R., Wessely, S., McManus, S., & Abel, K.M. (2020). Mental health before and during the COVID-19 pandemic: A longitudinal probability sample survey of the UK population. *The Lancet Psychiatry, 7*(10), 883–892. http://dx.doi.org/10.1016/S2215-0366(20)30308-4

Pitchforth, J., Fahy, K., Ford, T., Wolpert, M., Viner, R., & Hargreaves, D. (2019). Mental health and well-being trends among children and young people in the UK, 1995–2014: Analysis of repeated cross-sectional national health surveys. *Psychological Medicine, 49*(8), 1275–1285. https://doi.org/10.1017/S0033291718001757

Price, J. H., & Khubchandani, J. (2019). The changing characteristics of African-American adolescent suicides, 2001–2017. *Journal of Community Health, 44*(4), 756–763. https://doi.org/10.1007/ s10900-019-00678-x

Shevlin, M., Murphy, S., Mallett, J., Stringer, M., & Murphy, J. (2013). Adolescent loneliness and psychiatric morbidity in Northern Ireland. *British Journal of Clinical Psychology, 52,* 230–234. https://doi.org/10.1111/bjc.12018

Somrongthong, R., Wongchalee, S., & Laosee, O. (2013). Depression among adolescents: A study in a Bangkok slum community. *Scandinavian Journal of Caring Sciences, 27,* 327–334. https://doi.org/10.1111/j.1471-6712.2012.01037.x

Twenge, J. M., Cooper, A. B., Joiner, T. E., Duffy, M. E., & Binau, S. G. (2019). Age, period, and cohort trends in mood disorder indicators and suicide-related outcomes in a nationally representative dataset, 2005–2017. *Journal of Abnormal Psychology, 128*(3), 185–199. https://doi. org/10.1037/abn0000410

Vancampfort, D., Stubbs, B., Firth, J., Van Damme, T., & Koyanagi, A. (2018). Sedentary behavior and depressive symptoms among 67,077 adolescents aged 12–15 years from 30 low- and middle-income countries. *The International Journal of Behavioral Nutrition and Physical Activity, 15*(1). https://doi.org/10.1186/s12966-018-0708-y

World Health Organization. (2009). Global health risks: Mortality and burden of disease attributable to selected major risks. https://apps.who.int/iris/handle/10665/44203

Zhou, S. J., Zhang, L. G., Wang, L. L., Guo, Z. C., Wang, J. Q., Chen, J. C., Liu, M., Chen, X., & Chen, J. X. (2020). Prevalence and socio-demographic correlates of psychological health problems in Chinese adolescents during the outbreak of COVID-19. *European Child & Adolescent Psychiatry, 29*(6), 749–758. https://doi.org/10.1007/s00787-020-01541-4

Zhou, J., Yuan, X., Qi, H., Liu, R., Li, Y., Huang, H., Chen, X., & Wang, G. (2020). Prevalence of depression and its correlative factors among female adolescents in China during the coronavirus disease 2019 outbreak. *Global Health, 16*(1). https://doi.org/10.1186/s12992-020-00601-3

Zubrick, S. R., Hafekost, J., Johnson, S. E., Lawrence, D., Saw, S., Sawyer, M., Ainley, J., & Buckingham, W. J. (2016). Suicidal behaviors: Prevalence estimates from the second Australian Child and Adolescent Survey of Mental Health and Well-being. *The Australian and New Zealand Journal of Psychiatry, 50*(9), 899–910. https://doi.org/10.1177/0004867415622563

Seen and Heard – a creative piece by young people (18–25 years old), as part of the work of the YOULEAD Research Group, National University of Ireland, Galway, Ireland, and Fregoli Theatre Company, Galway, Ireland in collaboration with SpunOut.ie

Waiting, and waiting and waiting for help
Suffering and waiting

Available at: https://www.youtube.com/watch?v=Wuz-XE8hCao&feature=youtu.be

10 Early intervention in psychosis

Gary Donohoe
National University of Ireland Galway

Karen O'Connor
RISE Early Intervention in Psychosis, Ireland

Introduction

Youth mental health disorders are a major cause of disability (WHO, 2008), accounting for 45 per cent of the total burden of disability in those aged between 10–25 years old (Gore et al. 2011). Because the onset of mental ill-health peaks in late adolescence/early adulthood, it can enormously impact the most productive years of life (Kessler et al. 2005). Consequently, it is calculated to pose the single greatest threat to the GDP of both developed and developing nations in the next 20 years (Bloom et al. 2011).

Given these health, social and economic impacts, investing in the area of youth mental health has been described as a 'no-brainer' in terms of prevention of future burden of disease in adulthood, and relieving the current disease burden among young people (McGorry et al. 2007). This is supported by evidence from health economics studies that investment in children and youth to promote their mental health and resilience provides a greater rate of return than for later investment (Heckman 2006). Maximizing the return on current and future investment necessitates access to a strong evidence base that can inform treatment provision decisions.

This chapter will draw on the growing body of evidence supporting the value of early intervention in the treatment of young people with emerging serious mental health disorders. To do so, it will focus in particular on the development of early intervention service for psychosis as a model for understanding the development of mental health services for young people with serious mental health difficulties. By considering the evidence to support the various approaches to treatment – biological, psychological, social and occupational, we hope to highlight some of the issues that have been addressed, as well as those that remain to be addressed. In so doing, we highlight the need for integrated treatments that aim not just to reduce clinical symptom severity but also to support the recovery of social and occupational function more broadly.

Implementation of early intervention services: an international perspective

Early Intervention in Psychosis (EIP) service development began nearly three decades ago, with the establishment of the Early Psychosis Prevention and Intervention Centre in Melbourne Australia (1992), the Birmingham EIP service (1994), the Prevention and Early Intervention in Psychosis Programme in London, Ontario (1996), the Treatment and Intervention in Psychosis Study programme in Norway (1997), the Recognition and Prevention programme in New York (1998), and the Lambeth Early Onset service (2000) in London (Omer et al. 2010; Power, 2019).

The past two decades have seen EIP services being introduced across England, Canada, Australia, New Zealand, Denmark, parts of Italy and USA, as well as many other individual examples in Europe, Iceland, South America, Mexico, Scandinavia, Singapore, Hong Kong, South Korea, India and Japan (Csillag et al. 2016; Csillag et al. 2018; McGorry et al. 1996; McGorry et al. 2010; Niendam et al. 2019; Power, 2019; Ruggeri et al. 2015).

The data emerging from these services demonstrates that it is possible to improve access, reduce Duration of Untreated Psychosis (DUP), improve outcomes including reduced severity of positive and negative symptoms, depression, anxiety, increased functioning, and lower rates of suicide (Bertelsen et al. 2007; Marshall et al. 2005; Nordentoft et al. 2014).

Central to the EIP service model are specialised multidisciplinary teams who carry reduced caseloads, apply an assertive outreach approach to engagement and follow-up, and provide a comprehensive array of evidence-based interventions (Nordentoft et al. 2014). EIP services' clinical interventions are not restricted to pharmacological interventions but also include psychoeducation, psychological interventions, family-based interventions, educational and vocational supports, and physical health interventions. Comorbidity such as a personal experience of complex trauma, substance misuse/addiction, and/or depression/anxiety is common in first episode psychosis (FEP) and needs to be addressed early and in an integrated manner (Csillag et al. 2018; Upthegrove et al. 2014; Upthegrove et al. 2015). EIP services strive to support and include family members from the outset.

Care is delivered in a collaborative, recovery-orientated way, with the person experiencing psychosis central to the care planning process. EIP services embody a culture of hope and realistic optimism to service users, their families and the public.

In countries where the widespread implementation of EIP services has been successful, several factors have been identified as important (Csillag et al. 2018). These include champions at multiple healthcare system levels and society who promote the evidence of clinical, economic benefit associated with EIP services. These champions include researchers, clinicians, service users and family members who can raise awareness of early psychosis, illustrate the challenges of treatment as usual and give voice to the lived experience of EIP care. Combining clinical and economic evidence with the service user and family narratives can have a very significant impact. The capacity to embed EIP services within publicly funded healthcare systems and a capacity to apply central coordination in countries where there is regional variability have been identified as key elements that facilitate EIP service implementation (Csillag et al. 2018), helping to maintain fidelity to the EIP service model.

However, other countries have experienced significant barriers to EIP service development. Among the factors which have been identified as contributing to this include: a lack of political interest or understanding; limited public understanding of psychosis and the challenges experienced by people with psychosis; and little advocacy from non-clinician service users, families and other health professionals (Csillag et al. 2018). Structural challenges in the healthcare system, e.g. focus on institutionalisation and constraints in public finances, are identified barriers that can make EIP service implementation more challenging.

Given the weight of evidence that has emerged over the past 30 years supporting the positive impact EIP services can have on outcomes for young people, it is no surprise that opportunities to identify and intervene earlier in other areas of mental health are being researched and developed (Addington et al. 2020; Berk et al. 2007; Fineberg et al. 2019; Vieta et al. 2018). These developments are underpinned by several key theories, including that illness progression follows a well-established developmental path or stages of illness, and that the early stages of illness in particular represent a critical period for successful intervention.

Theories informing service: Staging models of psychosis and the 'critical period' concept

Clinical staging models attempt to approach diagnosis and treatment options on the basis of illness progression. This approach is well established in the treatment of physical health disorders such as cancer, where the selection of appropriate interventions is informed by the developmental characteristics of the identified tumour. The main benefit of this approach is treating illness not as static, but rather as an emergent phenomenon with a longitudinal course. In mapping this course, a key idea of the staging model is that quantifying the extent, progression and effects on individual well-being will be informative about prognosis (McGorry et al. 2008).

As outlined in several key reviews of the area (Fusar-Poli et al. 2013; McGorry et al. 2018) the stages of psychosis have been variously described in terms of (1) at risk or ultra-high risk, (2) first-episode psychosis, (3) early psychosis (first five years post-diagnosis) and (4) chronic stages of illness. The term 'At-Risk Mental State' (ARMS) and 'ultra-high risk' (UHR) are used to denote individuals who meet several important criteria of risk for developing psychosis as measured by scales such as the CAARMS (Yung et al. 2005) and the SIPS/SOPS (McGlashan et al. 2001). By comparison, the term 'prodromal' has been used to retrospectively describe changes in function in the months prior to a first episode of psychosis, after illness has been diagnosed (McGorry et al. 2008).

The periods prior to, during and immediately after a first episode of psychosis are often enormously stressful for individuals diagnosed and their families. Symptoms can be difficult to understand and initial interactions with clinical services can be anxiety provoking, particularly if requiring an involuntary admission. Diagnosis of a first episode of psychosis depends on the presence of positive symptoms, for example auditory and visual hallucinations and delusions (delusions of reference, grandiose delusions) and negative symptoms (including alogia, anhedonia and avolition) in the presence or absence of affective disturbances. The diagnosis may be further qualified on the basis of whether or not it follows substance misuse (i.e. substance-induced psychosis). Further specification of whether these psychotic symptoms are consistent with a diagnosis of schizophrenia, schizoaffective disorder, bipolar or unipolar disorder with psychotic features is made longitudinally. For example, a diagnosis of schizophrenia is only made after a minimum of six months following initial diagnosis of a psychotic disorder.

Reducing duration of untreated psychosis (DUP) remains a key objective in the delivery of services. This stems from an abundance of evidence that accelerated diagnosis and treatment leads to improved outcomes both in terms of symptom management and functional recovery. A meta-analysis of determinants of recovery by Santesteban-Echarri and colleagues (2017) found that DUP, cognitive function and concurrent remission of positive and negative symptoms were each independently related to functional recovery. For duration of untreated illness, 18 of the 30 studies included observed that longer DUP was associated with poorer outcomes, despite significant differences between the studies reviewed.

The evidence that a longer duration of an untreated disorder is associated with poorer outcomes in psychosis is related to the idea of a 'critical period' for intervention (Birchwood & Macmillan, 1993). Informed by studies such as McGorry and colleagues' (1993) EPPIC study of early intervention outcomes, Birchwood's concept of a critical period reflected the belief that patients had both more to gain (in terms of recovery) from specialist services and more to lose (in terms of disability and relapse) if these services were prematurely withdrawn during the first five years after diagnosis. This concept was at the heart of the establishment of the early intervention services for psychosis in the UK in the late 1990s and early 2000s. Of note, simply attending clinical services was not sufficient to reduced DUP. Birchwood and colleagues (2013) found that the strongest predictor of a long DUP is ever having been treated in a CAMHS service, with the suggestion here that psychosis onset seems to be particularly poorly recognised and treated in these services. While few would now argue about the value of early intervention and reduced DUP, the idea of a critical period has been challenged in at least one important regard – the precise duration of the critical period. Some reports now suggest that stepping down interventions after the initial 2–5 years results in a slowing (or even reversal) of initial gains in recovery (Nordentoft et al. 2014). What does this say about the critical stage concept? Perhaps that while early intervention is important, continued intervention is also important. While the economic implications of this suggestion are onerous, a key need for future service development will be to ensure the supports needed to sustain early recovery in the longer term are maintained.

Hitting the right target: Reducing duration of untreated illness, reducing symptoms, improving function

Psychosocial disability is a term that describes the social and economic consequences of disability related to mental ill-health, affecting most aspects of an individual's ability to participate fully in life, including attending college, holding down a job or building a social network (WHO, 2008). The combination of early onset and significant unemployment results in psychosis having a significant social and economic cost (Green, 2016), that largely explains psychosis being ranked as one of the top five leading causes of disability for 18- to 30-year-olds. While antipsychotic treatment is effective for ameliorating clinical symptoms in 75 per cent of cases, it has less impact on social and occupational function (Santestaban-Echarri et al. 2017). As a consequence, successfully addressing functional recovery in psychosis has become a significant clinical and research focus.

A recent study by Hodgekins and colleagues (2015) investigated trajectories of social recovery following a diagnosis of first-episode psychosis in individual attention early intervention for psychosis services in the UK. Using a statistical approach known as latent class growth analysis, which seeks to identify general patterns of outcome over time (in this case, 12 months), the authors identified three main patterns of outcomes: one group (representing 66 per cent of individuals) who showed an initial low level of social functioning that remained low at the 12-month follow-up; a second group (27 per cent) who showed low social functioning initially but who improved over the 12-month period, and a small (7 per cent) third group who showed a reduction in function over time. In summary, these data suggest that even with better quality services, a majority of attendees struggled to make gains in social recovery. The likelihood of falling into this 'poor recovery' category was predicted by male gender, ethnic minority status, younger age at onset, increased negative symptom severity and poorer premorbid adjustment.

In addition to DUP and concurrent symptom severity described above, the importance of changes in cognitive function has also emerged as an important independent predictor of functional outcomes (Santesteban-Echarri et al. 2017; Stouten et al. 2017). These are present well before the onset of psychosis, they increase following a first episode of psychosis, and remain impaired during the chronic stage of the disorder (Green 2016). Several questions remain about the role of cognitive function in predicting functional outcome, including whether cognitive function predicts functional outcomes once clinical symptom severity is controlled for.

We recently conducted a meta-analysis of cross-sectional and longitudinal studies in early psychosis to address whether cognitive function in early psychosis predicts social and occupational outcomes (Cowman et al. 2021). The data reviewed – based on 46 studies comprising 3,767 participants – was unequivocal. Of nine cognitive domains investigated, all were related to functional recovery, both cross-sectionally and longitudinally. Importantly, the amount of variance explained by individual cognitive abilities remained significant even when the effects of clinical symptom severity was accounted for. Among these, general cognitive ability and social cognition were most strongly associated with both concurrent and long-term functioning, with effect sizes in the medium range. The largest single effect observed was for social cognition, with evidence from longitudinal studies that this aspect of cognition explained, approximately 19 per cent of variation in functional outcomes.

A number of conclusions follow from these data. Firstly, that measurement of functional outcomes is required to adequately track and monitor improvement in social and functional outcomes. Secondly, that a comprehensive clinical assessment needs to include symptom severity, cognitive function and other factors likely to determine psychosocial outcomes. Thirdly, that effectively targeting the factors involved in cognitive function require multicomponent therapies, with components including a focus on cognitive function. This is discussed in greater detail below (see Family-based interventions).

Pharmacological treatments

Antipsychotic medications are not recommended in the 'at-risk mental state' group because of a limited evidence base, high sensitivity to side effects, and stigmatisation (Fusar-Poli et al. 2013).

Antipsychotic medications are a first-line treatment in psychosis and most people experiencing a first episode of psychosis will benefit from pharmacological intervention (Huhn et al. 2019). All of the antipsychotic drugs in use for the treatment of psychosis have broad safety windows and proven efficacy in large and well-controlled trials (Huhn et al. 2019). All antipsychotic medications currently available for use block the dopamine type-2 receptor which underlies their antipsychotic effect (Kapur and Remington, 2001). Antipsychotic medications also bind to other receptors in the brain, and their relative propensity to bind to different receptors can result in unwanted side effects. Some antipsychotic medications also have anxiolytic and antidepressant properties (Liu et al. 2014; Merideth et al. 2012).

Antipsychotic naive young people experiencing a first episode of psychosis are more sensitive to pharmacological effects of medication (Barnes et al. 2020). As a group, they typically respond to treatment more quickly and at lower doses. They are also more prone to side effects. Atypical antipsychotics are the first line pharmacological treatment in first-episode psychosis, and the general mantra in EIP services is 'start low and go slow'. Medication experiences at the beginning of treatment can have a long-lasting impact on future attitudes towards medication, compliance and outcomes (Barnes et al. 2020). As such, it is important that clinicians support young people and their families to understand the potential benefits and also the potential side effects associated with different antipsychotic medications. Psychoeducation is vital, and ideally, treatment decisions should tend towards the young person being equipped to make their own medication choices.

When making collaborative decisions on medication choices, it is worth distinguishing between the treatment of an acute psychotic episode and maintenance treatment (Morrison et al. 2020). In the acute phase, the focus of treatment is on the prompt relief of symptoms and distress. Some of the side effects of antipsychotic medication that are problematic in the long term, e.g. sedation and increased appetite, can be helpful in the acute phase where insomnia, distress and loss of appetite are common. Benzodiazepines and hypnotics can be a useful adjunct to treatment in the acute phase of psychosis. However, in the maintenance phase of treatment, the emphasis is on avoiding side effects so that a young person is more likely to adhere to treatment in the longer term (Morrison et al. 2020). Non-adherence to medication is the best predictor of relapse in psychosis and failure of insight to return is the best predictor of non-adherence among those aged 21–32 years old (Alvarez-Jimenez et al. 2012), further underlying the importance of psychoeducation and building a strong therapeutic alliance with young people experiencing psychosis.

The relative efficacy of antipsychotic medications does not vary significantly (Huhn et al. 2019; Zhu et al. 2017). Except when there is treatment resistance, then clozapine is superior to all other antipsychotic medication. Treatment resistance is defined as the persistence of psychotic symptoms despite two trials of antipsychotic medication at an adequate dose for an adequate duration with documented adherence (Howes et al. 2016). With sustained assertive treatment, over 80 per cent of people with a first episode of psychosis achieve remission of symptoms within six months (Kahn et al. 2018). Full remission takes time but will occur in the majority of young people. Antipsychotic treatment should be tailored towards the needs of the individual. Individualised care often involves trial and error, with feedback and adjustment. Side effects must be monitored closely and addressed aggressively. Discontinuation of medication carries a high risk of relapse over the first three years. However, a high antipsychotic load may be associated with poorer long-term functional outcomes.

About 15 per cent of those presenting with a first episode of psychosis will present with mania and psychosis. Mania responds to lithium, valproate, carbamazepine and antipsychotic medication. Antipsychotic medications have a relatively quick onset of action and currently atypical antipsychotics are considered first-line treatment for acute mania (Cipriani et al. 2011; Grande et al. 2016). Depression and anxiety disorders are common comorbidities in first-episode psychosis (Upthegrove et al. 2014). It is important these disorders are identified and treated appropriately.

Psychological treatments for early psychosis

As discussed above, there has been considerable evolution in thinking about what constitutes the right target for treatment in early psychosis, with an exclusive focus on symptom reduction gradually giving way to a broader focus on social recovery. Psychosocial interventions targeting clinical features of early psychosis over the past 20 years have consisted primarily of CBT for psychosis. Recent meta-analyses of these interventions suggest somewhat limited evidence in support of this approach, however. For example, a recent Cochrane meta-analyses of global outcomes following CBT (based on n = 60 studies and approximately 6,000 individuals) for psychosis across the lifespan indicates only small benefits in terms of global clinical state, no benefits in terms of relapse or social function, and no significant advantage over other psychosocial interventions (Jones et al. 2018). In terms of specific clinical symptoms, the evidence is marginally better. Following an older study of the effects of CBT on positive symptoms showing a small but significant effect (effect size [ES]-0.3; Zimmerman et al. 2005), more recent studies suggest that benefits are greatest for auditory delusions (ES = 0.4) whereas effects on delusions were non-significant after controlling for heterogeneity of results (Van Der Gaag et al. 2014). Similarly, Mehl et al. (2015) found that CBT was non-superior to other psychological interventions for delusions. Meta-analysis of CBT for negative symptoms has not been more encouraging (Fusar-Poli et al. 2015), with the suggestion that evidence of significant effects from older studies is not replicated in recent/better quality studies.

By comparison with these reviews showing modest benefits across the lifespan, is the evidence of the efficacy of CBT any stronger in early psychosis? The evidence here is still emerging. A recent review by Devoe and colleagues (2019), comparing CBT vs other psychosocial interventions among youth, reported a modest advantage of CBT to other psychosocial treatments, becoming non-significant at either 6 or 12 months following treatment. One might object here though, given the critical period discussion above, that any treatment effects might diminish following cessation. One might also argue that when CBT is provided as part of multi-component early interventions, patient benefits clearly outstrip treatment as usual (Correll et al. 2018). As evidence continues to build across early intervention services the unique contribution of CBT in reducing symptoms will no doubt become clearer.

When psychosocial treatments in early psychosis are measured in terms of social recovery, the relative benefits of individual treatments become clearer. We (Frawley et al. 2021) recently completed a meta-analysis of psychosocial interventions targeting social function. In total, 31 studies involving 2,811 participants were included in our analysis. Studies were categorised by psychosocial intervention type as follows: Cognitive Behavioural Therapy (CBT), Family-Based Therapy (FBT), Supported Employment, Cognitive Remediation Training (CRT) and Multi-Component psychosocial interventions. Of these, CRT – a behavioural training-based intervention that aims to improve cognitive processes (attention, memory, executive function, social cognition or meta-cognition) with the goal of durability and generalisation – has become a significant research focus in early psychosis, second only to CBT. Across interventions, psychosocial interventions were broadly associated with improvements in social and occupational function. Effect sizes varied by intervention type, stage of illness (at-risk mental state vs first episode vs early psychosis), length and duration of treatment, and measure used. Of note here was the difference in strength of association between these. For instance, of the two most widely studied psychosocial interventions in early psychosis, CRT was associated with a significant improvement in social recovery whereas the association between CBT and social cognition was non-significant. In some respects, this is perhaps unsurprising, given that a principal focus of CRT interventions is social recovery, whereas the CBT studies reviewed were primarily focused on symptom reduction. Of note, one CBT study that specifically targeted social recovery rather than symptom severity (Fowler et al. 2018) was an exception. Patients in the intervention arm of this study showed significant benefits in terms of social engagement as measured by time use, for example the amount of time spent doing various activities, such as paid work, household and family care, personal care, voluntary work, social life, travel and leisure activities.

Family-based interventions and individual placement supports (IPS), both of which are discussed next, were also significantly associated with improved social function. However, the number of individual studies of IPS and family-based interventions that reported social and occupational outcomes in early psychosis were small (three studies of each), thus precluding meta-analysis of their effects.

Family-based interventions

Family members of young people attending mental health services often report feeling side-lined and excluded from assessment, care planning and interventions. Family-centred care is central to EIP services' ethos and has been identified as a critical ingredient to their efficacy (Addington et al. 2013). Tenets which should underlie family-centred care in early psychosis services include: (1) a collaborative working relationship between the family and the clinical team starting at the assessment stage and continuing through out treatment course, (2) early assessment of family support needs by the EIP team, and (3) families being informed about and offered evidence-based individual family interventions and carer-focused interventions as early as possible post-diagnosis (Health Service Executive, 2019). Confidentiality and sharing of information are managed by the EIP team so as to respect the rights and wishes of the service user while also considering the need for appropriate information, support and interventions to assist families to support their family member experiencing psychosis.

Group psychoeducation for families provides families with the knowledge and confidence they need to work collaboratively with the EIP clinical team to support the service user. This approach's benefit has been confirmed in a number of studies (Claxton et al. 2017; McWilliams et al. 2010). Group psychoeducation programmes for families have been demonstrated to decrease the risk of relapse and rehospitalisation, reduce carer burden and improve family engagement with clinical teams (Breitborde et al. 2009).

Research also supports whole-family interventions, whether delivered in single-family formats like behavioural family therapy (Fadden, 2009) or in multi-family group work to two or three families at once (McFarlane, 2016). Whole-family interventions should consist of at least ten sessions over three months to one year, and include the service user whenever possible (McFarlane, 2016; National Institute for Health and Care Excellence [NICE], 2014). Other evidence-based whole-family interventions are the Somerset Model (Burbach & Stanbridge, 2006), and Systemic Family Therapy (Carr, 2016). The UK's NICE guidelines (2014) recommend that in addition to whole-family interventions, carer-focused interventions should be provided to all families. These carer-focused interventions include support, information, and skills groups for families. These groups do not necessarily include the young person themselves. Carer-focused interventions can be particularly useful for families when the young person has disengaged from services or where there is a lack of consent for a whole-family intervention.

Family peer-support services have been developed in many early intervention services with great effect (see Chapter 12). These services refer to informal, informational and emotional support provided to family members by other families who themselves have experience of psychosis. This support is typically provided at family/carer support groups. However, it can also occur at an individual family to family level. There is emerging evidence for family peer-support services, which suggest that they can be a very acceptable and effective means of supporting families to develop their understanding of psychosis, recovery, medications, relapse prevention and comorbidities. There is also evidence that family peer-support services can reduce isolation and the experience of stigma (Day et al. 2017; Duckworth & Halpern, 2014; Leggatt, 2007).

Educational and employment supports

Individuals with lived experience of psychosis often report that they place the goals of completing their education and gaining employment above addressing their clinical symptoms (Ramsay et al. 2012). This mirrors the data for individuals with mental health disorders generally, 70–90 per cent of whom identify education and work as an important goal (Grove, 1999; Secker et al. 2001). Despite these stated goals, the trajectory of young people living with psychosis to complete their education and transition into employment remains low, and typically reported at approximately 20 per cent (Rinaldi et al. 2010; Waghorn et al. 2012). Related to this, clinicians often report feeling they had little relevant training in helping people return to work, and limited confidence in the vocational services currently available (Marwaha et al. 2009). To address these difficulties, and under the umbrella of the supported employment model, the Individual Placement and Support model (IPS; Killackey et al. 2008) has been integrated into clinical guidelines and is now implemented in several early intervention services.

The overarching philosophy of IPS is that anyone is capable of partaking in paid, competitive employment with careful consideration of job type, job environment and with effective supports available. This approach has eight guiding principles, prioritising the following: the individual's job preferences; approaching employers with the individual's needs in mind; competitive employment; provision of ongoing time-unlimited support; integration within the mental health treatment team; and finally, that job searches begin directly on entry into the IPS programme ('place and train' rather than 'train and place'). IPS is typically provided as part of a wider early intervention service, making the disentanglement of the effect on function difficult. Moreover, intervention components of IPS overlap to an extent with psychological and family therapies in terms of psychoeducation, problem-solving skills, goal formulation and notably a community-based, practical approach to recovery (see also Chapter 12 on family engagement). Three studies to date have evaluated the efficacy of IPS in terms of social recovery (Killackey et al. 2008; Killackey et al. 2019; Rosenheck et al. 2017); all three studies report significant improvement following outcome. The largest of these, a study of n = 146 FEP individuals (Killacky et al. 2019) reported that the likelihood of being in open employment for six months was 71 per cent for those enrolled in IPS arm of the study vs 48 per cent in the control condition.

Conclusions and future directions

As noted above, older psychosocial interventions had focused principally on reducing the severity and untreated duration of clinical symptoms, on the basis that this would provide the best chance of illness recovery. This approach has only been partly supported by research evidence, resulting in a broader treatment focus that targets social and occupational function more directly. There is now broad evidence to support the efficacy of psychosocial interventions for improving social and occupational function in the early stages of psychosis. Furthermore, the currently available data suggests that delivering psychosocial interventions in community-based (rather than clinic-based) settings is a key consideration. Community-based, assertive outreach – irrespective of treatment type – appears to have a greater impact on function in the early psychosis population. Moving from clinic-based interventions towards providing treatment in the person's everyday milieu (e.g. in college, or other places they frequent) and with involvement of key community stakeholders appears a key ingredient for effective and collaborative interventions. Continuing to study community-based rather than clinic-based interventions represents an important study focus for future research.

A personalised treatment approach that matches therapeutic interventions to individual needs appears critical to meeting the complex needs in the early stages of psychosis. Multi-component interventions, capable of being tailored to the needs of the individual, are likely to have greatest potential to impact a range of psychosocial treatment targets in a more-than-the-sum-of-the-parts manner. This would appear in large part to reflect their capacity to provide what matters most to a given individual at a given time and in their changing circumstances. Given this, future research will need to make use of innovative trial methodologies that are capable of comparing alternative combinations of intervention components, rather than more traditional 'head-to-head' trials.

In estimating the contribution of individual psychosocial intervention types, both treatment intensity and duration were observed to moderate efficacy. For example, our meta-analysis (Frawley et al. 2021) observed that interventions of a six-month duration (or >30 sessions) were found to have a greater impact on social and occupational functioning compared to those six months or fewer. In the context of the critical period concept, it is likely that early intervention provides the start to recovery, rather than the whole story. Of course, many people will emerge from successful treatment of a first episode without further intervention being required. But many will not. And even if, for pragmatic (economic) reasons, early intervention only targets the first two years, establishing a pathway to obtaining sufficient treatment supports thereafter is likely to be necessary to recovery in the medium term. Research that maps alternative treatment pathways based on individual need will provide important data for alternatives to the currently funded 'one-size-fits-all' (i.e. two to three years) duration of care.

In conclusion, the value of multicomponent treatments in early psychosis appears to be well founded, particularly when delivered in accessible community-based settings. Many of the lessons learned from the development of early interventions for psychosis are likely to be relevant to the development of youth mental health services broadly, and particularly for those with more severe mental health difficulties.

Further reading

Malla, A., & McGorry, P. (2019). Early intervention in psychosis in young people: a population and public health perspective. American journal of public health, 109(S3), 181–184.

McGorry, P. (2019). Building the momentum and blueprint for reform in youth mental health. The Lancet Psychiatry, 6(6), 459–461.

Correll, C. U., Galling, B., Pawar, A., Krivko, A., Bonetto, C., Ruggeri, M., Craig, T. J., Nordentoft, M., Srihari, V. H., Guloksuz, S., Hui, C. L. M., Chen, E. Y. H., Valencia, M., Juarez, F., Robinson, D. G., Schooler, N. R., Brunette, M. F., Mueser, K. T., Rosenheck, R. A., … & Kane, J. M. (2018). Comparison of early intervention services vs treatment as usual for early-phase psychosis: a systematic review, meta-analysis, and meta-regression. JAMA psychiatry, 75(6), 555–565.

References

Addington, J., Liu, L., Farris, M. S., Goldstein, B. I., Wang, J. L., Kennedy, S. H., Bray, S., Lebel, C., & MacQueen, G. (2020). Clinical staging for youth at-risk for serious mental illness: A longitudinal perspective. *Early Intervention in Psychiatry, 15*(5), 1188–1196. https://doi.org/10.1111/eip.13062

Addington, D. E., McKenzie, E., Norman, R., Wang, J., & Bond, G. R. (2013). Essential evidence-based components of first-episode psychosis services. *Psychiatric Services, 64*(5), 452–457.

Alvarez-Jimenez, M., Priede, A., Hetrick, S. E., Bendall, S., Killackey, E., Parker, A. G., McGorry, P. D., & Gleeson, J. F. (2012). Risk factors for relapse following treatment for first episode psychosis: A systematic review and meta-analysis of longitudinal studies. *Schizophrenia Research, 139*(1–3), 116–128.

Barnes, T. R., Drake, R., Paton, C., Cooper, S. J., Deakin, B., Ferrier, I. N., Gregory, C. J., Haddad, P. M., Howes, O. D., Jones, I., Joyce, E. M., Lewis, S., Lingford-Hughes, A., MacCabe, J. H., Owens, D. C., Patel, M. X., Sinclair, J. M., Stone, J. M., Talbot, P. S., ... & Yung, A. R. (2020). Evidence-based guidelines for the pharmacological treatment of schizophrenia: Updated recommendations from the British Association for Psychopharmacology. *Journal of Psychopharmacology, 34*(1), 3–78.

Berk, M., Conus, P., Lucas, N., Hallam, K., Malhi, G. S., Dodd, S., Yatham, L. N., Yung, A. & McGorry, P. (2007). Setting the stage: From prodrome to treatment resistance in bipolar disorder. *Bipolar Disorders, 9*(7), 671–678.

Bertelsen, M., Jeppesen, P. I. A., Petersen, L., Thorup, A., Le Quach, P., Christensen, T. Ø., Krarup, G., Jorgensen, P., & Nordentoft, M. (2007). Suicidal behaviour and mortality in first-episode psychosis: The OPUS trial. *The British Journal of Psychiatry, 191*(S51), 140–146.

Birchwood, M., & Macmillan, F. (1993). Early intervention in schizophrenia. *Australian and New Zealand Journal of Psychiatry, 27*(3), 374–378.

Birchwood, M., Connor, C., Lester, H., Patterson, P., Freemantle, N., Marshall, M., Fowler, D., Lewis, S., Jones, P., Amos, T., Everard, L., & Singh, S. P. (2013). Reducing duration of untreated psychosis: Care pathways to early intervention in psychosis services. *The British Journal of Psychiatry, 203*(1), 58–64.

Bloom, B., Cohen, R. A., & Freeman, G. (2011). Summary health statistics for US children. *National Health Interview Survey, 2010.*

Breitborde, N. J., Woods, S. W., & Srihari, V. H. (2009). Multifamily psychoeducation for first-episode psychosis: A cost-effectiveness analysis. *Psychiatric Services, 60*(11), 1477–1483.

Burbach, F., & Stanbridge, R. (2006). Somerset's family interventions in psychosis service: An update. *Journal of Family Therapy, 28*(1), 39–57.

Carr, A. (2016). How and why do family and systemic therapies work?.*Australian and New Zealand Journal of Family Therapy, 37*(1), 37–55.

Cipriani, A., Barbui, C., Salanti, G., Rendell, J., Brown, R., Stockton, S., Purgato, M., Spineli, L. M., Goodwin, G. M., & Geddes, J. R. (2011). Comparative efficacy and acceptability of antimanic drugs in acute mania: A multiple-treatments meta- analysis. *The Lancet, 378*(9799), 1306–1315.

Claxton, M., Onwumere, J., & Fornells-Ambrojo, M. (2017). Do family interventions improve outcomes in early psychosis? A systematic review and meta-analysis. *Frontiers in Psychology, 8*, 371.

Correll, C. U., Galling, B., Pawar, A., Krivko, A., Bonetto, C., Ruggeri, M., Craig, T. J., Nordentoft, M., Srihari, V. H., Guloskuz, S., Hui, C. L. M., Chen, E. Y. H., Valencia, M., Juarez, F., Robinson, D. G., Schooler, N. R., Brunette, M. F., Mueser, K. T., Rosenheck, R. A., ... & Kane, J. M. (2018). Comparison of early intervention services vs treatment as usual for early-phase psychosis: A systematic review, meta- analysis, and meta-regression. *JAMA Psychiatry, 75*(6), 555–565.

Cowman, M., Holleran, L., Lonergan, E., O'Connor, K., Birchwood, M., & Donohoe, G. (2021). Cognitive predictors of social and occupational functioning in early psychosis: A systematic review and meta-analysis of cross-sectional and longitudinal data. *Schizophrenia Bulletin, 47*(5), 1243–1253. https://doi.org/10.1093/schbul/sbab033

Csillag, C., Nordentoft, M., Mizuno, M., Jones, P. B., Killackey, E., Taylor, M., Chen, E., Kane, J., & McDaid, D. (2016). Early intervention services in psychosis: From evidence to wide implementation. *Early Intervention in Psychiatry, 10*(6), 540–546.

Csillag, C., Nordentoft, M., Mizuno, M., McDaid, D., Arango, C., Smith, J., Lora, A., Verma, S., Di Fiandra, T., & Jones, P. B. (2018). Early intervention in psychosis: From clinical intervention to health system implementation. *Early Intervention in Psychiatry, 12*(4), 757–764.

Day, K., Starbuck, R., & Petrakis, M. (2017). Family group interventions in an early psychosis program: A re-evaluation of practice after 10 years of service delivery. *International Journal of Social Psychiatry, 63*(5), 433–438.

Devoe, D. J., Farris, M. S., Townes, P., & Addington, J. (2019). Attenuated psychotic symptom interventions in youth at risk of psychosis: A systematic review and meta- analysis. *Early Intervention in Psychiatry, 13*(1), 3–17.

Duckworth, K., & Halpern, L. (2014). Peer support and peer-led family support for persons living with schizophrenia. *Current Opinion in Psychiatry, 27*(3), 216–221.

Fadden, G. (2009). Family interventions in psychosis. *Clinical Psychology in Practice, 17*, 199–208.

Fineberg, N. A., Dell'Osso, B., Albert, U., Maina, G., Geller, D., Carmi, L., Sireau, N., Walitza, S., Grassi, G., Pallanti, S., Hollander, E., Brakoulias, V., Menchon, J. M., Marazziti, D., Ioannidis, K., Apergis-Schoute, A., Stein, D. J., Cath, D. C., Veltman, D. J., ... & Zohar, J. (2019). Early intervention for obsessive compulsive disorder: An expert consensus statement. *European Neuropsychopharmacology, 29*(4), 549–565.

Fowler, D., Hodgekins, J., French, P., Marshall, M., Freemantle, N., McCrone, P., Everard, L., Lavis, A., Jones, P. B., Amos, T., Singh, S., Sharma, V., & Birchwood, M. (2018). Social recovery therapy in combination with early intervention services for enhancement of social recovery in patients with first-episode psychosis (SUPEREDEN3): A single-blind, randomised controlled trial. *The Lancet Psychiatry, 5*(1), 41–50.

Frawley, E., Cowman, M., Lepage, M., & Donohoe, G. (2021). Social and occupational recovery in early psychosis: A systematic review and meta-analysis of psychosocial interventions. *Psychological Medicine*, 1–12. DOI:10.1017/S003329172100341X

Fusar-Poli, P., Borgwardt, S., Bechdolf, A., Addington, J., Riecher-Rossler, A., Schultze- Lutter, F., Keshavan, M., Wood, S., Ruhrmann, S., Seidman, L. J., Valmaggia, L., Cannon, T., Velthorst, E., De Haan, L., Cornblatt, B., Bonoldi, I., Birchwood, M., McGlashan, T., Carpenter, W., & Yung, A. (2013). The psychosis high-risk state: A comprehensive state-of-the-art review. *JAMA Psychiatry, 70*(1), 107–120.

Fusar-Poli, P., Papanastasiou, E., Stahl, D., Rocchetti, M., Carpenter, W., Shergill, S., & McGuire, P. (2015). Treatments of negative symptoms in schizophrenia: Meta-analysis of 168 randomized placebo-controlled trials. *Schizophrenia Bulletin, 41*(4), 892–899.

Gore, F. M., Bloem, P. J., Patton, G. C., Ferguson, J., Joseph, V., Coffey, C., ... & Mathers, C. D. (2011). Global burden of disease in young people aged 10–24 years: A systematic analysis. *The Lancet, 377*(9783), 2093–2102.

Grande, I., Berk, M., Birmaher, B., & Vieta, E. (2016). Bipolar disorder. *Lancet, 387*(10027), 1561–1572.

Grove, B. (1999). Mental health and employment: Shaping a new agenda. *Journal of Mental Health, 8*, 131–140.

Green, M. F. (2016). Impact of cognitive and social cognitive impairment on functional outcomes in patients with schizophrenia. *The Journal of Clinical Psychiatry, 77*(suppl 2), 8–11.

Health Service Executive (HSE) National Clinical Programme. (2019). HSE National Clinical Programme for Early Intervention in Psychosis – Model of Care Executive Summary. https://www.hse.ie/eng/about/who/cspd/ncps/mental health/psychosis/resources/hse-early-intervention-in-psychosis-model-of-care-executive-summary-june-2019.pdf

Heckman, J. J. (2006). Skill formation and the economics of investing in disadvantaged children. *Science, 312*(5782), 1900–1902.

Hodgekins, J., Birchwood, M., Christopher, R., Marshall, M., Coker, S., Everard L., Lester H., Jones. P., Amos T, Sharma,V., Freemantle N., & Fowler, D. (2015). Investigating trajectories of social recovery in individuals with first-episode psychosis: A latent class growth analysis. *British Journal of Psychiatry*, 207(6), 536–543.

Howes, O. D., McCutcheon, R., Agid, O., de Bartolomeis, A., van Beveren, N. J., Birnbaum, M. L., Bloomfield, M. A., Bressan, R. A., Buchanan, R. W., Carpenter, W. T., Castle, D. J., Citrome, L., Daskalakis, Z. J., Davidson, M., Drake, R. J., Dursun, S., Ebdrup, B. H., Elkis, H., Falkai, P., ... & Correll, C. U. (2016). Treatment-Resistant Schizophrenia: Treatment Response and Resistance in Psychosis (TRRIP) Working Group Consensus Guidelines on Diagnosis and Terminology *American Journal of Psychiatry*, 174(3), 216–229.

Huhn, M., Nikolakopoulou, A., Schneider-Thoma, J., Krause, M., Samara, M., Peter, N., Arndt, T., Bäckers, L., Rothe, P., Cipriani, A., Davis, J., Salanti, G., & Leucht, S. (2019). Comparative efficacy and tolerability of 32 oral antipsychotics for the acute treatment of adults with multi-episode schizophrenia: A systematic review and network meta-analysis. *The Lancet*, 394(10202), 939–951.

Jones, C., Hacker, D., Xia, J., Meaden, A., Irving, C. B., Zhao, S., Chen, J., & Shi, C. (2018). Cognitive behavioural therapy plus standard care versus standard care for people with schizophrenia. *Cochrane Database of Systematic Reviews*, 2018, Issue 11. Art. No.: CD008712. DOI: 10.1002/14651858.CD008712.pub3

Kahn, R. S., van Rossum, I. W., Leucht, S., McGuire, P., Lewis, S. W., Leboyer, M., Arango, C., Dazzan, P., Drake, R., Heres, S., Díaz-Caneja, C. M., Rujescu, D., Weiser, M., Galderisi, S., Glenthój, B., Eijkemans, M. J. C., Fleischacker, W. W., Kapur, S., Sommer, I. E., ... & Wilson, D. (2018). Amisulpride and olanzapine followed by open-label treatment with clozapine in first-episode schizophrenia and schizophreniform disorder (OPTiMiSE): A three-phase switching study. *The Lancet Psychiatry*, 5(10), 797–807.

Kapur, S., & Remington, G. (2001). Dopamine D(2) receptors and their role in atypical antipsychotic action: Still necessary and may even be sufficient. *Biological Psychiatry*, 50(11), 873–883.

Kessler, R. C., Berglund, P., Demler, O., Jin, R., Merikangas, K. R., & Walters, E. E. (2005). Lifetime prevalence and age-of-onset distributions of DSM-IV disorders in the National Comorbidity Survey Replication. *Archives of General Psychiatry*, 62(6), 593–602.

Killackey, E., Jackson, H. J., & McGorry, P. D. (2008). Vocational intervention in first-episode psychosis: Individual placement and support v. treatment as usual. *The British Journal of Psychiatry*, 193(2), 114–120.

Killackey, E., Allott, K., Jackson, H. J., Scutella, R., Tseng, Y. P., Borland, J., Proffitt, TM., Hunt, S., Kay-Lambkin, F., Chinnery, G., Baksheev, G., Alvarez-Jimenez, M., McGorry, P. D., & Cotton, S. M. (2019). Individual placement and support for vocational recovery in first-episode psychosis: Randomised controlled trial. *The British Journal of Psychiatry*, 214(2), 76–82.

Leggatt, M. S. (2007). Minimising collateral damage: Family peer support and other strategies. *Medical Journal of Australia*, 187(S7), S61–S63.

Liu, Y., Zhou, X., Qin, B., Del Giovane, C., Zhang, Y., & Xie, P. (2014). Efficacy, quality of life, and acceptability outcomes of atypical antipsychotic augmentation treatment for treatment-resistant depression: Protocol for a systematic review and network meta-analysis. *Systematic Reviews*, 3, 133.

Marshall, M., Lewis, S., Lockwood, A., Drake, R., Jones, P., & Croudace, T. (2005). Association between duration of untreated psychosis and outcome in cohorts of first-episode patients: A systematic review. *Archives of General Psychiatry*, 62(9), 975–983.

Marwaha, S., Balachandra, S., & Johnson, S. (2009). Clinicians' attitudes to the employment of people with psychosis. *Social Psychiatry and Psychiatric Epidemiology*, 44(5), 349.

McFarlane, W. R. (2016). Family interventions for schizophrenia and the psychoses: A review. *Family Process*, 55(3), 460–482.

McGlashan, T. H., Miller, T. J., Woods, S. W., Hoffman, R. E., & Davidson, L. (2001). Instrument for the assessment of prodromal symptoms and states. In *Early intervention in psychotic disorders* (pp. 135–149). Springer.

McGorry, P. (1993). Early psychosis prevention and intervention centre. *Australasian Psychiatry, 1*(1), 32–34.

McGorry, P. D., Edwards, J., Mihalopoulos, C., Harrigan, S. M., & Jackson, H. J. (1996). EPPIC: An evolving system of early detection and optimal management. *Schizophrenia Bulletin, 22*(2), 305–326.

McGorry, P. D., Purcell, R., Hickie, I. B., & Jorm, A. F. (2007). Investing in youth mental health is a best buy. *Medical Journal of Australia, 187*(S7), S5–S7.

McGorry, P. D., Killackey, E., & Yung, A. (2008). Early intervention in psychosis: Concepts, evidence and future directions. *World Psychiatry, 7*(3), 148.

McGorry, P., Johanessen, J. O., Lewis, S., Birchwood, M., Malla, A., Nordentoft, M., Addington, J., & Yung, A. (2010). Early intervention in psychosis: Keeping faith with evidence-based healthcare. *Psychological Medicine, 40*(3), 399–404.

McGorry, P. D., Hartmann, J. A., Spooner, R., & Nelson, B. (2018). Beyond the 'at risk mental state' concept: Transitioning to transdiagnostic psychiatry. *World Psychiatry, 17*(2), 133–142.

McWilliams, S., Egan, P., Jackson, D., Renwick, L., Foley, S., Behan, C., Fitzgerals, E., Fetherston, A., Turner, N., Kinsella, A., & O'Callaghan, E. (2010). Caregiver psychoeducation for first-episode psychosis. *European Psychiatry, 25*(1), 33–38.

Mehl, S., Werner, D., & Lincoln, T. M. (2015). Does Cognitive Behavior Therapy for psychosis (CBTp) show a sustainable effect on delusions? A meta-analysis. *Frontiers in Psychology, 6,* 1450.

Merideth, C., Cutler, A. J., She, F., & Eriksson, H. (2012). Efficacy and tolerability of extended release quetiapine fumarate monotherapy in the acute treatment of generalized anxiety disorder: A randomized, placebo controlled and active-controlled study. *International Clinical Psychopharmacology, 27*(1), 40–54.

Morrison, A. P., Pyle, M., Maughan, D., Johns, L., Freeman, D., Broome, M. R., Husain, N., Fowler, D., Hudson, J., MacLennan, G., Norrie, J., Shiers, D., Hollis, C., Birchwood, M., Bhogal, R., Bowe, S., Byrne, R., Clacey, J., Davies, L., … & Yung, A. (2020). Antipsychotic medication versus psychological intervention versus a combination of both in adolescents with first-episode psychosis (MAPS): A multicentre, three-arm, randomised controlled pilot and feasibility study. *The Lancet Psychiatry, 7*(9), 788–800.

National Institute for Health & Care Excellence (NICE) (2014). Psychosis and schizophrenia in adults: Prevention and management. https://www.nice.org.uk/guidance/cg178/resources/psychosis-and-schizophrenia-in-adults-prevention-and-management-pdf-35109758952133

Niendam, T. A., Sardo, A., Savill, M., Patel, P., Xing, G., Loewy, R. L., Dewa, C. S., & Melnikow, J. 2019). The rise of early psychosis care in California: An overview of community and university-based services. *Psychiatric Services, 70*(6), 480–487.

Nordentoft, M., Rasmussen, J. O., Melau, M., Hjorthôj, C. R., & Thorup, A. A. (2014). How successful are first episode programs? A review of the evidence for specialized assertive early intervention. *Current Opinion in Psychiatry, 27*(3), 167–172.

Omer, S., Behan, C., Waddington, J. L., & O'Callaghan, E. (2010). Early intervention in psychosis: Service models world-wide and the Irish experience. *Irish Journal of Psychological Medicine, 27*(4), 210–214.

Power, P. (2019). Early intervention services for psychosis in Ireland: Are we there yet? *Irish Journal of Psychological Medicine, 36*(4), 243–248.

Ramsay, C. E., Stewart, T., & Compton, M. T. (2012). Unemployment among patients with newly diagnosed first-episode psychosis: Prevalence and clinical correlates in a US sample. *Social Psychiatry and Psychiatric Epidemiology, 47*(5), 797–803.

Rinaldi, M., Killackey, E., Smith, J., Shepherd, G., Singh, S. P., & Craig, T. (2010). First episode psychosis and employment: A review. *International Review of Psychiatry, 22*(2), 148–162.

Rosenheck, R., Mueser, K. T., Sint, K., Lin, H., Lynde, D. W., Glynn, S. M., Robinson, D. G., Schooler, N. R., Marcy, P., Mohamed, S., & Kane, J. M. (2017). Supported employment and education in comprehensive, integrated care for first episode psychosis: Effects on work, school, and disability income. *Schizophrenia Research, 182*, 120–128.

Ruggeri, M., Bonetto, C., Lasalvia, A., Fioritti, A., de Girolamo, G., Santonastaso, P., Pileggi, F., Neri, G., Ghigi, D., Giubilini, F., Miceli, M., Scarone, S., Cocchi, A., Torresani, S., Faravelli, C., Cremonese, C., Scocco, P., Leuci, E., Mazzi, F., ... & Group, G. U. (2015). Feasibility and Effectiveness of a Multi-Element Psychosocial Intervention for First-Episode Psychosis: Results From the Cluster-Randomized Controlled GET UP PIANO Trial in a Catchment Area of 10 Million Inhabitants. *Schizophrenia Bulletin, 41*(5), 1192–1203.

Santesteban-Echarri, O., Paino, M., Rice, S., González-Blanch, C., McGorry, P., Gleeson, J., & Alvarez-Jimenez, M. (2017). Predictors of functional recovery in first-episode psychosis: A systematic review and meta-analysis of longitudinal studies. *Clinical Psychology Review, 58*, 59–75.

Secker, J., Grove, B., & Seebohm, P. (2001). Challenging barriers to employment, training and education for mental health service users: The service user's perspective. *Journal of Mental Health, 10*(4), 395–404.

Stouten, L. H., Veling, W., Laan, W., van der Helm, M., & van der Gaag, M. (2017). Psychosocial functioning in first-episode psychosis and associations with neurocognition, social cognition, psychotic and affective symptoms. *Early Intervention in Psychiatry, 11*(1), 23–36.

Upthegrove, R., Ross, K., Brunet, K., McCollum, R., & Jones, L. (2014). Depression in first episode psychosis: The role of subordination and shame. *Psychiatry Research, 217*(3), 177–184.

Upthegrove, R., Chard, C., Jones, L., Gordon-Smith, K., Forty, L., Jones, I., & Craddock, N. (2015). Adverse childhood events and psychosis in bipolar affective disorder. *British Journal of Psychiatry, 206*(3), 191–197.

Van der Gaag, M., Valmaggia, L. R., & Smit, F. (2014). The effects of individually tailored formulation-based cognitive behavioural therapy in auditory hallucinations and delusions: A meta-analysis. *Schizophrenia Research, 156*(1), 30–37.

Vieta, E., Salagre, E., Grande, I., Carvalho, A. F., Fernandes, B. S., Berk, M., Birmaher, B., Tohen, M., & Suppes, T. (2018). Early intervention in bipolar disorder. *American Journal of Psychiatry, 175*(5), 411–426.

Waghorn, G., Saha, S., Harvey, C., Morgan, V. A., Waterreus, A., Bush, R., ... & McGrath, J. J. (2012). 'Earning and learning' in those with psychotic disorders: The second Australian national survey of psychosis. *Australian & New Zealand Journal of Psychiatry, 46*(8), 774–785.

World Health Organization. (2008). *The global burden of disease: 2004 update.* World Health Organization.

Yung, A. R., Yung, A. R., Pan Yuen, H., Mcgorry, P. D., Phillips, L. J., Kelly, D., Dell'olio, M., Francey. D. M., Cosgrave, E. M., Killackey, E., Stanford, C., Godfrey, K., & Buckby, J. (2005). Mapping the onset of psychosis: The comprehensive assessment of at-risk mental states. *Australian & New Zealand Journal of Psychiatry, 39*(11–12), 964–971.

Zhu, Y., Krause, M., Huhn, M., Rothe, P., Schneider-Thoma, J., Chaimani, A., Li, C., Davis, J. M., & Leucht, S. (2017). Antipsychotic drugs for the acute treatment of patients with a first episode of schizophrenia: A systematic review with pairwise and network meta-analyses. *Lancet Psychiatry, 4*(9), 694–705.

Zimmermann, G., Favrod, J., Trieu, V. H., & Pomini, V. (2005). The effect of cognitive behavioral treatment on the positive symptoms of schizophrenia spectrum disorders: A meta-analysis. *Schizophrenia Research, 77*(1), 1–9.

11 Youth participation in mental health services

Aileen O'Reilly, Siobhan McGrory, Karen Butler
The National Centre for Youth Mental Health, Ireland

Melissa Keller-Tuberg, Magenta Simmons
Orygen, Australia

The purpose of the mental health system is to empower young people to be agents of their own mental health. It follows that the system itself should be designed and delivered in partnership with us. Giving those it seeks to serve a voice in policy, research and clinical programmes is absolutely essential for those programmes to work.

Melissa Keller-Tuberg[3]

Introduction

A child's right to participate is most famously protected by Article 12 of the 1989 United Nations Convention on the Rights of the Child (UNCRC), which establishes the right of every child to freely express their views in matters affecting them, and the subsequent right for those views to be given due weight. Internationally, participation has been highlighted as important in policy, planning and service delivery (UNICEF, 2003; World Health Organization [WHO], 2018). However, it is only recently that the importance of *youth* involvement in mental health services has been advocated for (Hawke et al. 2018; James, 2007; Monson & Thurley, 2011; World Economic Forum [WEF], 2020). Consequently, youth participation in service development and delivery, community engagement, research and policy are features of many newer youth mental health services (Hawke et al. 2019; Hetrick et al. 2017). Here, the term youth refers to 12–25-year-olds, reflecting international trends in service provision for young people, research in this area (Hetrick et al. 2017), and international policy definitions (United Nations [UN], 2013).

It is critical that any consideration of young people's mental health recognises that their participation is central to building a comprehensive understanding of

---

[3] Melissa Keller-Tuberg is a member of Orygen's Youth Research Council; Karen Butler is a member of Jigsaw's Youth Advisory Panel. In addition to co-authoring this chapter their own views on youth participation are highlighted throughout the chapter.

young people's needs and how best to meet these needs. This chapter, written in collaboration with two youth advocates, considers youth participation specifically in relation to youth mental health service development, provision and reform. First, information on the definitions and models of youth participation is provided. Next, the reasons for implementing a participation model and barriers and facilitators to implementation are outlined, drawing on two examples of youth participation in action from Jigsaw: The National Centre for Youth Mental Health, Ireland, and Orygen, Australia. These case studies provide insights into the realities, challenges and opportunities for participation in youth mental health services. After this, the available evidence on youth participation is summarised. The chapter ends with some key considerations for stakeholders interested in supporting youth participation in mental health services in a meaningful and systematic way.

What is youth participation?

The language of participation can be vague and contradictory, and terms like 'partnership', 'participation', 'shared decision-making', 'involvement', 'engagement' and 'inclusion' are often used interchangeably when discussing the involvement of young people in services (Day, 2008; McPherson, 2010). After assessing 14 definitions of youth participation, Farthing (2012: 73) described it as 'a process where young people, as active citizens, take part in, express views on and have decision-making power about issues that affect them.' In this chapter we use the term 'participation' and this definition to describe youth involvement in mental health services, as we feel it best reflects our experiences and the literature in this area. Further, in line with practice in this area, our use of the term encompasses the participation of young people with lived experience of mental ill-health; engagement with mental health services; and/or an interest in, and commitment to, youth mental health.

In addition to challenges defining youth participation, it is an area of policy, research and practice that is heralded but relatively under-theorised (Cahill & Dadvand, 2018; Malone & Hartung, 2010). Nonetheless, a number of models for thinking about and guiding youth participation have been proposed, the most well-known of which are summarised in Table 11.1. As this table shows, many make distinctions between levels of participation according to the degree of power that is shared or transferred by parties. The oldest model, Hart's (1992) Ladder of Participation, separates participation into eight levels that reflect the degree to which authority and control is shared between adults and young people. Shier's (2001) Pathways to Participation model expands on Hart's model, and proposes five levels of participation, but also acknowledges that organisational support is required for effective youth participation. However, both models have been criticised for assuming participation can be placed in hierarchical order and failing to recognise the importance of situations, cultures and context (Barber, 2009; Head, 2011). Treseder's Degrees of Participation (1997) addresses this by proposing five non-hierarchical levels of participation, and suggests that the appropriate level is the one that best fits the needs of those involved. Similarly,

Table 11.1 Summary of youth participation models

Name	Levels/ Elements	Youth involvement	Description
Hart's Ladder of Participation (1992)	8	No	• Levels of participation range from low levels (1–3), where young people are placed in predetermined roles and have no opportunity to influence but may be involved in manipulative, decorative, or tokenistic ways, to higher levels (4–8). At the highest level, young people are fully in control, with support from adults.
Shier's Pathways to Participation (2001)	5	No	• Levels progress from young people being listened to towards being supported to express themselves, influencing decision-making, and, at the highest level, sharing power with responsibility for decision-making. • Organisational support is required for effective participation, which relies on openings (commitment to listening and supporting decision-making), opportunities and obligations (i.e., the requirement of staff to act).
Treseder's Degrees of Participation (1997)	5	No	• Non-hierarchical model depicting different degrees of participation in a circle. This includes engaging young people in adult directed tasks (assigned but informed), and engaging young people as directors with high levels of responsibility (youth initiated and directed). • Considers different levels of participation as equally valid depending on circumstances.
Lundy's Model of Child Participation (2007)	4	Insights gathered from 1,064 students	• Non-hierarchical model focused on four elements of the rights provisions in Article 12, UNCRC: (i) space to take part, (ii) voice to contribute opinions, (iii) audience to have opinions heard, and (iv) influence to shape decisions.

Lundy's (2007) model depicts four interrelated elements to participation and recognises the fluid nature of decision-making processes in its construction. This model is widely acknowledged as being of significant value in interpreting Article 12 of the UNCRC, both in theory and in practice (O'Donnell, 2016).

In addition to these models, there is a plethora of other less well-known typologies of participation, including the Clarity Model of Participation (Lardner, 2001), the Typology of Youth Participation and Empowerment (TYPE) Pyramid

(Wong et al. 2010), the McCain Model of Youth Engagement (Heffernan et al. 2017), and P7 Model (Cahill & Dadvand, 2018). All help to break down the complexity of participation, and have been powerful tools in advocating for change (Day, 2008; Tisdall, 2010). They have also informed a wide range of toolkits for services and young people. Yet, most are adult-developed, which raises a fundamental question about how youth participation is conceptualised. Additionally, young people have articulated criticisms of the models, including that they are not helpful in measuring or explaining their participation in decision-making, and that the language and terminology is adult-oriented and insufficiently contextualised (Charles & Haines, 2014; Malone & Hartung, 2010). As a result, commentators have identified a need to develop a theory or model of participation that fully captures the complexity of this field, although there has been little progress in this regard (Malone & Hartung, 2010; Tisdall, 2010).

Purpose and value of youth participation

Typically, youth participation in mental health services has involved engaging young people via defined participation structures to inform service design and delivery. This is critical as young people have unique developmental needs, and experiences of mental ill-health and help-seeking different to adults (Ennis & Wykes, 2013; Hetrick et al. 2017). More recently, there has been a move towards involving young people in youth mental health research and policy related activities (Faithfull et al. 2019; Heffernan et al. 2017; Simmons et al. 2020). Although there is limited youth-specific evidence for partnerships[4] in mental health research, the perspectives of young people can improve the quality and meaning of research activities such as: prioritising research topics and questions, study design and methodological approaches; and the translation of research into practice, and dissemination of findings (Faithfull et al. 2019; Hawke et al. 2018; Simmons et al. 2020). The level of youth participation in research varies from young people taking part as active informants, through stages of greater participation, where young people are engaged (or employed) as co-researchers or primary researchers (Bradbury-Jones & Taylor, 2015).

Young people with lived experience of mental health challenges have also been involved in peer work roles to support other young people accessing youth mental health services. Peer workers can help engage young people and make them feel more involved in making decisions about their own mental healthcare (Simmons et al. 2018). In many countries, the peer workforce is the fastest growing workforce in mental health; for example, in Australia it features as a key solution to mental health reform (Fava et al. 2020). While youth peer support has traditionally been conceptualised as youth participation (Monson & Thurley, 2011), the increasing professionalisation of peer workers (qualified, trained employees with a defined role and associated responsibilities) means they should be regarded as a distinct workforce (McMahon, 2019). (See also Chapter 12 for an account of peer support for families.)

---

[4] The term 'partnership' is typically used to describe youth participation in research, to distinguish it from the involvement of research participants in a study

Through the various modes of participation, young people can develop their confidence, acquire new skills, and learn more about organisations and policy, thereby improving their education and employment opportunities, their knowledge about mental health, and providing the opportunity to meet new people and help communities (Checkoway, 2011; Coates & Howe, 2014; Collin et al. 2009; Howe et al. 2011; Ramey & Rose-Krasnor, 2015). Participation can also foster resilience in young people, giving them a sense of belonging and connectivity, and have a positive impact on their mental health (Oliver et al. 2006). At an organisational level, youth input is vital to improving the quality of services, which even in high-income countries are often part of a fragmented mental health system that is underfunded and under-resourced (Collin et al. 2009; Howe et al. 2011). Challenges in youth mental health are often complex and nuanced, and young people can contribute their unique perspectives to tackle complex problems with creative solutions. Young people bring with them a contemporaneous understanding of what it is like to be a young person today, and are best able to plan for what young people in the future may need from a mental health service (James, 2007). Moreover, what it is like to be a young person in any given point in time can change rapidly (e.g. rise of social media, meme culture, impact of socio-political climate); thus, including the voices of young people is an ideal way to capture what it means to be a young person at a particular time (International Youth Foundation, 2012).

Barriers and facilitators to youth participation

As a relatively new approach, there has been significant emphasis on the challenges and enablers for youth participation. Notably, this has indicated that appropriate resources are required to maximise the contribution of young people (Barry, 2014; Howe et al. 2011). Howe et al. (2011) propose that young people should be appropriately remunerated for their participation, thereby ensuring their input is seen as valued and equal. A supportive environment and organisational culture can also have a significant impact on the success of youth participation strategies (Barry, 2014; Worrall-Davies, 2008). The relationship between adults and young people is another key facilitator for participation (Ramey & Rose-Krasnor, 2015). There is evidence that open and frequent communication underpins a dynamic and productive relationship between young people and staff (Collin et al. 2012). Supporting skills and knowledge development is essential, as young people need training to enable their participation and may be considering how their engagement is related to their personal and professional development, while adults also need to recognise the need for their own skills development when it comes to meaningful collaboration.

Clarity around the purpose of participation is equally important, as disengagement can occur if organisations are unclear with young people about the purpose of their participation, or ask for their views repeatedly and do not take action (Collin et al. 2009; Fenton et al. 2020; Kirby et al. 2003; Worrall-Davies, 2008). Practitioners should regularly check the level of involvement desired by young people and provide flexibility for them to move fluidly between various levels of participation, depending on their circumstances, experiences and interests (Kirby et al. 2003). Indeed, time has been identified as a critical challenge for participation, especially when young people have competing interests including school/college and work, and this is often a reason why young people who become involved in participatory activities are middle class, well educated and articulate (Collin et al. 2009). Ensuring representativeness, gender parity and diversity is an ongoing difficulty for many services (Fenton et al. 2020; Roe & McEvoy, 2011; Un-Habitat and the Focal Point on Youth [UNDESA], 2013). Consideration of the developmental stage of adolescence and negotiating consent is another challenge and, consequently, many participation structures are designed for young people aged 16 and above.

Although newer youth mental health services have been established with youth participation as part of the genesis of each service (O'Reilly et al. 2021; Rickwood et al. 2019), in most cases youth participation structures are applied to existing services or created in those with very limited tradition of youth involvement. In such circumstances, it is especially important to consider and be transparent about the power dynamics between existing, older staff members and young people, and the degree to which young people can be involved in, and influence, decision-making (Fenton et al. 2020). It is also important for services to reflect on how to build on the knowledge generated by youth participation, both within and across programmes, and to retain that expertise when young people 'age out' of participation structures (e.g. through alumni programmes).

> *I've been a 'lived-experience advisor' on a project which left me feeling like the project wanted to 'try out' youth participation but weren't aware of what best practice looked like. I wasn't reimbursed for meetings, even though all other attendees were paid. I didn't get a position description or regular updates, which limited my ability to give feedback, and made me unsure about my role. There was no allocated meeting time for me to discuss ideas ... instead, I had to 'pipe up' among other discussions, and it was difficult to get a word in. When I did make suggestions, I was subtly challenged or told that 'things are already finalised'. I felt pretty disillusioned, as if I was the token young person they could say they had spoken to but hadn't meaningfully engaged with.*
>
> Melissa Keller-Tuberg

Implementing a youth participation model

Case study 1: Orygen

Orygen is the world's largest organisation dedicated to youth mental health research, policy, education and clinical care, and it works collaboratively with young people to develop, implement and evaluate its programmes and services. Using a youth-adult participation model, Orygen aspires to work with young people at all organisational levels and functional domains. Fundamentally, Orygen's youth participation strategy is guided by the best-practice principles of providing well-supported, meaningful and mutually beneficial engagement opportunities. The current strategy is the product of a long history of redesign, and at its core is the desire and capacity to self-evaluate and reform (Simmons et al. 2020). Below is a snapshot of the strategy's core national and regional programmes in 2020. However, the true scope of the organisation's youth participation strategy is international, with recent programmes and partnerships being established on a global scale.

On a national level, engagement with young people primarily takes place with two national youth councils: the Youth Advisory Council (YAC) and Youth Research Council (YRC). Each comprises approximately nine young Australians aged 16–25 years old, of varying genders and sexual identities, cultural backgrounds, lived experiences with mental illness and caregiving, geographic localities, interests and expertise. Over a two-year tenure, the councils meet separately via monthly teleconferences, and together in bi-annual, in-person meetings. In order to ensure that young people are able to participate, members are reimbursed for their time and have face-to-face meeting expenses fully covered. While both councils are situated to influence organisational decision-making processes from the top down, they have different roles and responsibilities. The YAC was established to advise on the overall implementation of Orygen's youth participation strategy and provide project-specific advice to policy and advocacy programmes. For example, the council recently initiated a motion to establish gender-inclusive bathrooms at Orygen's on-site facility. Additionally, a subgroup of the YAC is involved in advising on the organisation's social media and communications to ensure that it is relevant and appropriate for youth audiences. The Youth Research Council (YRC) provides research-specific advice with respect to research projects' design and methodology, data analysis, recruitment, risk management, dissemination and translational activities. Further, a handful of YRC representatives are members of Orygen's ethics committee, where they evaluate project protocols and related documentation and ensure that research projects are youth friendly prior to ethics approval. YAC and YRC members are also invited to apply for additional ad hoc opportunities, such as contributing to governmental policy papers, national campaigns and media interview requests.

As council members, we are encouraged to keep up to date with the organisation outside of our regular duties, challenge the status quo and speak up when differences in opinion between staff members and young people arise. For example, in 2020, a YRC member highlighted how Orygen was systematically failing to provide adequate interpretation and translation services for culturally and linguistically diverse participants... The YRC member then facilitated a webinar and workshop where staff and young people brainstormed what cultural safety in research at Orygen should look like. The recommendations made are currently being addressed, and action items will soon be submitted to the Director of Research and Executive Board for review. This is just one example where a young person has spurred positive organisational change from the top down. Although nothing happens overnight, and sometimes it feels like there's lots of bureaucratic hoops to jump through, I genuinely feel that our opinions are valued and our voices make a difference.

Melissa Keller-Tuberg

Whereas the YAC and YRC operate on a national level, separate programmes facilitate collaborative decision-making processes from the ground up. Orygen is the lead agency for several community-based, early-intervention youth mental health *headspace* centres, which offer holistic allied health, medical and related (e.g. substance use, vocational support) assessment and care. Each centre works alongside a local Youth Advisory Group (YAG) who advise on clinical and research programmes and engage with local communities to reduce stigma and promote hope and help-seeking. In a similar fashion, Orygen's specialist mental health services are delivered in collaboration with a youth Platform team comprising past and present clients. This group engages in a range of clinical and community-focused activities such as service feedback, consumer advocacy and peer-support, staff interviews and training. Both the YAGs and Platform teams are empowered to design and implement their own independent activities in addition to their regular duties.

Orygen's youth participation model provides an example of how young people can be engaged to ensure that mental health services, policy and research programmes are appropriate and responsive to the needs of the international, national and local community. Importantly, Orygen's approach recognises that the needs and priorities of both the organisation and the young people it serves change. In this sense, effective youth participation is a moving target, and engagement strategies evolve accordingly. For example, volunteers have identified the need to strengthen the organisation's ties with Australian Indigenous and Torres Strait Islander communities. In response, a mixed youth and adults' First Nations of Australia Advisory Group (FNAAG) was recently established within Orygen to oversee initiatives and policies which affect these communities. Above all, the model demonstrates that with ongoing refinement, it is possible to successfully support youth participation across all areas and levels of a youth mental health organisation.

Case study 2: Jigsaw: The National Centre for Youth Mental Health, Ireland

Jigsaw is Ireland's leading youth mental health charity and focuses on delivering services, influencing change and strengthening communities to create an Ireland where every young person's mental health is valued and supported. Jigsaw provides primary care therapeutic sessions for young people aged 12–25 years old across a network of 14 services; implements community-based programmes aimed at better informing, supporting, educating and empowering young people and those around them; offers a wide range of online mental health supports; and undertakes pioneering research and robust evaluation, leading to transformative evidence (O'Reilly et al. 2021).

Young people have always been at the heart of the Jigsaw service model and, from the outset, the organisation made a commitment to listening and responding to what young people were saying about their mental health needs. Jigsaw views participation as a process, and places emphasis on supporting young people to ensure they are meaningfully involved in a way that best meets their needs. To facilitate youth participation, each of the 14 Jigsaw services has a Youth Advisory Panel (YAP) comprised of volunteers aged 16–25 years old. The YAP invites membership from any young person in the community with an interest in mental health. The aim of the YAP is to ensure that service policy and provision is youth-centred and meeting the needs of young people. For example, YAP members sit on recruitment panels for staff interviews, advise on the design of service hubs and promotional materials, and often lead and develop projects within services.

YAP members receive an induction programme as well as bi-annual check-ins which enable staff to identify strengths or areas for development, and provide young people with the opportunity to consider their capacity to remain on the YAP. Jigsaw allows for a pause in participation, which affords young people an opportunity to step back from participation duties for a period of up to three months. There are typically 12 YAP meetings annually and each young person is expected to commit to at least six. This process acknowledges young people's need for flexibility, and is further facilitated by staff holding meetings during times that suit young people (e.g. evenings, weekends). YAP members are regularly offered the opportunity to participate in training covering a diverse range of topics such as mental health and group facilitation skills. Young people at Jigsaw are reimbursed for travel, but otherwise receive no financial incentive. Instead, local services host YAP appreciation events, to recognise and show gratitude for the work of the YAP in whatever form young people and staff choose.

A typical YAP meeting at Jigsaw takes place on a Friday evening or Saturday afternoon, and lasts approximately three hours. After a settling-in period we eat, get comfortable, and take a few minutes to have a casual catch-up with friends. Once everyone has settled in, attention shifts to the agenda. The meeting begins with a service update from our Youth and Community Engagement Worker, who might speak to wait times, number of appointments, or share news from National Office. This helps to inform our work, and gives us the opportunity to ask questions or raise concerns. We then typically move on to the programme of work. In some circumstances, the meeting takes the form of a training session, where we receive a presentation from staff or an external body and engage in a series of interactive activities. Regardless of format, the halfway point of every meeting is marked with a 'picnic lunch', which gives us a break, allows us to bond, and often facilitates further discussion of key issues. Meeting minutes are circulated after. We keep in touch between meetings using our group chat where we can share updates, further ideas, or sign up for additional ad hoc opportunities.

Karen Butler

At a national level, Jigsaw has a group of youth advocates who regularly represent the organisation at conferences and events and in the media. Within youth mental health promotion, young people are involved in informing and co-creating workshops and programmes; plans are in place to train them, as community champions, to deliver workshops to other young people. Young people are members of the organization's Youth Research Council (YRC) and research ethics committee, sit on interview panels, and contribute to public affairs campaigns and publications. Representatives also sit with Jigsaw's Board of Directors and on the Board Subcommittees. In addition, youth participation is embedded in Jigsaw's therapeutic services which are fundamentally person-centred in their orientation. Young people are centrally involved in their assessment and intervention plans, and satisfaction data are routinely gathered from young people to inform service delivery. An online service user forum is planned to ensure that the views of young people who have used Jigsaw services are informing future developments.

> While Jigsaw is an amazing organisation to be involved in, there have been instances where youth voice and bureaucracy have clashed. One example was Jigsaw's response to Blackout Tuesday, a social media campaign aimed at bringing attention to the Black Lives Matter movement. Jigsaw had not made any public commitment to this campaign. Each of the YAP members in my local service wrote to the leadership team articulating our feelings on the matter, with many of us expressing that Jigsaw's lack of acknowledgement of this campaign would affect many young people. As a result, Jigsaw promoted its commitment to the movement on social media and have put this into practice by joining the Irish Network Against Racism (INAR).
>
> Karen Butler

The benefits of youth participation in Jigsaw have been significant. Young people have ensured that services, policies and initiatives are youth friendly and responsive, and that the work of the organisation is credible, transparent and accountable. Early in 2020, Jigsaw partnered with Ireland's Department of Children, Equality, Disability, Integration and Youth (DCEDIY) to review and further improve the organisation's approach to youth participation. Following a comprehensive mapping of current practice, structured against the four areas of the Lundy (2007) model of participation, Jigsaw has decided to evolve practice towards a more fundamental rights-based approach and the obligations set out in Article 12 of the UNCRC. This will support the organization to more clearly define youth participation practice and how to better harness the voices and contributions of young people in decision-making, beyond, as well as within, Jigsaw.

Evidence on youth participation

A key challenge for participation is ensuring it is not tokenistic, but rather meaningful, effective and sustainable (Sinclair, 2004). Although there is currently no consensus on the best way to assess various dimensions of young people's participation (Bohnert et al. 2010), Lansdown (2006) suggests three elements should be considered when exploring how young people's participation is measured and evaluated:

(1) *scope*: to what degree participation has been achieved, (2) *quality*: the extent by which participatory processes comply with recognised standards for good practice, and (3) *impact*: the impact on young people, organisations and the wider community.

Often, there is a focus on measuring the scope/breadth of young people's participation, which typically involves measuring number of activities, their frequency, duration and/or attendees (Bohnert et al. 2010). More recently, there has been an emphasis on examining the quality of young people's involvement in particular initiatives, and their psychological engagement (Ramey et al. 2015; Ramey et al. 2018; Tiffany et al. 2012). High-quality engagement, which refers to sustained involvement in an activity outside of oneself, is believed to result from structural elements, such as having supportive staff, facilities, learning opportunities, voice in decision-making and individual engagement with programmes (Pancer et al. 2002; Tiffany et al. 2012). However, very few – if any – suitable measures of quality of youth participation exist, and research has rarely considered how young people's demographic or background characteristics influence the quality of their engagement. Further, questions are increasingly being asked about the impact of young people's participation (Crowley & Skeels, 2010; Thomas, 2010). It is proposed that studies evaluating effectiveness should examine the personal/social development of participation, such as changes in knowledge and skills, evaluate the effects of participation on organisational development, and assess the impact on society (Checkoway, 2011; Kirby et al. 2003).

Unfortunately, there is insufficient research on youth participation in mental health services (WEF, 2020). The available evidence largely describes individual outcomes for young people, as described earlier in this chapter. Less commonly, participation from members of minority groups and lessons from implementation of youth participation initiatives in mental health services have been articulated (Canas, 2019; Simmons et al. 2020). Youth engagement is least developed with respect to the articulation of outcomes at the organisational level, although this is partly due to the diversity of contexts where youth participation happens, and the scarcity or low applications of theoretical models to inform this work (Canas, 2019). Indeed, a systematic review examining youth involvement in secondary mental health services (Worrall-Davies & Marino-Francis, 2008) found no evidence of change in mental health services resulting from youth participation, but this review was limited to a small number of papers. Future research is required to address these gaps. This should facilitate young people's involvement on the monitoring, reporting and evaluation of instruments, strategies and programmes, and provide agency to young people as much as possible. It has also been suggested that any research/evaluation should be incorporated into existing systems and processes, to avoid becoming too onerous, and be considered as part of a wider learning culture (Brady, 2017; Johnson, 2010). It is important that research/evaluation provides flexibility for young people, and is rigorous but creative.

Recommendations for mental health services

There are a number of recommendations we can make to services interested in facilitating youth participation, to avoid tokenism, disillusionment and disengagement from young people:

1. Expectations and the purpose of participation should be discussed and agreed by all stakeholders at the outset, and reviewed as appropriate. Ideally, an existing model or framework of youth participation should be used to guide these conversations.
2. There should be a defined structure to enable participation and resources (including time, budget and dedicated staff) to support this group. Young people should be offered flexibility within these structures.
3. Consideration of how to create a warm and engaging environment for young people and facilitate their participation is important.
4. There should be some reflection on developmental stage, diversity and accessibility when recruiting young people for participation structures.
5. Training may be required for staff and young people, and supports for young people to assist with their personal and professional development.
6. A culture of participation, which may require change among senior management, staff and in policy, is crucial. Changing organisational culture may be complex and should take a top-down, bottom-up approach. Youth participation champions may help in this regard.
7. It is critical there is clear communication with young people, and feedback, so they feel valued and that their contributions are having impact. Ongoing reflection and evaluation is required.
8. There is a need to be mindful of the power dynamics that exist between staff members and young people.
9. Some assessment of the scope/breadth, quality and impact of young people's participation should be conducted, ideally in partnership with young people, and embedded in a wider learning culture within an organisation.
10. Finally, reflecting on ways of keeping young people engaged when they age out of participation structures, to maximise knowledge and further support young people in their development is important.

Conclusion

Young people between 10–24 years old account for almost a quarter of the total global population (Gupta, 2014). Many young people become involved in participation initiatives within mental health services because they want to make a difference, and sometimes this is driven by personal experience. As an emerging field of study, there is a need for a collective and better understanding of youth participation in mental health services, and the influence of participation on organisational outcomes (Checkoway & Gutierrez, 2006; UNDESA, 2013). Regardless, organisations must approach youth participation with a genuine desire and openness to value, listen and respond to the ideas of the young people they seek to serve. Each organisation should find the structure and environment that works best for them and the young people they are working with. Once this is in place, young people can often go a long way to address and guide the organisation in potential questions or obstacles that may arise.

Further reading

Brady, L.M. (Ed.). (2020). Embedding young people's participation in health services: New approaches. Bristol University Press.

Percy-Smith, B., & Thomas, N. (Eds.). (2010). *A handbook of children and young people's participation.* Routledge.

References

Barber, T. (2009). Participation, citizenship, and well-being: Engaging with young people, making a difference. *Young, 17*(1), 25–40. https://doi.org/10.1177/110330880801700103

Barry, J. (2014). *An investigation of youth participation in an Irish youth mental health service: Staff and young people's perspectives* (Unpublished Master's thesis). Dublin Institute of Technology: Dublin, Ireland.

Bohnert, A.M., Fredricks, J., & Randall, E. (2010). Capturing unique dimensions of youth organized activity involvement: Theoretical and methodological considerations. *Review of Educational Research, 80,* 576–610. https://doi.org/10.3102/0034654310364533

Bradbury-Jones, C., & Taylor, J. (2015). Engaging with children as co-researchers: Challenges, counter-challenges and solutions. *International Journal of Social Research Methodology, 18*(2), 161–173. https://doi.org/10.1080/13645579.2013.864589

Brady, L. M. (2017). Rhetoric to reality: An inquiry into embedding young people's participation in health services and research. PhD thesis, University of the West of England. Available from: http://eprints.uwe.ac.uk/29885

Cahill, H., & Dadvand, B. (2018). Re-conceptualising youth participation: A framework to inform action, *Children and Youth Services Review, 95,* 243–253. https://doi.org/10.1016/j.childyouth.2018.11.001

Canas, E. (2019). Working with Youth as Stakeholders in Mental health system Transformation: An Institutional Ethnography of a Service Organization in ACCESS Open Minds. Electronic Thesis and Dissertation Repository. 6327. https://ir.lib.uwo.ca/etd/6327

Charles, A., & Haines, K. (2014). Measuring young people's participation in decision making: What young people say. *International Journal of Children's Rights, 22,* 641-659. https://doi.org/10.1163/15718182-55680022

Checkoway, B. (2011). What is youth participation? *Children and Youth Services Review, 33*(2), 340–345. https://doi.org/10.1016/j.childyouth.2010.09.017

Checkoway, B., & Gutierrez, L. (2006) *Youth Participation and community change.* Routledge.

Coates, D., & Howe, D. (2014). The importance and benefits of youth participation in mental health settings from the perspective of the headspace Gosford Youth Alliance in Australia. *Children and Youth Services Review, 46,* 294–299.

Collin, P., Rahilly, K., Stephens-ReIcher, J., Blanchard, M., Herman, H., & Burns, J. (2009). *Inspire Foundation 2009 youth participation evaluation. Meaningful participation for promoting mental health and well-being of young Australians.* Inspire Foundation.

Collin, P., Rahilly, K., Stephens-Reicher, J. C., Blanchard, M., Herrman, H., & Burns, J. (2012). Complex connections: Meaningful youth participation for mental health promotion. *Youth Studies Australia, 31*(1), 36–47.

Crowley, A., & Skeels, A. (2010). Getting the measure of children and young people's participation: An exploration of practice in Wales. In S. Redsell & A. Hastings (Eds.), *Listening to children and young people in healthcare consultations* (pp 184–192). Radcliffe Publishing.

Day, C. (2008), Children's and young people's involvement and participation in mental health-care. *Child and Adolescent Mental Health, 13*, 2–8. https://doi.org/10.1111/j.1475-3588. 2007.00462.x

Ennis, L., & Wykes, T. (2013). Impact of patient involvement in mental health research: Longitudinal study. *British Journal of Psychiatry, 203*(5), 381–386. DOI: 10.1192/bjp.bp.112.119818.

Faithfull, S., Brophy, L., Pennell, K., & Simmons, M. B. (2019). Barriers and enablers to meaningful youth participation in mental health research: Qualitative interviews with youth mental health researchers. *Journal of Mental Health, 28*(1), 56–63. https://doi.org/10.1080/09638237.2 018.1521926

Farthing, R. (2012). Why youth participation? Some justifications and critiques of youth participation using New Labour's youth policies as a case study. *Youth & Policy, 109*, 71–97.

Fava, N., Simmons, M. B., Anderson, R., Zbukvic, I., & Baker, D. (2020). *Side by side: Supporting youth peer work in mental health services.* Orygen.

Fenton, S. J., Carr, S., Boyden, L., Molloy, J., Moyse, H., Rathore, I., Skinner, B., Tresadern, C., Virgo, H., Williams, B., & Campbell, N. (2020). Valuing youth involvement in mental health service design and delivery. In L. Theodosiou, P. Knightsmith, P. Lavis, & S. Bailey (Eds.), *Children and young people's mental health: Early intervention, ongoing support and flexible evidence-based care* (pp. 163–178). Pavilion Publishing and Media Ltd.

Gupta, M. D. (2014). *The power of 1.8 billion: Adolescents, youth and the transformation of the future.* United Nations Population Fund.

Hart, R. A. (1992) *Children's Participation: From Tokenism to Citizenship.* UNICEF International Child Development Centre.

Hawke, L. D., Relihan, J., Miller, J., McCann, E., Rong, J., Darnay, K., Docherty, S., Chaim, G., & Henderson, J. L. (2018). Engaging youth in research planning, design and execution: Practical recommendations for researchers. *Health Expectations, 21*(6), 944–949. https://doi. org/10.1111/hex.12795

Hawke, L. D., Mehra, K., Settipani, C., Relihan, J., Darnay, K., Chaim, G., & Henderson, J. (2019). What makes mental health and substance use services youth friendly? A scoping review of literature. *BMC Health Services Research, 19*(1), 257. https://doi.org/10.1186/s12913-019-4066-5

Head, B. W. (2011). Why not ask them? Mapping and promoting youth participation. *Children and Youth Services Review, 33*(4), 541–547. https://doi.org/10.1016/j.childyouth.2010.05.015

Heffernan, O. S., Herzog, T. M., Schiralli, J. E., Hawke, L. D., Chaim, G., & Henderson, J. L. (2017). Implementation of a youth-adult partnership model in youth mental health systems research: Challenges and successes. *Health Expectations, 20*(6), 1183–1188. https://doi.org/10.1111/hex.12554

Hetrick, S. E., Bailey, A. P., Smith, K. E., Malla, A., Mathias, S., Singh, S., O'Reilly, A., Verma, S. K., Benoit, L., Fleming, T. M., Moro, M. R., Rickwood, D. J., Duffy, J., Eriksen, T., Illback, R., Fisher, C. A., & McGorry, P. (2017). Integrated (one-stop shop) youth healthcare: Best available evidence and future directions. *Medical Journal of Australia, 207*(10), S5–S18. https://doi.org/10.5694/mja17.00694

Howe, D., Batchelor, S., & Bochynska, K. (2011). Finding our way: Youth participation in the development and promotion of youth mental health services on the NSW Central Coast. *Advances in Mental Health*, 20–28. https://doi.org/10.5172/jamh.2011.10.1.20

International Youth Foundation. (2012). *Opportunity for Action: Preparing youth for 21st century livelihoods.* https://www.iyfnet.org/sites/default/files/Opportunity_ for_ Action.pdf

James, A. M. (2007). Principles of youth participation in mental health services. *Medical Journal of Australia, 187*(7), S57. DOI: 10.5694/j.1326-5377.2007.tb01339.x

Johnson, V. (2010). Rights through evaluation and understanding children's realities. In B. Percy-Smith, & N. Thomas (Eds.), *A handbook of children and young people's participation: Perspectives from theory and practice* (pp. 154–163). Routledge.

Kirby, P., Lanyon, C., Cronin, K., & Sinclair, R. (2003). *Building a culture of participation: Involving children and young people in policy, service planning, delivery and evaluation.* National Children's Bureau.

Lansdown, G. (2006). International developments in children's participation: Lessons and challenges. In Tisdall E. K. M., Davis, J., Hill M., and Prout A. (Eds.), *Children, young people and social inclusion: Participation for what?* The Policy Press.

Lardner, C. (2001). Youth participation: A new model. http://www.clarity-scotland.pwp.blueyonder.co.uk/docs/downloads/model_ of_participation.pdf

Lundy, L. (2007) 'Voice' is not enough: Conceptualising Article 12 of the United Nations Convention on the Rights of the Child. *British Educational Research Journal, 33*(6), 927–942. https://doi.org/10.1080/01411920701657033

Malone, K, & Hartung, C. (2010). Challenges of participatory practice with children. In B. Percy-Smith & N. Thomas (Eds.), *A handbook of children and young people's participation: Perspectives from theory and practice* (pp. 24–39). Routledge.

McMahon, J. (2019). *Towards professionalisation: A project to undertake a feasibility study into the establishment of a member based organization for the peer workforce in Australia.* Private Mental Health Consumer Carer Network.

McPherson, A. (2010). Involving children: Why it matters. In Redsell S., & Hastings A. (Eds.), *Listening to children and young people in healthcare consultations* (pp. 15–29). Radcliffe Publishing

Monson, K., & Thurley, M. (2011). Consumer participation in a youth mental health service. *Early Intervention in Psychiatry, 5*(4), 381–88. https://doi.org/10.1111/j.1751-7893.2011.00309.x

O'Donnell, A. (2016). Child participation structures in Ireland: implementation of agency rights in the UNCRC. Master's thesis. Universite de Geneve.

Oliver, K.G., Collin, P., Burns, J. & Nicholas, J. (2006). Building resilience in young people through meaningful participation. *Australian e-Journal for the Advancement of Mental Health, 5*(1). https://researchonline.jcu.edu.au/3691/1/3691_Oliver_et_al_2006.pdf

O'Reilly, A., O'Brien, G., Moore, J., Duffy, J., Longmore, P., Cullinan, S., & McGrory, S. (2021). Evolution of Jigsaw–a National Youth Mental Health Service. *Early Intervention in Psychiatry, 16*(5), 561–67. DOI: 10.1111/eip.13218

Pancer, S. M., Rose-Krasnor, L., & Loiselle, L. D. (2002). Youth conferences as a context for engagement. *New Directions for Youth Development, 96*, 47–64. https://doi.org/10.1002/yd.26

Ramey, H. L., & Rose-Krasnor, L. (2015). The new mentality: Youth–adult partnerships in community mental health promotion. *Children and Youth Services Review, 50*, 28–37. https://doi.org/10.1016/j.childyouth.2015.01.006

Ramey, H. L., Rose-Krasnor, L., Busseri, M. A., Gadbois, S., Bowker, A., & Findlay, L. (2015). Measuring psychological engagement in youth activity involvement. *Journal of Adolescence, 45*, 237–249. https://doi.org/10.1016/j.adolescence.2015.09.006

Ramey, H. L., Lawford, H. L., Rose-Krasnor, L., Freeman, J., & Lanctot, J. (2018). Engaging diverse Canadian youth in youth development programs: Program quality and community engagement. *Children and Youth Services Review, 94*, 20–26. DOI: 10.1016/j.childyouth.2018.09.023

Roe, S., & McEvoy, O. (2011). *An audit of children and young people's participation in decision-making.* https://www.drugsandalcohol.ie/16278/1/DOC_childandyppart_decisionmaking.pdf

Rickwood, D., Paraskakis, M., Quin, D., Hobbs, N., Ryall, V., Trethowan, J., & McGorry, P. (2019). Australia's innovation in youth mental healthcare: The headspace centre model. *Early Intervention in Psychiatry, 13*(1), 159–166. https://doi.org/10.1111/eip.12740

Shier, H. (2001). Pathways to participation: openings, opportunities and obligations. *Children & Society, 15*(2), 107–117. https://doi.org/10.1002/chi.617

Simmons, M. B., Fava, N., Faliszewski, J., Browne, V., Chinnery, G., van der El, K., Hodges, C., Pennell, K., & Brushe, M. (2020). Inside the black box of youth participation and engagement: Development and implementation of an organization-wide strategy for Orygen, a national youth mental health organization in Australia. *Early Intervention in Psychiatry.* https://doi.org/10.1111/eip.13033

Simmons, M. B., Coates, D., Batchelor, S., Dimopoulos-Bick, T., & Howe, D. (2018). The CHOICE pilot project: Challenges of implementing a combined peer work and shared decision-making programme in an early intervention service. *Early Intervention in Psychiatry, 12*(5), 964–971. https://doi.org/10.1111/eip.12527

Sinclair, R. (2004). Participation in practice: Making it meaningful, effective and sustainable. *Children & Society, 18*(2), 106–118. https://doi.org/10.1002/chi.817

Thomas, N. (2010). Towards a theory of children's participation. *International Journal of Children's Rights, 15*(2007) 199–218. https://doi.org/10.1163/092755607X206489

Tiffany, J. S., Exner-Cortens, D., & Eckenrode, J. (2012). A new measure for assessing youth program participation. *Journal of Community Psychology, 40*(3), 277–291. https://doi.org/10.1002/jcop.20508

Tisdall, K.M. (2010). Governance and participation. In B. Percy-Smith & N. Thomas (Eds.), *A handbook of children and young people's participation: Perspectives from theory and practice* (pp. 318–329). Routledge.

Treseder, P. (1997) *Empowering children and young people training manual: Promoting involvement in decision-making.* Save the Children UK.

Un-Habitat and the Focal Point on Youth [UNDESA]. (2013). *Youth participation.* https://www.un.org/esa/socdev/documents/youth/fact-sheets/youth-participation.pdf.

United Nations [UN]. (2013). *Definition of youth [fact sheet].* Available from: https://www.un.org/esa/socdev/documents/youth/fact-sheets/youth-definition.pdf [Accessed 15 May 2020].

UNICEF. (2003). The state of the world's children 2003. https://www.unicef.org/publications/files/pub_sowc03_en.pdf

Wong, N. T., Zimmerman, M. A., & Parker, E. A. (2010). A typology of youth participation and empowerment for child and adolescent health promotion. *American Journal of Community Psychology, 46*(1–2), 100–114. https://doi.org/10.1007/s10464-010-9330-0

World Economic Forum [WEF]. (2020). A global framework for youth mental health: Investing in future mental capital for individuals, communities and economies. Available on https://www.weforum.org/reports/a-global-framework-for-youth-mentalhealthdb3a7364df/mentalhealth-approaches

World Health Organization [WHO]. (2018). *Engaging young people for health and sustainable development: Strategic opportunities for the World Health Organization and partners.* https://apps.who.int/iris/handle/10665/274368.

Worrall-Davies, A. (2008). Barriers and facilitators to children's and young people's views affecting CAMHS planning and delivery. *Child and Adolescent Mental Health, 13*(1), 16–18. https://doi.org/10.1111/j.1475-3588.2007.00456.x

Worrall-Davies, A., & Marino-Francis, F. (2008). Eliciting children's and young people's views of child and adolescent mental health services: A systematic review of best practice. *Child and Adolescent Mental Health, 13*(1), 9–15. https://doi.org/10.1111/j.1475-3588.2007.00448.x

Quotation from the parent of an adolescent who participated in Daráine Murphy's (2022) Doctoral Dissertation, University College Dublin:

'You have this hope and your desires for your children and suddenly it gets knocked out in terms of like I don't want my son feeling like this, you know, I don't want my son to have struggle and to go through these things. But at the same token this is part of his makeup. Emm so I would [say] our job [...] over the last two years [is]: (a) to support him though it and (b) trying to build that resilience in him'

12 | Family engagement and support

Daráine Murphy
University College Dublin, Ireland

Caroline Heary
National University of Ireland, Galway, Ireland

Eilis Hennessy
University College Dublin, Ireland

Susan Preece
Orygen, Australia

Introduction

Families are central to the lives of most young people and in times of distress may have an important role in the help-seeking process as well as in providing ongoing support. However, the role of the family has been conceptualised in a variety of different ways and through various lenses. Historically, families have frequently been seen as contributing to the cause of the mental disorder, sustaining the problem and/or contributing to relapse (Bland & Foster, 2012). This perspective contributed to stigma and shame both for the young person and other family members. An alternative and more inclusive perspective considers the involvement of families in mental health services as paramount in improving the experience and outcomes for the young person and also their family (Coates, 2016).

More recently there is a growing understanding that family may be able to offer a unique perspective on a young person's mental disorder and draw on knowledge and resources that will help recovery. It is also more widely recognised that families are dealing with a range of concerns about the young person and that family members need to be equipped with information and skills on how to provide help and support (Rickwood et al. 2014). There is also growing evidence that engaging families in youth mental health treatment has measurable positive outcomes. For example, it has reduced the incidence of relapse, improved adherence to treatment, improved family relationships and increased young people's well-being and social adjustment (Pitschel-Walz et al. 2001). Despite the acknowledged importance of taking a family perspective from the point of contact through intake, assessment and service provision, very often families feel excluded from the process (Boulter & Rickwood, 2013).

This chapter will provide a rationale for the importance of including families in the young person's recovery by looking at the value of family engagement for the young person as well as the other members of the family. The chapter provides an introduction to the literature on fostering families' initial engagement in services and, in turn, on ways to support and retain families in services (e.g. via psychoeducation, peer support and how to manage the family relationship and the young person's confidentiality). Finally, the importance of self-care for the parents, something that is often overlooked, will be highlighted with some questions for clinicians to use to encourage parents to think about their own self-care.

Family engagement

Family engagement typically refers to a wide range of activities that are intended to encourage and facilitate families to take an active role in supporting a young person with a mental health difficulty (Waid & Kelly, 2019). It can include activities designed to encourage professional help-seeking, and then to support continued engagement with therapy; it also includes encouraging family members to attend to, and be aware of, their own needs, strengths and resources (Waid & Kelly, 2020) and to contribute to shared decision-making about treatment (Hayes et al. 2021). Foster et al. (2016) refer to 'family-focused practice' rather than 'family engagement' but identify a similarly broad range of activities. They also note that 'family' is defined in different ways in the literature, at times referring primarily to parents and, in other studies, including siblings and extended family.

The important role that families can have in supporting young people is evident from research which has shown that between 28 per cent and 75 per cent of adolescents drop out of services prematurely and those who need services the most, including those with the most severe difficulties and low-income minority families, are at the greatest risk for dropping out of services (de Haan et al. 2013; Johnson et al. 2008). However, family engagement goes beyond attendance and retention in services. Families can also have a positive effect when they actively participate in a young person's treatment, respond to any requests of the practitioner and engage in efforts to support a young person outside of treatment. Foster et al. (2016) identify four principles that underpin family-focused practice: (1) families have a key role in supporting recovery; (2) families can be empowered to address and meet the needs of a family member with a mental health difficulty; (3) individuals with mental health difficulties can be supported via their family; (4) relationships with clinicians are important.

The experience and knowledge that families bring to a young person's treatment are very important. Family members know the young person's developmental history, are aware of adverse experiences and offer a unique perspective regarding their strengths, resourcefulness and abilities. Therefore, efforts should be made to engage and retain families in the young person's treatment in order to get the best outcomes. Waid & Kelly's (2020) review of the literature identified a number of barriers at an individual, service and community level which impact on the likelihood of families engaging with services. One such barrier is family awareness and attitudes towards mental health, help-seeking and mental health treatment. Research has shown that if parents are supportive and encourage their adolescent to seek help, they are subsequently more likely to obtain professional help (Gulliver et al. 2010). Financial difficulties, lack of time, conflicting work schedules, lack of transport and family obligations can also act as barriers to family engagement (Waid & Kelly, 2020). Community-level barriers include limited availability of services in a geographical area and community attitudes and stigma towards mental health; this is something that is particularly relevant in rural areas (Waid & Kelly, 2020).

At a service level the scheduling and referral process, flexibility and availability of services and provider competency/specialist availability can all impact on family engagement. If services have long wait times, no after-hours services, high turnover or under-qualified staff this can impact on the families' overall perception of the service, thus impacting on engagement. Services that take a family- and youth-centred approach that address the needs of the family at the outset have been found to have greater levels of engagement (Muir et al. 2012; Poon et al. 2019). When engaging families, it is important to look beyond retaining those who are already linked in with services and to ensure that some families are not missing out, for example, those from seldom heard backgrounds including minority ethnic groups. Minority groups are significantly less likely to seek help for mental health difficulties, experience more barriers when attempting to access services and are more likely to receive poorer quality care (Moore, 2018). This can be due in part to a lack of culturally sensitive mental health services for these individuals because of practitioners' lack of exposure to the families' culture or lack of awareness of potential cultural differences. Cultural adaptation of services can play an important role in the engagement of minority youth and their families (Moore, 2018).

Family engagement may also involve more than asking families to support a treatment regime determined by mental health professionals. Collaborative care planning is an increasingly important tool in recovery-oriented mental healthcare and the provision of personalised care. A care plan is developed by professionals in partnership with service users and their carers (Simpson et al. 2016). However, very little research has been conducted into the processes of care planning for youth. A recent review of families' experiences of care planning for adult mental health service users suggests that meaningful collaborative partnerships are absent in many contexts (Doody et al. 2017). However, we are not aware of any published research on the role of families in the care-planning process in adolescent mental health services.

Engaging families at a broader organisational level can be facilitated by building mechanisms and structures for the voice of families to influence policy and service development; partnering with family advocacy groups; and building meaningful and lasting relationships with families. The training of staff on family engagement can increase capacity for a wide range of inclusive practices. Actions taken at an organisation level can also include training and support for family members to take on advisory, mentoring or advocacy roles (Ontario Centre of Excellence for Child and Youth Mental Health, 2016).

With a growth in emphasis on health service engagement with the families of young people, there is a growing body of research on the effectiveness of different interventions to increase engagement for families of adolescents and young adults (Kim et al. 2012). For example, Szapocznik et al. (1988) used a form of therapist-led family intervention called Strategic Structural Systems Engagement (SSSE) to engage Latino adolescent drug users and their families in therapy. The goal of the intervention was to identify and reduce interactions that prevent family members from engaging with treatment. The intervention was successful at increasing both initial attendance and continuing engagement. Donohue et al. (1999) compared two interventions (a parent-only intervention and an intensive parent and youth intervention) for engaging families of youth diagnosed with substance use and conduct disorder. The parent-only intervention involved a telephone call prior to scheduling an appointment which outlined what was involved in treatment and the benefits to the family and the young person. Parents who received the intensive parent and youth intervention received the same phone call but more effort was put into building rapport with the parent. The parent also had an opportunity to discuss any concerns that they had about treatment. The intensive intervention resulted in greater attendance at the first appointment and more frequent attendance at appointments overall.

Evidence of the merits of family engagement has resulted in national and state policies increasingly emphasising the role of family in treatment for young people with mental health difficulties. For example, the Chief Psychiatrist's Guide from the Victoria State Government (2018) in Australia outlines practical ways for clinicians to engage families in a young person's treatment including: inviting family members to attend case-management meetings; collaborating with family members on developing and implementing treatment care and discharge plans; recognising the significant role that parents can play in a person's recovery; and the importance of support for all family members. Similar moves to promote greater participation of families in care planning exist across the UK (Department of Health, UK, 2008; Welsh Assembly Government, 2012). In Ireland, the most recent mental health policy recommends that individualised recovery-oriented plans are co-produced with service users and families, where appropriate, for all users of specialist mental health services (Department of Health, 2020).

Before concluding this section, it is important to note that the work designed to foster family engagement in child and adolescent mental health services has a strong applied focus, but there are few theoretical frameworks underpinning this work. One notable exception is the work of Olin and colleagues (Olin et al. 2010). These authors developed a Parent Empowerment Programme (PEP) based on explicit recognition of empowerment as a process and the need to support parents as active agents of change. The authors developed PEP, based on a strong theoretically driven approach called the Parents as Agents of Change model. This framework is built on an integrated theory of behaviour change and identifies the four key determinants of parents' intentions to engage in mental health treatment for their child as: (1) beliefs and the perceived value of initiating and participating in treatment; (2) social norms or pressure such as whether others in one's close circle are supportive of treatment; (3) attitudes towards mental health difficulties; and (4) self-efficacy.

A key principle of this approach is recognising parents' role in the help-seeking process. Using this framework, family advocates (typically parents of children with mental health difficulties who help other parents of children with similar difficulties) can identify what factors influence parents' intention to engage and participate in their child's care and identify strategies to address any barriers they face. The authors propose that this conceptual model can guide much-needed research efforts to assess the impact of family support services and empowerment-based approaches. Evaluation of this theory-based training programme has been found to improve the knowledge and self-efficacy of family peer advocates (Hoagwood et al. 2018).

To conclude, in recent years we have seen a paradigmatic shift towards more inclusive family policies and services internationally. The American Academy of Child and Adolescent Psychiatry AACAP (2009) advocates for the importance of families, youth and professionals working collaboratively to support individualised, strengths-based and culturally competent care. Families can play a key role in their child's care from the point of assessment, treatment planning, implementation, monitoring and outcome evaluation (AACAP, 2009). Inclusive mental health policies, system-wide supports, family engagement service models, and family capacity and readiness to engage are necessary to foster family, youth and health professional collaboration. Engaging young people and their families in services can improve outcomes for the young person but can also be an important source of support for parents, as we will highlight below. Evaluation of inclusive family practice is also needed. This is particularly the case for system-level initiatives designed to support family engagement given the scant research in this area.

Impact on the family

When adolescents and young adults experience a mental health difficulty it can have an impact on the overall family unit and each family member. The impact begins with the initial onset of symptoms and diagnosis as parents may recognise that their hopes and aspirations for their child may have to change. Parents very often go through stages of grieving and have to reframe their expectations for their child's future (Geraghty et al. 2011; Sin et al. 2017). However, for some parents, the onset of mental health difficulties in an adolescent can actually strengthen existing family relationships. Kuhn et al. (2014) note that, in practice, the relationship between family functioning and adolescent mental health is likely to be 'bi-directional and transactional' (p. 128), meaning that family well-being is influenced by the young person's well-being and vice versa.

There is a wealth of evidence that ongoing care for a relative with a mental health difficulty can put family members at greater risk of poor psychological and physical health (Angold et al. 1998; Geraghty et al. 2011), particularly if the young person alternates between periods of recovery and relapse. Families often report that they feel as if they are 'walking on eggshells' and the recovery journey is like being 'on a rollercoaster'. This can result in family members feeling exhausted, and carer fatigue is common especially if the mental health difficulty doesn't resolve quickly. In addition, parents may have to take leave from work or, in exceptional situations, may have to give up their job altogether to care for the young person (Ferrey et al. 2016). Parents may also have to take on responsibilities they had previously relinquished (for example, having a young adult return to live at home after living independently) and return to an earlier, more dependent form of the parent-child relationship such as monitoring medication, taking the young person to appointments and providing financial assistance, among others (McCann et al. 2011). Managing the family dynamic can also be challenging for parents, particularly if there are younger siblings who are unaware of what is going on.

In the past, parents were often blamed or judged for bad parenting when their child experienced a mental health difficulty (McFarlane, 2016). With more research highlighting the biological basis of mental disorders, and emphasis being placed on the key role of parents in the process of recovery, this has dispelled notions that parents are to blame. However, many parents still feel a sense of responsibility for their child's distress (Corrigan and Miller, 2004; Geraghty et al. 2011). For example, Curtis et al. (2018) found parents of young people who self-harm reported feelings of guilt and shame, doubts about their ability to parent effectively and fears of exacerbating self-harm. The discovery of self-harm can also lead to changes in parenting strategies and uncertainty on how to address the situation. Families fear they may provoke relapse or a suicide attempt if they put boundaries on a young person's behaviour.

Although the majority of studies on family engagement in young people with mental health difficulties focus on parents, there is a growing recognition that siblings also feel loss and grief about the mental ill-health of their brother or sister but might display that differently to parents. Siblings may also resent the perceived loss of parental time and attention. Although some studies published in the last five years have sought to understand the experiences of siblings, in most cases the focus has been on the specific circumstances of having a sibling with schizophrenia or psychosis. This means that very little is known about the experiences of siblings in families where there is a young person with a mental health difficulty or a non-psychotic mental disorder. Notwithstanding this rather narrow focus, we believe that it is important to highlight these research findings as they emphasise the importance of considering the experiences of siblings as part of the family.

Some insight into the experiences of siblings is provided by the findings of research by Sin et al. (2012) which noted that siblings of young people with psychosis found themselves taking on multiple roles within the family including providing emotional support, gathering and sharing illness-related information, monitoring symptoms and even supervising medication. They also documented a range of emotional responses reported by siblings including embarrassment (especially among the youngest siblings), resentment, guilt, stress and the feeling of having 'lost' the sibling they had prior to the onset of the illness. However, their accounts were not all negative and many reported feeling positive about improved family communications and feeling closer to their family. Graves et al. (2020) also highlighted positive experiences including the sense of solidarity within the family. Although not well documented, research by Bowman et al. (2017) and Sin et al. (2012) point to the relevance of gender, age and birth order as influences on sibling experiences.

Although the volume of research is not large, it is clear that serious mental disorders impact siblings and not just parents. It is also clear that siblings can have a positive supportive role either to their parents or to their ill sibling. However, more research is needed in order to better understand the kinds of supports that siblings of different ages need. Service providers should consider the roles that siblings may play and their need for developmentally appropriate psychoeducation, respite, education support and diversion activities (Baker et al. 2019).

Research findings documenting the range of challenges and concerns that families face serve to emphasise that family members need support too, and some of these are documented in the sections that follow.

Family psychoeducation

Often when a young person is initially diagnosed with a serious mental disorder, for example schizophrenia, the family's only knowledge about the illness may come from the media and will usually be negative. Psychoeducation helps to de-mystify the terminology for families. Families also have indicated that they see psychoeducation as giving them an opportunity to increase their understanding of the young person's illness, providing them with coping strategies and ensuring they feel supported as the young person accesses services (Leggatt, 2007). Family psychoeducation describes interventions designed to engage, inform and educate family members so that they feel empowered to help their family member experiencing mental ill-health (Anderson et al. 1980). It is commonly recommended for families with a member diagnosed with schizophrenia, major depression and bipolar disorder (McFarlane et al. 2003). The psychoeducational approach recognises that a mental disorder is only partially remediable by medication, and that families can have a significant role in their relative's recovery (McFarlane et al. 2003). It can incorporate cognitive behavioural and supportive therapeutic approaches, utilises a consultative framework and shares some common characteristic with structural family therapy (McFarlane, 2016).

A small number of family psychoeducation interventions have been designed for parents of adolescents and there are reasons to be cautiously optimistic about their value. For example, pilot research by Sanford et al (2006) evaluated an intervention that provided psychoeducation that aimed to increase families' knowledge about adolescent depression, understanding of the experience of depression and its impact on the family, to strengthen family communication and to enhance effective coping, problem solving, and management relapses. Overall, the programme was found to be successful in improving the parent-adolescent relationship and the adolescents' social functioning. A similarly positive outcome was reported by O'Donnell et al. (2017) who evaluated a programme specifically designed for parents of young people diagnosed with bipolar disorder. The intervention focused on a range of topics including medication adherence, relapse prevention, communication and problem solving. Adolescents assigned to the family-focused intervention reported improvements in the quality of family relationships and overall well-being compared to controls. However, an RCT by Bernal et al. (2019), comparing a psychoeducation intervention (TEPSI) as part of cognitive-behavioural therapy (CBT) to CBT alone with parents of adolescents who have major depressive disorder found no difference between the treatment (TEPSI) and control groups.

Peer support

Despite the value of psychoeducation for families, it cannot necessarily address all their needs. For example, parents can often feel isolated when managing a young person's mental health difficulty and navigating a complex healthcare system on their own. In order to address these wider concerns a range of additional family supports have been designed to support and empower families. Family peer support (also as known as a Parent Support Providers, Family Peer Advocates, Family Support Partners, Family Navigators) is usually provided by a parent who has lived experience of navigating the mental health system with their own child and has a good understanding of what the family is experiencing (Visa and Harvey 2019). Peer support differs from psychoeducation interventions described earlier, which are usually delivered by mental health professionals with the aim of supporting the young person's clinical outcomes. Peer support, on the other hand, is focused on providing support to the parents themselves to improve coping skills, reduce stress and to promote parental self-care (Hoagwood et al. 2010).

Emotional support and advocacy, identified by Hoagwood et al. (2010) as key components of family support, are most often employed in peer-delivered programmes. The aim is to ensure that parents do not feel isolated when managing their adolescent's difficulty and to decrease feelings of shame, guilt and helplessness. Peer support may also include an instrumental component linking parents to community-based services like transportation, childcare and social services. Finally, the advocacy component aims to empower parents by providing information about their rights and entitlements so parents can advocate for their adolescent in services (Hoagwood et al. 2010; Kuhn & Laird, 2014).

Unlike clinician-led family support (e.g. psychoeducation), peer-support programmes are less likely to have been empirically evaluated (and those that are evaluated rarely employ a RCT design). One programme that has been evaluated is Parent Connectors (Kutash et al. 2013). This nine-month programme was designed to improve outcomes for parents of adolescents with emotional difficulties. A family peer-support worker engaged with parents to empower them to see the benefit of engaging in their child's mental health services. A range of positive outcomes were reported with the greatest benefits for parents who were experiencing the most strain.

Self-care

Self-care refers to the performance of activities necessary to achieve, maintain or promote physical, mental and emotional health; it includes having the required level of social support and meeting one's social and psychological needs (Godfrey et al. 2011). The topic of self-care for parents of adolescents and young adults with mental health difficulties or mental disorders has received very little attention despite evidence that parents are likely to experience heightened stress and a range of other negative effects (Wingrove & Rickwood, 2019). Thus, we know very little about the extent to which this group of parents engage in self-care or how best to promote self-care and reduce the risk that they will feel overwhelmed

Table 12.1 Domains of self-care for parents

Domains to consider	Questions
Social support	Do you have people to support YOU? Friends? Family members?
Physical health	Have you checked up on your physical health lately? When did you last visit your GP?
Mental health	Would you consider some counselling? Would it help to have some training in reducing stress?
Communication	How is your communication with your adolescent/young adult?
Sleep	How are you sleeping? Do you have regular bed times?
Eating	Is your eating OK? Too little or too much?
Financial	How are you going financially? Have you checked whether there are financial supports available to you?
Social life/fun	Do you have a social life, hobbies, interests?
Learning/staying involved	Are you informed about mental health issues? Do you know where to find out more?

by their responsibilities. However, anecdotally, there are reports that family members (particularly the primary carer) can be resistant to the idea of carer self-care and may even regard any thoughts of it as 'selfish'. This can stem from a belief that if the service can 'fix' their loved one then life will go back to normal and that in the interim their focus should be on caring for their loved one, not about their own well-being.

In the absence of research on self-care among parents of young people with mental health difficulties, it is nonetheless possible to speculate on their self-care needs by drawing on a very small number of studies into research on self-care among other groups of parents. For example, Miller, A. E. et al. (2019) noted that the self-care needs of some foster parents may include a greater focus on nutrition and exercise, whereas others may need to focus on emotional self-awareness. Miller, J. J et al. (2019) reported that adoptive parents with better health and greater financial stability were more likely to engage in self-care than those with poorer health or less financial stability. It is very likely that parents of young people with mental health difficulties or mental disorders may have similar self-care needs and may face very similar barriers but more research is needed to identify these needs and any barriers that need to be overcome.

Miller, A. E. et al. (2019) note that professionals have a role in prompting parents to consider self-care and in providing information about how self-care can be implemented. However, they also need to consider that not all parents will have the resources necessary for some forms of self-care. Table 12.1 above indicates some of the domains of self-care that parents might be prompted to consider and the questions that professionals can ask.

There is now sufficient evidence from a wide range of studies on the stresses associated with family caring responsibilities, that self-care should be taken seriously in order to avoid parents becoming overwhelmed. However, there is still a need for more research to improve understanding of the specific needs of the parents of adolescents and young adults and to provide guidance to professionals on how best to offer advice. In any such research it will be most important to ensure that the needs of mothers and fathers are considered as the small number of studies conducted to date on parents' self-care needs have noted that we know almost nothing about fathers because they are far less likely to participate in research than mothers.

Information sharing

Throughout this chapter we have emphasised the importance of family as a source of support for an adolescent or young adult who is experiencing a mental health difficulty or a mental disorder. However, the nature and extent of support provided by the family is likely to vary significantly with the age of the young person, the type and severity of the difficulties they are experiencing, as well as their relationships with family. For example, the age at which young people can seek treatment independently of their parents varies between countries (European Union, 2017; McNarry, 2014), and those who are below the age for independent help-seeking will necessarily have parent/guardian involvement at the outset. For older adolescents and young adults, the nature of family support and their definition of family may be quite different. Partners may also become more involved as key sources of support.

Once the young person is engaging independently with a service provider there will be a need for professionals to find a balance between the family's need for information to assist them in their supporting role and the young person's right to privacy (Pinfold et al. 2007). A review of families' experiences of care planning in adult mental health services highlighted the complexities that confidentiality poses, often creating an impasse between families and mental health professionals (Doody et al. 2017). Several organisations have developed frameworks and guidance for professionals to help them achieve this balance between the rights of the young person and the needs of family members including Baker et al. (2019) in Australia, and Pinfold et al. (2007) in the UK. Key principles of these frameworks typically include having family, professionals and the young person come together to discuss information sharing; providing psychoeducation to help families understand the young person's experience; and providing families with information on the support options available to them. It is also always important to keep in mind that adolescence and early adulthood are times of significant social change with many transitions (e.g. moving out of home, starting employment) and a growing sense of independence, so the nature of the support needed is likely to change regularly and this needs to be considered. However, open engagement with families can help them to feel that they can be supportive to the young person and can allow them to adapt as circumstances change.

Need for further research

It is important to note that the majority of research on family engagement is focused on families of young people with the most serious diagnosed mental disorders (e.g. psychosis) and who have engaged with mental health services. Much less is known about the impact on family members of other mental disorders such as anxiety or depression. The experience of coping with a young family member who is depressed may be disruptive and distressing, particularly if professional support is difficult to access. It is even possible that the experience could have long-term consequences for family functioning that persists beyond the young person's recovery. To date, however, very little research has been conducted on the consequences of these situations on the family and how they cope.

In Chapter 8, Ndetei and colleagues emphasise the key role of families in supporting young people with mental health problems in Kenya and a recent systematic review by Pederson et al. (2019) has synthesised the findings of family interventions to support youth mental health in LMIC. Although the focus of the review was much broader than family engagement, nonetheless, the elements most commonly identified in the interventions overlap with studies that have focused on promoting family engagement in HIC including psychoeducation for caregivers, support networking, maintenance and relapse prevention. In the great majority of these studies there was a significant positive effect in the intervention group on youth mental health and well-being, as well as parenting behaviours and family functioning. Of importance in terms of the sustainability of such interventions is the fact that the majority were delivered by trained non-specialists, a feature of intervention delivery in LMICs that Healy et al. (2018) have identified as particularly valuable for scaling up mental health programmes. However, more high-quality research is needed as Pederson et al. (2019) note that only half of the studies in their review were rated as good quality.

A further gap in the research literature relates to the needs of families from minority cultural, ethnic and religious backgrounds and the design of culturally appropriate supports for these families. Such research may need to focus on how best to provide information on accessing mental health services and making information available in a medium that facilitates access (e.g. via local community/religious groups or through schools).

Further research is also needed on peer support and self-care. We have already noted the lack of research on peer support despite the fact that good quality research may provide insights into the kinds of training that peer-support workers need and the optimal types of support that can be provided. Self-care is also under-researched and what research exists typically focuses on the negative outcomes associated with lack of self-care (e.g. caregiver fatigue).

Conclusions

A notable shift has occurred internationally towards more family-centred and family-inclusive practices in youth mental healthcare. However, there is much work to be done in terms of evaluating family engagement initiatives. There is growing evidence that families have a key role to play in supporting young people with mental health difficulties and with diagnosed mental disorders. When the positive role that families can play in supporting and maintaining therapeutic intervention and recovery is recognised by professionals, the outcomes for young people are overwhelmingly positive. However, having a family member with a mental health difficulty can be challenging and families need support and advice to manage the ongoing demands. There is need for more research on family engagement including more research in LMICs on peer support and self-care.

Further reading

Baker, D., Burgat, L. & Stavely, H. (2019). *We're in this together: Family inclusive practice in mental health services for young people.* Melbourne: Orygen.

Logan, D. E., & King, C. A. (2001). Parental facilitation of adolescent mental health service utilization: A conceptual and empirical review. *Clinical Psychology: Science and Practice, 8*(3), 319.

Murphy, D., Heary, C., Hennessy, M., O'Reilly, M. D., & Hennessy, E. (2022). A Systematic Review of Help-Seeking Interventions for Parents of Adolescents. *Journal of Adolescent Health.* 70, 16–27.

Slade et al. (2007). Best practice when service users do not consent to sharing information with carers. *British Journal of Psychiatry, 190,* 148–155.

References

American Academy of Child and Adolescent Psychiatry. (2009). *Family and Youth Participation in Clinical Decision-Making.* https://www.aacap.org/AACAP/Policy_Statements/2009/Family_and_Youth_Participation_in_Clinical_Decision_Making.aspx

Anderson, C. M., Hogarty, G. E., & Reiss, D. J. (1980). Family treatment of adult schizophrenic patients: A psycho-educational approach. *Schizophrenia Bulletin, 6*(3), 490–505.

Angold, A., Farmer, E. M. Z., Costello, E. J., Burns, B. J., Stangl, D., & Messer, S. C. (1998). Perceived parental burden and service use for child and adolescent psychiatric disorders. *American Journal of Public Health, 88*(1), 75–80. https://doi.org/10.2105/AJPH.88.1.75

Baker, D., Burgat, L., & Stavely, H. (2019). *We're in this together: Family inclusive practice in mental health services for young people.* Melbourne: Orygen.

Bernal, G., Rivera-Medina, C. L., Cumba-Avilés, E., Reyes-Rodríguez, M. L., Sáez-Santiago, E., Duarté-Vélez, Y., Nazario, L., Rodríguez-Quintana, N., & Rosselló, J. (2019). Can cognitive-behavioral therapy be optimized with parent psychoeducation? A randomized effectiveness trial of adolescents with major depression in Puerto Rico. *Family Process, 58*(4), 832–854. https://doi.org/10.1111/famp.12455

Bland, R., & Foster, M. (2012). Families and mental illness: Contested perspectives and implications for practice and policy. *Australian Social Work, 65*(4), 517–534.

Boulter, E., & Rickwood, D. (2013). Parents' experience of seeking help for children with mental health problems. *Advances in Mental Health, 11*(2), 131–142.

Bowman, S., Alvarez-Jimenez, M., Wade, D., Howie, L., & McGorry, P. (2017). The positive and negative experiences of caregiving for siblings of young people with first episode psychosis. *Frontiers in Psychology, 8,* 730. doi: 10.3389/fpsyg.2017.00730

Coates, D. (2016). Client and parent feedback on a Youth Mental Health Service: The importance of family inclusive practice and working with client preferences. *International Journal of Mental Health Nursing, 25*(6), 526–535. https://doi.org/10.1111/inm.12240

Corrigan, P. W., & Miller, F. E. (2004). Shame, blame, and contamination: A review of the impact of mental illness stigma on family members. *Journal of Mental Health, 13*(6), 537–548. https://doi.org/10.1080/09638230400017004

Curtis, S., Thorn, P., Mcroberts, A., Hetrick, S., Rice, S., & Robinson, J. (2018). Caring for young people who self-harm: A review of perspectives from families and young people. *Mdpi.Com.* https://doi.org/10.3390/ijerph15050950

de Haan, A. M., Boon, A. E., de Jong, J. T. V. M., Hoeve, M., & Vermeiren, R. R. J. M. (2013). A meta-analytic review on treatment dropout in child and adolescent outpatient mental health-care. *Clinical Psychology Review 33*(5) (pp. 698–711). Pergamon. https://doi.org/10.1016/j.cpr.2013.04.005

Department of Health (2008). *Refocusing the care programme approach. Policy and positive practice guidance.* Department of Health.

Department of Health (2020) *Sharing the Vision: A Mental Health Policy for Everyone.* Department of Health Dublin

Donohue, B., Azrin, N. H., Lawson, H., Friedlander, J., Teichner, G., & Rindsberg, J. (1999). Improving initial session attendance of substance abusing and conduct disordered adolescents: A controlled study. *Journal of Child and Adolescent Substance Abuse, 8*(1), 1–13. https://doi.org/10.1300/J029v08n01_01

Doody, O., Butler, M.P., Lyons, R., & Newman, D. (2017). Families' experiences of involvement in care planning in mental health services: An integrative literature review. *Journal of Psychiatric and Mental Health Nursing, 24*, 412–430.

European Union Agency for Fundamental. Minimum age requirements related to the rights of the child in the EU. https://fra.europa.eu/en/publications-and-resources/data-and-maps/minag?-dataSource=MINAG_en_62756&media=png&width=740&topic=group05&question=MINAG_HE01&plot=MAP&subset=NONE&subsetValue=NONE&answer=MINAG_HE01&year=2017. Published 2017. Accessed January 19, 2021.

Ferrey, A. E., Hughes, N. D., Simkin, S., Locock, L., Stewart, A., Kapur, N., Gunnell, D., & Hawton, K. (2016). The impact of self-harm by young people on parents and families: A qualitative study. *BMJ Open, 6*(1), e009631. doi:10.1136/bmjopen-2015-009631

Foster, K., Mayberry, D., Reupert, A., Gladstone, B., Grant, A., Ruud, T., Falkov, A., & Kowalenko, N. (2016). Family-focused practice in mental health care: An integrative review, *Child & Youth Services, 37*(2), 129–155, DOI: 10.1080/0145935X.2016.1104048

Geraghty, K., Mccann, K., King, R., & Eichmann, K. (2011). Feature Article_ 730 253..262 Sharing the load: Parents and carers talk to consumer consultants at a child and youth mental health inpatient unit. *Wiley Online Library, 20*(4), 253–262. https://doi.org/10.1111/j.1447-0349.2011.00730.x

Godfrey, C. M., Harrison, M. B., Lysaght, R., Lamb, M., Graham, I. D., & Oakley, P. (2011). Care of self–care by other–care of other: The meaning of self-care from research, practice, policy and industry perspectives. *International Journal of Evidence-Based Healthcare, 9*(1), 3–24. doi:10.1111/j.1744-1609.2010.00196.x

Graves, J. M., Marsack-Topolewski, C. N., & Shapiro, J. (2020). Emerging adult siblings of individuals with schizophrenia: Experiences with family crisis. *Journal of Family Issues, 41*(11), 2002–2021. DOI:10.1177/0192513X20905327

Gulliver, A., Griffiths, K. M., & Christensen, H. (2010). Perceived barriers and facilitators to mental health help-seeking in young people: A systematic review. *BMC Psychiatry, 10*(1), 113. https://doi.org/10.1186/1471-244X-10-113

Hayes, D., Edbrooke-Childs, J., Town, R., Wolpert, M., & Midgley, N. (2021). A systematic review of shared decision making interventions in child and youth mental health: Synthesising the use of theory, intervention functions, and behaviour change techniques. *European Child & Adolescent Psychiatry,* 1–14. https://doi.org/10.1007/s00787-021-01782-x

Healy, E. A., Kaiser, B. N., & Puffer, E. S. (2018). Family-based youth mental health interventions delivered by nonspecialist providers in low- and middle-income countries: A systematic review. *Families, Systems, & Health, 36*(2), 182–187. doi:10.1037/fsh0000334.

Hoagwood, K. E., Cavaleri, M. A., Olin, S. S., et al. (2010). Family support in children's mental health: A review and synthesis. *Clinical Child and Family Psychology Review, 13*, 1–45.

Johnson, E., Mellor, D., & Brann, P. (2008). *Differences in dropout between diagnoses in child and adolescent mental health services.* https://doi.org/10.1177/1359104508096767

Kim, H. S., Munson, M. R., & McKay, M. M. (2012). Engagement in mental health treatment among adolescents and young adults: A systematic review. *Child and Adolescent Social Work Journal, 29*(3), 241–266. https://doi.org/10.1007/s10560-012-0256-2

Kuhn, E. S., & Laird, R. D. (2014). Family support programs and adolescent mental health: Review of evidence. Adolescent Health, Medicine and Therapeutics, 5, 127–142. http://dx.doi.org/10.2147/AHMT.S48057

Kutash, K., Duchnowski, A. J., Green, A. L., & Ferron, J. (2013). Effectiveness of the Parent Connectors program: Results from a randomized controlled trial. *School Mental Health*, 5(4), 192–208.

Leggatt, M. S. (2007). Minimising collateral damage: Family peer support and other strategies. *Medical Journal of Australia, 187*(S7), S61–S63.

Mccann, T. V., Lubman, D. I., & Clark, E. (2011). First-time primary caregivers' experience accessing first-episode psychosis services. *Early Intervention in Psychiatry, 5*(2), 156–162. https://doi.org/10.1111/j.1751-7893.2010.00246.x

McFarlane, W. R. (2016). Family interventions for schizophrenia and the psychoses: A review. *Family Process, 55*(3), 460–482. https://doi.org/10.1111/famp.12235

McFarlane, W. R., Dixon, L., Lukens, E., & Lucksted, A. (2003). Family psychoeducation and schizophrenia: A review of the literature. *Journal of Marital and Family Therapy, 29*(2), 223–245. https://doi.org/10.1111/j.1752-0606.2003.tb01202.x

McNary, A. (2014). Consent to treatment of minors. *Innovations in Clinical Neuroscience, 11*(3–4), 43–45. http://www. ndaa.org/pdf/Minor C

Miller, A. E., Green, T. D., & Lambros, K. M. (2019). Foster parent self-care: A conceptual model. *Children and Youth Services Review, 99*, 107–114. doi.org/10.1016/j.childyouth.2019.01.014

Miller, J. J., Niu, C., Womack, R., & Shalash, N. (2019). Supporting adoptive parents: A study on personal self-care. *Adoption Quarterly, 22*(2), 157–171. doi.org/10.1080/10926755.2019.1627451

Moore, K. L. (2018). Mental health service engagement among underserved minority adolescents and young adults: A systematic review. *Journal of Racial and Ethnic Health Disparities, 5*(5), 1063–1076. https://doi.org/10.1007/s40615-017-0455-9

Muir, K., Powell, A., & McDermott, S. (2012). 'They don't treat you like a virus': Youth-friendly lessons from the Australian National Youth Mental Health Foundation. *Health & Social Care in the Community, 20*(2), 181–189. https://doi.org/10.1111/j.1365-2524.2011.01029.x

O'Donnell, L. A., Axelson, D. A., Kowatch, R. A., Schneck, C. D., Sugar, C. A., & Miklowitz, D. J. (2017). Enhancing quality of life among adolescents with bipolar disorder: A randomized trial of two psychosocial interventions. *Journal of Affective Disorders, 219*, 201–208. https://doi.org/10.1016/j.jad.2017.04.039

Olin, S. S., Hoagwood, K. E., Rodriguez, J., Ramos, B., Burton, G., Penn, M., Crowe, M., Radigan, M., & Jensen, P. S. (2010). The application of behavior change theory to family-based services: Improving parent empowerment in children's mental health. *Journal of Child and Family Studies, 19*, 462–470.

Ontario Centre of Excellence for Child and Youth Mental Health. (2016). *Evidence in-sight: BEST practices in engaging families in child and youth mental health.* https://www.cymh.ca/modules/ResourceHub/?id=071CBA9D-C9A9-497A-9919-7E6960285D3A

Pedersen, G. A., Smallegange, E., Coetzee, A., Hartog, K., Turner, J., Jordans, M. J., & Brown, F. L. (2019). A systematic review of the evidence for family and parenting interventions in low- and middle-income countries: Child and youth mental health outcomes. *Journal of Child and Family Studies, 28*(8), 2036–2055. doi.org/10.1007/s10826-019-01399-4

Pinfold, V., Rapaport, J., & Bellringer, S. (2007). Developing partnerships with carers through good practice in information sharing. *Mental Health Review Journal, 12*(2), 7–14.

Pitschel-Walz, Q., Leucht, S., Bduml, J., Kissling, W., & Engel, R. (n.d.). *The Effect of Family Interventions on Relapse and Rehospitalization in Schizophrenia – A Meta-analysis.* https://academic.oup.com/schizophreniabulletin/article/27/1/73/1828973

Poon, A. W. C., Harvey, C., Fuzzard, S., & O'Hanlon, B. (2019). Implementing a family-inclusive practice model in youth mental health services in Australia. *Early Intervention in Psychiatry, 13*(3), 461–468. https://doi.org/10.1111/eip.12505

Rickwood, D., Anile, G., Telford, N., Thomas, K., Brown, A., & Parker, A. (2014). Service innovation project component 1: Best practice framework. Melbourne: headspace.

Sanford, M., Boyle, M., Mccleary, L., Miller, J., Steele, M., Duku, E., & Offord, D. (2006). A pilot study of adjunctive family psychoeducation in adolescent major depression: Feasibility and treatment effect. *Journal of the American Academy of Child and Adolescent Psychiatry, 45*, 386–395. https://doi.org/10.1097/01.chi.0000198595.68820.10

Simpson, A., Coffey, M., Hannigan, B., Barlow, S., Cohen, R. L., Jones, A., Faulkner, A., Thornton, A., Všetečková, J., Haddad, M. and Marlowe, K (2016). Cross-national comparative mixed-methods case study of recovery-focused mental healthcare planning and co-ordination: Collaborative Care Planning Project (COCAPP). *Health Services and Delivery Research, 5*(4). DOI: 10.3310/hsdr05260

Sin, J., Moone, N., & Wellman, N. (2005). Developing services for the carers of young adults with early-onset psychosis: Listening to their experiences and needs. *Journal of Psychiatric and Mental Health Nursing, 12*(5), 589–597. https://doi.org/10.1111/j.1365-2850.2005.00883.x

Sin, J., Moone, N., Harris, P., Scully, E., & Wellman, N. (2012). Understanding the experiences and service needs of siblings of individuals with first-episode psychosis: A phenomenological study. *Early Intervention in Psychiatry, 6*(1), 53–59. doi:10.1111/j.1751-7893.2011.00300.x

Sin J., Gillard, S., Spain, D., Cornelius, V., Chen, T., & Henderson, C. (2017). Effectiveness of psychoeducational interventions for family carers of people with psychosis: A systematic review and meta-analysis. *Clinical Psychology Review, 56*, 13–24. https://doi.org/10.1016/j.cpr.2017.05.002

Staudt, M. (2007). Treatment engagement with caregivers of at-risk children: Gaps in research and conceptualization. *Journal of Child and Family Studies, 16*(2), 183–196. https://doi.org/10.1007/s10826-006-9077-2

Szapocznik, J., Perez-Vidai, A., Brickman, A. L., Foote, F. H., Santisteban, D., Hervis, O., & Kurtines, W. M. (1988). Engaging adolescent drug abusers and their families in treatment: A strategic structural systems approach. *Annual Review of Addictions Research and Treatment, 1*(C), 331–336. https://doi.org/10.1037//0022-006x.56.4.552

Victoria State Government (2018). Working together with families and carers. Chief Psychiatrist's guideline. https://www2.health.vic.gov.au/about/key-staff/chief-psychiatrist/ chief-psychiatrist-guidelines.

Visa, B., & Harvey, C. (2019). Mental health carers' experiences of an Australian Carer peer support program: Tailoring supports to carers' needs. *Health & Social Care in the Community, 27*(3), 729–739. DOI: 10.1111/hsc.12689

Waid, J., & Kelly, M. (2020). Supporting family engagement with child and adolescent mental health services: A scoping review. *Health and Social Care in the Community, 28*(5), 1333–1342. https://doi.org/10.1111/hsc.12947

Welsh Assembly Government (2012). Code of Practice to Parts 2 and 3 of the Mental Health (Wales) Measure 2010. Welsh Assembly Government, Cardiff.

Wingrove, C. & Rickwood, D. (2019). Parents and carers of young people with mental ill-health: What factors mediate the effect of burden on stress?, *Counselling Psychology Quarterly, 32*(1), 121–134. DOI: 10.1080/09515070.2017.1384362

Quotation from a young person with social anxiety disorder who participated in Cal McDonagh's (2020) Doctoral Dissertation, University College Dublin:

'It meant a lot to me because [...] there was something that was worth hearing about. It wasn't something that I was just like a nuisance, or I wasn't just like attention-seeking or weird. That it was serious and ... that people would actually listen to me.'

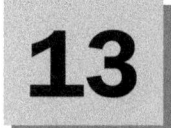

13 Service structure models

Sarah Hetrick
University of Auckland, New Zealand

Alan Bailey
University of Melbourne, Australia

Alex Parker
Victoria University, Melbourne, Australia

Introduction

In the last decade several models of youth mental health service delivery have emerged in different parts of the world that exemplify the key elements of the International Declaration on Youth Mental Health (Coughlan et al. 2013) and the World Economic Forum's *A Global Framework for Youth Mental Health* (2020). This chapter will briefly introduce some models that are in line with the principles of the International Declaration on Youth Mental Health (Coughlan et al. 2013) and the World Economic Forum's Global Framework for Youth Mental Health (2020).

Background

Mental health disorders are the leading cause of disability and poor outcomes in young people, who bear the major burden of mental health disorders (GBD 2019 Diseases and Injuries Collaborators, 2020; Gore et al. 2011). The contribution to the global burden of disease is because of the investment in young people with a view to them becoming socially and economically productive, with mental disorders therefore potentially disrupting the most productive years of life. The onset of mental disorders peaks in adolescence and early adulthood with 35 per cent of disorders emerging before 14 years old, 48 per cent before 18 years old, and 62.5 per cent before 25 years old (Solmi et al. 2021). In addition, a large proportion of young people may experience subthreshold mental health problems, stress and distress that also have tremendous impact on their well-being and functioning (Pascoe et al. 2019). Young people have experienced considerable insecurity in recent decades with rapid technological innovation, significant and frequent economic recessions, climate change (including catastrophic climate events), and recently the COVID-19 pandemic, an extreme version of a series of threatening health and well-being incidents over the last several decades. At the same time, this age group have experienced relatively poor access to a range of services to address these needs. Some reports suggest that up to 75 per cent of young people with mental health difficulties may not access a service and, even when they do, they may not engage in the service in a way that results in benefit (Cosgrave et al. 2008).

Specific and significant prevention and intervention that is early, responsive to broad needs, sustained and recovery focused is urgently required. This represents significant policy and service-delivery reform. This must be underpinned by a strengths-based approach that acknowledges protective factors such as having positive relationships with peers, family and other people in the community; supportive family environments; good emotional and mental well-being; strong cultural identity; physical health; active engagement in their community; and adequate levels of economic well-being, education and employment. In order for this to be meaningfully achieved it is increasingly acknowledged that the structural and social determinants of health must be addressed (Welsh et al. 2015). The World Health Organization's Commission on Social Determinants of Health conceptualframeworkhighlightsthatthesocio-political(socialandpublicpolicy),socio-economic (macro-economic policies) and socio-cultural environment (colonisation, racisms, discrimination) influences an individual's socio-economic position (income, education, occupation). These structural and social determinants interact with individual factors, resulting in inequity in health outcomes, including mental health (Solar & Irwin, 2010) (see also Chapter 3 on the structural and social factors influencing youth mental health). Addressing these factors and the influence they have on mental health outcomes for young people is critical in reform.

Various significant pieces of work have been progressed that form the basis of this required service reform. This includes early work by the World Health Organization (World Health Organization, 2012) and Orygen, an internationally renowned mental health research and clinical centre of excellence in Australia, to establish guiding principles for youth mental health services. The principles highlight the need for an evidence-informed continuum of care and easy transition between services to ensure timely access to what is needed, when it is needed. Services must be 'youth friendly', ensure youth participation across service development and delivery (see also Chapter 11), and appropriate autonomy and self-determination, via approaches such as shared decision-making (Simmons et al. 2010), in the context of understanding the developmental stage of a young person. Family-sensitive practice means that, where appropriate and relevant, families are involved (see also Chapter 12). Services must be responsive to diverse cultural and ethnic backgrounds and ensure equity in access and care. Assertive and comprehensive treatment for those with severe and complex mental disorders, and provision of a comprehensive range of services relevant for a holistic recovery-focused approach, are highlighted as important (Hughes et al. 2017).

International Declaration on Youth Mental Health

The International Declaration on Youth Mental Health (the 'International Declaration') was documented in 2013 on the basis of a Youth Mental Health Summit held in 2010 in Killarney, Ireland, that included a range of stakeholders, and importantly, young people themselves (Coughlan et al. 2013). The International Declaration sets out a vision, core principals and targets for youth mental health service provision. The objectives include: (1) reductions in mortality, including mortality due to suicide; (2) increased mental health literacy for young people (see Chapter 7), their families and communities so that there is an improved understanding of youth mental health in communities; (3) training in youth mental health approaches and interventions so that those who need support are recognised and provided with support that has a focus on resiliency, hope and recovery; (4) universally available and accessible youth-focused mental health specialist services that are strengths based and ensure equitable outcomes; and (5) meaningful youth and family participation in service development.

Global Framework for Youth Mental Health

In 2019 the World Economic Forum partnered with Orygen to develop a framework to guide service delivery as a response to the Forum's prioritisation of action on mental health. The Global Framework for Youth Mental Health (the 'Framework') sets out the economic imperative to ensure early and responsive youth mental health services. The Framework builds on the above key pieces of work. It was developed on the basis of evidence and extensive international stakeholder consultation, which included the meaningful involvement of young people in the development of the Framework. The aim was for the Framework to be internationally relevant and to guide local implementation (including strong local involvement) of youth mental health service delivery.

The Framework consists of eight guiding principles for youth mental health service delivery:

1. Rapid, easy and affordable access
2. Youth-specific care
3. Awareness, engagement and integration
4. Early intervention
5. Youth partnership
6. Family engagement and support
7. Continuous improvement
8. Prevention

Together, the International Declaration and the Framework, along with guiding principles from the WHO and Orygen, provide a roadmap for youth-responsive services. In summary, youth mental health services should be accessible to young people including being community based and in youth-friendly locations. They should be comfortable and welcoming places for youth to be, with the focus on decreasing stigma and discrimination. Cost should be removed as a barrier; hours of operation should suit young people and self-referral must be acceptable. There should be trained staff who understand the unique developmental features of this age group, and how to support youth appropriately. Mental health and social care must be integrated into general or primary care (World Health Organization, 2001, 2012b), and there should be integration with secondary and tertiary care so that while primary care might be leveraged as a point of access, there is immediate access to specialist care if it is needed. In both primary care and specialist care, the service provision must be specifically responsive to the needs of youth. There must be a continuity of care across these services, and other relevant services, ensuring holistic care that addresses the whole range of needs that a young person might present with. This includes being mindful and responsive to all phases of development within this broad youth age group with good transition into adult services if and when required. The basis of service delivery should be evidence based and the focus must be on outcomes that not only include the resolution of symptoms but also participation in education, vocation, meaningful relationships and activities and the community. The culture of service provision must be strengths based and focused on hope and recovery ensuring respect and eliminating systemic and structural racism and discrimination, as well as interpersonal racism and discrimination directed towards service users. Services should integrate digital and face-to-face services. The meaningful engagement of young people and their families in design and the ongoing delivery of these services is essential. In summary, services should be culturally safe and responsive, evidence based, integrated and offer holistic care.

International models of youth mental health service delivery

As identified in a comprehensive review of these services in 2017 (Hetrick et al. 2017), real-world implementation of youth mental health services on the basis of this roadmap might look different in different settings. Indeed, there are a number of initiatives that have developed internationally, which demonstrate variation in terms of the nature of integration, accessibility, youth participation and particulars of service provision. This is not surprising given their evolution within a particular historical, philosophical, cultural, fiscal and political context that give rise to differences in the way these services are deployed. Integration across mental health and social care can be implemented in a number of ways: for example via the operation of one youth centre where all staff are trained to provide all services, or via co-location where separate services are housed under one roof. It can also mean that services operate with an integrated referral, medical record and single treatment plan. Further, whatever approach is used, it is essential that young people are not pushed between pillar and post and lost somewhere in between.

The vast majority of these services have only been established since 2000, with the exception of New Zealand's Youth One Stop Shops (YOSSs), which was established as a concept in 1994, and the Adolescent Health Service in Israel in 1993. The review highlighted the variation in the age services included as 'youth'; some were only for those up to 18, the majority were for those up to the age of 24, and in one case the service was provided for those up to age 30. While all of the services included at least some range of service, some were specifically described as focusing on mental health, while the YOSS network in New Zealand was described by their stakeholders that they were not explicitly a mental health service (NZ YOSS) with their origins in a youth developmental model within a Maori (Indigenous people of New Zealand) holistic model of health. Even within networks of services, there was variation in terms of the services available within any one service centre. Interventions delivered across youth mental health services therefore tend not to be well-defined and may be delivered inconsistently across services.

Accessibility was operationalised as including walk-in and self-referral options, being located centrally or close to public transport and offering appointments outside of normal school and business hours. Some services described having a 'shop front', which typically is the use of café style street frontage. This is designed to address the fact that young people are attuned to stigma with regard to mental health difficulties and prefer signage that does not alert people to the service being clinical or mental health focused. Some of the larger networks of youth mental health services have used branding to its full advantage which, when linked to a good communication strategy (marketing), can increase accessibility.

Ideally the environment is purpose-built for youth, or fitted out to be youth friendly, which typically means having an informal, relaxed and non-clinical aesthetic. The environment might be decorated/designed by youth to ensure it is attractive, and might include café features like music, availability of coffee and tea, wi-fi and computer access, and activities. Peer or layperson first point of contact may be used as a way to provide a warm entry to service. A drop-in element has often been included in the design of these services. Permanent youth reference groups are often a feature and some services provide youth peer support, which is highly valued by young people.

There has been some work done internationally to evaluate these services. They appear to have increased access to care for young people, and there is evidence that there are some young people who would not have otherwise accessed any type of health or mental healthcare if a youth mental health service had not been available. Because of the way these services are funded and deployed, the types of evaluations that are undertaken mean that data on impact or outcome are often not available. Where data are available, there is some indication that a timely service (shorter wait time) can be provided. Young people report these services to be helpful. While measured in different ways there are many reports indicating positive outcomes in terms of improved mental health, including for some of the most adverse of outcomes of mental health difficulties (suicidal ideation and self-harm). There are also many reports indicating improved functioning as a result of receiving support from a youth mental health service, including improvement in school or work engagement, in confidence and self-esteem, and physical health.

Typically, youth mental health services are offering only relatively brief interventions, but there is some indication that levels of improvement are higher when more treatment sessions are received. Typically designed to support those with mild to moderate difficulties, these services nevertheless are attracting those with severe and complex difficulties. What is important here is to ensure that there is appropriate resourcing and integration with secondary and tertiary care to ensure the needs of all young people who are presenting to these services are addressed. At the same time, specialist services need to ensure the principles of youth mental health care provision are integrated into their service models and practices, which will further support seamless care for young people.

Across the youth mental health services that have been described in the literature to date, there are some features young people have highlighted as important for ensuring they are accessible, acceptable and appropriate. These resonate with the International Declaration and the Framework, along with guiding principles from Orygen and include:

- the convenient and appropriate location of services (access to public transport was noted as useful)
- services that were youth friendly (staff and environment) and welcoming
- services staffed by young people
- when appointments were made in a timely way
- the low cost of services
- the maintenance of contact and outreach
- the maintenance of confidentiality and privacy
- the availability of a wide range of integrated services in one place with non mental health signage
- safe and appropriate interventions delivered in a positive, and strengths-based framework.

Specific examples of models of youth mental health service

headspace

Australia's National Youth Mental Health Foundation – *headspace* – was established in 2006 with funding from the Australian Federal Government. The *headspace* initiative was developed in response to the urgent need to provide more effective, engaging and accessible mental healthcare services for young people (McGorry et al. 2007). While the services delivered by *headspace* have expanded since its establishment to include an online platform (*eheadspace*), mental health promotion (*headspace* schools), *headspace* interactive website and psychosis treatment programmes (*headspace* early psychosis), the national network of *headspace* centres are the core of the initiative. *headspace* centres are integrated primary care services that provide early intervention for mental health problems for young people aged 12–25 years old. Starting with 10 *headspace* centres in 2007, the initiative has been scaled up to over 130 centres in operation throughout Australia, in a mix of metro/urban, regional and rural locations (Rickwood, Paraskakis et al. 2019). Each centre aims to deliver integrated services to respond to the mental health, general health, alcohol and other drug, and work and study concerns and needs of young people.

headspace centres aim to build the capacity of the local services in the areas in which they are located. The funding model provides for core *headspace* centre staff to work with mental health services, general practitioners, community-based health and well-being services, local schools and educational services, and youth services, to provide additional supports for young people while they are receiving mental health treatment at *headspace*. On the whole, mental health treatment is provided by the Better Access Scheme within Australia's Medicare Benefits Schedule, where private allied health practitioners (e.g. psychologists, social workers, occupational therapists, etc.) deliver fee-for-service treatment sessions within *headspace* centres (McGorry et al. 2007). Young people are eligible for up to 10 psychological treatment sessions per annum; however, due to increased need and demand during the COVID-19 pandemic, an additional 10 sessions were available until June 2022. Described in detail by Rickwood, Paraskakis et al. (2019), the *headspace* centre model has 16 core components that address service provision and system enablers. These include youth participation (treatment planning, service development and governance); participation of family and friends in supporting young people; community awareness; enhanced access by addressing known barriers to care; provision of early intervention and appropriate care; evidence-informed practice; providing integrated services, as well as supporting transitions to and from other services. Examples of supporting transitions may be liaising with school or employers, referral to tertiary services if required for complex care management, and for young people 'ageing out' of *headspace* and requiring access to adult mental healthcare.

Service and outcomes data from the *headspace* initiative are publicly available through independent evaluations, peer-reviewed publications by the *headspace* national evaluation team and academics associated with *headspace*, and by individual *headspace* centres that are affiliated with academic institutions. Combined, these data show that *headspace* has successfully increased the access of young people to youth mental health services, predominantly for mental health difficulties and situational problems such as bullying or relationship problems; (Rickwood, Telford et al. 2015), and has been able to reach marginalised young people, including those who identify as LGBTIQA+ and those who are disengaged from work or study (Hilferty et al. 2015). Results from a large file audit (n > 24,000) demonstrated that over a third of young people attending a *headspace* centre for treatment showed significant improvements in psychological distress and psychosocial functioning (Rickwood, Mazzer et al. 2015). These findings were replicated by the independent evaluation that showed around half of young people experienced a reduction in psychological distress, with 13 per cent demonstrating a clinically significant reduction (Hilferty et al. 2015).

The online mental health support and counselling service, *eheadspace*, was established in 2011 to address the high demand for youth mental health services that could not be met by in-person services (Rickwood, Wallace et al. 2019). The *eheadspace* service has increased access and reach for young people in regional or rural areas and for those who have a preference for online services. Recent *eheadpsace* service data indicates a steady increase in access and engagement, with over 35,000 young people using the service annually (*headspace*, 2020). Similar to the face-to-face *headspace* centres, young people predominantly access *eheadspace* for mental health difficulties (depression and anxiety) and situational problems, with a majority of females accessing the service, but also demonstrating access by LGBTIQA+ young people (*headspace*, 2020). The majority of young people are satisfied with the *eheadspace* service, with greater engagement with the service associated with greater satisfaction (Rickwood, Wallace et al. 2019).

Part of the challenge in delivering clinically meaningful outcomes is that most young people who seek assistance from a *headspace* centre report high to very high levels of psychological distress (Hilferty et al. 2015). The *headspace* model was originally designed and developed to provide early intervention for young people with mild to moderate common ('high prevalence') mental disorders. However, due to ongoing high demand of mental health and psychosocial services, this means that many *headspace* centres are offering services to young people with complex psychosocial and behavioural concerns, comorbid diagnoses and severe mental disorders (Filia et al. 2021; Hilferty et al. 2015). Additionally, waiting times continue to be a major concern, with an average wait time of almost one month for a first therapy appointment (*headspace*, 2019). In response, the Federal Government recently announced additional funding as part of a demand management and enhancement programme for *headspace* centres.

The *headspace* initiative, including *headspace* centres and the online *eheadspace* service, has been successful in increasing access to youth-friendly mental healthcare for young Australians, most of whom report a high level of satisfaction with the services they received (Rickwood et al. 2017). The model continues to be developed and refined, with the addition of specialised services to address early psychosis, national initiatives to offer more brief and timely interventions for those with milder presentations (see, for example, Schley et al. 2019) and continuous evaluation to improve service delivery and further understand the challenges to ensuring all young people can access and engage with appropriate and effective mental healthcare (Rickwood, Wallace et al. 2019).

Jigsaw model

Jigsaw: The National Centre for Youth Mental Health, Ireland is an early intervention mental health service (Illback & Bates, 2011). Similar to Australia's *headspace* model, Jigsaw provides targeted youth-specific mental health support to young people aged 12–25 years old, with 13 centres located in communities across Ireland. Jigsaw uses a model of primary healthcare and aims to support young people with mild to moderate mental health concerns. Around half of the young people who attend a Jigsaw service do so for a 'brief intervention', which Jigsaw defines as up to six sessions of therapeutic support with a mental health professional, and a quarter engage in 'brief contact' of one or two sessions for the provision of information or advice (O'Reilly et al. 2015).The final quarter of contacts are 'case consultations', providing mental health information and advice to parents, guardians, teachers or other individuals involved with a young person. The most common concerns for young people attending Jigsaw services are problems with their emotions and thoughts, with anxiety, depression, self-harming behaviour and anger issues among the main presentations. Again, similar to *headspace*, Jigsaw engages with a range of health and mental health services, education, other community and social services, youth and substance-use programmes in order to provide a collaborative approach to managing a young person's mental health and well-being.

Jigsaw offers online support in addition to its face-to-face services. The online support from mental health clinicians includes asking questions regarding mental health, joining moderated group chats, or engaging in one-to-one support. The Jigsaw services provide therapeutic support in the form of free sessions with a clinician and assisting a young person in connecting with other services or drawing on their supports from family, friends and community. Jigsaw clinicians are a range of allied health professionals, including psychologists, social workers, occupational therapists and mental health nurses. The Youth Advisory Panel (YAP) provides the youth voice to service delivery, engaging with other organisations, promoting mental health awareness and stigma reduction, and contributing to fundraising activities.

Evaluations of Jigsaw indicate a high satisfaction with the services, including from both young people and their families, and most young people believe that attending Jigsaw has assisted in managing their problems and has reduced their experience of psychological distress (O'Keeffe et al. 2015). Young people engaging with Jigsaw services reported high levels of psychological distress at the start of treatment, with the majority reporting clinically significant and reliable changes in the main outcome measure used by Jigsaw (CORE-10) (O'Keeffe et al. 2015).

The Jigsaw services have been shown to increase access to youth mental healthcare, that does not require a formal referral, and can offer timely support for those with mild to moderate mental health difficulties. In partnership with young people and based on further evaluations of outcomes, Jigsaw services aim to improve the effectiveness of the brief interventions offered to young people and to continue to build on the high levels of satisfaction of engaging with their services.

Youth One Stop Shop

The first Youth One Stop Shop in New Zealand was developed in 1994 by a Public Health Nurse in Whanganui. The services that were brought together included a general practitioner, the Family Planning Association, sexual health, child and adolescent mental health, and alcohol/drug services with regular clinics offered in the Youth Advice Centre (YAC). The following year, the 198 Youth Health Centre opened in Christchurch. The model for this service was based on a contract with the local health area authority. The service included a part-time doctor, nurse, counsellor, social worker, administrative staff and young people, all of whom were employed directly by the Youth Health Trust. Subsequently other Youth One Stop Shops have developed independently in other settings; they have been established and managed differently but do now exist within an umbrella group. Each one is unique and offers different services and operates under a different business model. The health sector, through District Health Boards (DHBs) and Primary Health Organizations (PHOs), has primarily funded Youth One Stop Shops although additional funding from other sources is individual to each shop.

A strengths-based and holistic youth development approach underpins the approach of the Youth One Stop Shops, which have implemented a wrap-around health and social care approach to service delivery. The aim is for the person to be at the centre of the care with individual needs addressed in a seamless and coordinated way. These wrap-around services are provided in community-based youth-friendly settings across these various Youth One Stop Shops, including general health/primary care, sexual and reproductive health, family planning, vaccinations, health promotion and education, counselling, mental health, and alcohol/other drug services. Health-promotion and non-health services are also key and included in service delivery are advocacy; social work and youth transition services; youth development programmes; mentoring programmes; information and advice on accommodation, training and education, and budgeting and employment. Some services offer secondary services – mostly sexual and reproductive health, mental health, alcohol/other drug services but also dental/oral care and diabetes clinics. Where it is required, referrals are made to other primary, community, secondary and tertiary services. Youth One Stop Shops have numerous formal and informal links with other sector services, as required for the provision of integrated care. General practitioner enrolment is encouraged for all clients and transitioning support is provided for those at the upper age limit for service. A recent study highlighted the work that goes into ensuring a wrap-around and seamless provision of care, which requires extensive and often complex information exchange and interaction with an enormous range and diversity of other agencies (Garrett et al. 2019). It was also noted that this work was inadequately resourced and represents a major risk for the successful sustained provision of service by Youth One Stop Shops.

The learnings from the Youth One Stop Shops include that the ability to relate to, and communicate with, young people is as important as qualifications in terms of employing staff. Young people are involved in recruitment of staff and are involved in, and represented on, government boards and management and service delivery roles, service planning and evaluation. Youth peer-support workers are a valuable resource as they actively engage with young people upon entry to the facility and help to create a welcoming environment while simultaneously providing information about the services. Depending on funding and resources, services are open between 27 and 45 hours (occasionally more) per week and are provided on-site, in schools or via mobile services and satellite clinics. Most services are free. The age range for service provision varies across Youth One Stop Shops but is mostly for 10- to 24-year-olds.

Youth One Stop Shops tend to be the preferred way young people access GP and sexual and reproductive health services; in one report 14 per cent (28/252) of clients surveyed said they access health services solely from Youth One Stop Shops (Communio, 2009). These clients tended to have higher health and/or social service needs. This preference was reported to be related to the cost, confidentiality and service flexibility, closely followed by the ability to drop in at a convenient location, as well as perceptions of non-judgmental, welcoming and safe staff who knew about youth-related issues. Young people were reported to appreciate the availability of a range of different services, reduced stigma due to non-specific signage (especially related to mental health services) and the youth-friendly focus from staff.

The importance of establishing and nurturing relationships with a range of health and disability and other (non-health) services and local communities is recognised by Youth One Stop Shops and is facilitated in most areas by good communication links that maintain funding, accountability and referral networks. A review of the Youth One Stop Shops identified linkages with in excess of 94 organisations, including funders, referrers or referees, services providers providing services through the Youth One Stop Shops and services providing staffing. Both formal and informal information exchange supports maintenance of these relationships. There are examples of sharing accommodation; co-location of services; collaboration on youth health or youth development community projects and events; training being provided by Youth One Stop Shops to other services; Youth One Stop Shops facilitating other organisations obtaining a youth perspective in service planning or collaboration; and consultation with Youth One Stop Shop staff as experts in the field.

Overall, the Youth One Stops Shops are focused on providing holistic care, including health, social, education, vocational and other services; providing a youth-centred environment; providing opportunities for youth development and community involvement; and developing partnerships and networks. The central tenet of operation is to promote local youth development.

Critique of the models and identification of next steps in service development and delivery

There are varying levels of national support and coordination evident in the delivery of these models internationally, with clear risks to sustainable service provision where this is not present. This also impacts on the appetite and capacity for evaluation and research functions, which has a direct impact on the ability to be continuously collecting information that can be used for ongoing quality improvement and evolution of the model to respond to need and the local context. Even where well supported and acknowledging that these types of interventions are not well suited to gold standard intervention research designs, there is room to continue to pursue an understanding of how these models of care impact on effectiveness of outcomes. This includes understanding impacts on those outcomes that young people believe are important demonstrations of well-being and ensuring that attention is paid to equity of outcomes across specific population groups. It also includes addressing consistency of service delivery in the context of an understanding of core and key components of, and approaches to, service delivery.

Conclusion

The peak onset of mental disorders is during adolescence and early adulthood; the potential for significant disruption to this important developmental period, therefore, demands a service model that is responsive to this age group. Specific, accessible and significant prevention and early intervention that responds to the needs of young people is critical to decrease the burden of mental disorders in this group. Significant work has progressed the field of youth mental health culminating in the Global Framework for Youth Mental Health that guides service delivery. There are now international models of youth mental health service delivery with a growing body of evaluation. These demonstrate benefits in terms of access, acceptability and outcomes, with a group of young people who, apart from these services, would not have accessed any service at all. It is consistently demonstrated in the literature that the quality of relationship with providers of service is critical to outcome and these types of services appear to be doing a good job of this. There is evidence that demand continues to outstrip availability, with national and coordinated support of these models of care impacting on sustainability. Increasing the quality of evaluation and research of these models of delivery will strengthen the field further and highlight key core components or approaches to service delivery, given notable variation in how models of youth mental health service delivery have been operationalised.

Further reading

Hetrick, S. E., Bailey, A. P., Smith, K. E., Malla, A., Mathias, S., Singh, S. P., McGorry, P. D. (2017). Integrated (one-stop shop) youth healthcare: Best available evidence and future directions. *Medical Journal of Australia, 207*(10), S5–S18.

Hughes, F., Hebel, L., Badcock, P., & Parker, A. G. (2017). Ten guiding principles for youth mental health services. *Early Intervention in Psychiatry, 12*(3), 513–519. https://doi.org/10.1111/eip.12429

Rickwood, D., Paraskakis, M., Quin, D., Hobbs, N., Ryall, V., Trethowan, J., & McGorry, P. D. (2019a). Australia's innovation in youth mental healthcare: The headspace centre model. *Early Intervention in Psychiatry, 13*(1), 159–166.

McGorry, P. (2007). The specialist youth mental health model: strengthening the weakest link in the public mental health system. Medical Journal of Australia. 187(s7): S53–S56.

References

Communio. (2009). *Evaluation of Youth One Stop Shops: Final Report v1.1*. https://www.health.govt.nz/system/files/documents/publications/youth-one-stop-shop-evaluation-report-v1.1.pdf

Cosgrave, E. M., Yung, A. R., Killackey, E., Buckny, J. A., Godfrey, K. A., Stanford, C. A., & McGorry, P. D. (2008). Met and unmet need in youth mental health. *Journal of Mental Health, 17*(6), 618–628.

Coughlan, H., Cannon, M., Shiers, D., Power, P., Barry, C., Bates, T., Birchwood, M., Buckley, S., Chambers, D., Davidson, S., Duffy, M., Gavin, B., Healy, C., Healy, C., Keeley, H., Maher, M., Tanti, C., & McGorry, P. (2013). Towards a new paradigm of care: The international declaration on youth mental health. *Early Intervention in Psychiatry, 7*(2), 103–108. DOI: 10.1111/eip.12048

Filia, K., Rickwood, D., Menssink, J., Gao, C., Hetrick, S., Parker, A., Hamilton, M., Hickie, I., Herrman, H., Telford, N., Sharmin, S., McGorry, P., & Cotton, S. (2021). Clinical and functional characteristics of a subsample of young people presenting for primary mental healthcare at headspace services across Australia. *Social Psychiatry and Psychiatric Epidemiology*, online ahead of print. DOI: 10.1007/s00127-020-02020-6

Garrett, S., Pullon, S., Morgan, S., & McKinlay, E. (2019). Collaborative care in 'Youth One Stop Shops' in New Zealand: Hidden, time-consuming, essential. *Journal of Child Healthcare, 24*(2), 180–194.

GBD 2019 Diseases and Injuries Collaborators. (2020). Global burden of 369 diseases and injuries in 204 countries and territories, 1990–2019: A systematic analysis for the Global Burden of Disease Study 2019. *The Lancet, 396*(10258), 1204–1222.

Gore, F. M., Bloem, P. J., Patton, G. C., Ferguson, J., Joseph, V., Coffey, C., Sawyer, S. M., & Mathers, C. D. (2011). Global burden of disease in young people aged 10–24 years: A systematic analysis. *The Lancet, 377*(9783), 2093-2102. https://doi.org/https://doi.org/10.1016/S0140-6736(11)60512-6

headspace. (2019). *Increasing demand in youth mental health: A rising tide of need*. https://headspace.org.au/assets/Uploads/Increasing-demand-in-youth-mentalh-a-rising-tide-of-need.pdf

headspace. (2020). *Year in review 2019–2020: headspace helping young people through challenging times*. https://headspace.org.au/assets/HSP10755_Year-in-Review-2020_FA05_DIGI.pdf

Hetrick, S. E., Bailey, A. P., Smith, K. E., Malla, A., Mathias, S., Singh, S. P., O'Reilly, A., Verma, S. K., Benoit, L., Fleming, T. M., Moro, M. R., Rickwood, D. J., Duffy, J., Erikson, T., Illback, R., Fisher, C. A., & McGorry, P. D. (2017). Integrated (one-stop shop) youth healthcare: Best available evidence and future directions. *Medical Journal of Australia, 207*(10), S5–S18. https://onlinelibrary.wiley.com/doi/abs/10.5694/mja17.00694

Hilferty, F., Cassells, R., Muir, K., Duncan, A., Christensen, D., Mitrou, F., Gao, G., Mavisakalyan, A., Hafekost, K., Tarverdi, Y., Nguyen, H., Wingrove, C., & Katz, I. (2015). *Is headspace making a difference to young people's lives? Final Report of the independent evaluation of the headspace program.* https://headspace.org.au/assets/Uploads/Evaluation-of-headspace-program.pdf

Hughes, F., Hebel, L., Badcock, P., & Parker, A. G. (2017). Ten guiding principles for youth mental health services. *Early Intervention in Psychiatry, 12*(3), 513–519. https://doi.org/10.1111/eip.12429

Illback, R., & Bates, T. (2011). Transforming youth mental health services and supports in Ireland. *Early Intervention in Psychiatry, 5*(1), 22–27. https://doi.org/DOI: 10.1111/j.1751-7893.2010.00236.x

McGorry, P. D., Tanti, C., Stokes, R., Hickie, I. B., Carnell, K., LIttlefield, L. K., & Moran, J. (2007). headspace: Australia's National Youth Mental Health Foundation — where young minds come first. *Medical Journal of Australia, 187*, S68–S70.

O'Reilly, A., Illback, R., Peiper, N., O'Keeffe, L., & Clayton, R. (2015). Youth engagement with an emerging Irish mental health early intervention programme (Jigsaw): Participant characteristics and implications for service delivery. *Journal of Mental Health, 24*(5), 283–88.

O'Keeffe, L., O'Reilly, A., O'Brien, G., Buckley, R., & Illback, R. (2015). Description and outcome evaluation of Jigsaw: An emergent Irish mental health early intervention programme for young people. *Irish Journal of Psychological Medicine, 32*(01), 71–77.

Pascoe, M., Hetrick, S., & Parker, A. (2019). The impact of stress on students in secondary school and higher education: A narrative review. *International Journal of Adolescence and Youth.* https://doi.org/10.1080/02673843.2019.1596823

Rickwood, D., Paraskakis, M., Quin, D., Hobbs, N., Ryall, V., Trethowan, J., & McGorry, P. D. (2019a). Australia's innovation in youth mental healthcare: The headspace centre model. *Early Intervention in Psychiatry, 13*(1), 159–166.

Rickwood, D., Wallace, A., Kennedy, V., O'Sullivan, S., Telford, N., & Leicester, S. (2019b). Young people' satisfaction with the online mental health service eheadspace: Development and implementation of a service satisfaction measure. *JMIR Mental Health, 6*(4), e12169.

Rickwood, D. J., Mazzer, K. R., Telford, N. R., Parker, A. G., Tanti, C. J., & McGorry, P. D. (2015). Changes in psychological distress and psychosocial functioning in young people accessing headspace centres for mental health problems. *Medical Journal of Australia, 202*(10), 537–541.

Rickwood, D. J., Nicholas, A., Mazzer, K., Telford, N., Parker, A. G., Tanti, C., & Simmons, M. B. (2017). Satisfaction with youth mental health services: Further scale development and findings from headspace – Australia's National Youth Mental Health Foundation. *Early Intervention in Psychiatry, 11*(4), 296–305.

Rickwood, D. J., Telford, N. R., Mazzer, K. R., Parkers, A. G., Tanti, C. J., & McGorry, P. D. (2015). The services provided to young people by headspace centres in Australia. *Medical Journal of Australia, 202*(10), 533–536.

Schley, C., Pace, N., Mann, R., McKenzie, C., McRoberts, A., & Parker, A. G. (2019). The headspace Brief Interventions Clinic: Increasing timely access to effective treatments for young people with early signs of mental disorders. *Early Intervention in Psychiatry, 13*(5), 1073–1082. https://doi.org/doi:10.1111/eip.12729

Simmons, M., Hetrick, S., & Jorm, A. (2010). Shared decision making: Benefits, barriers and current opportunities for application. *Australasian Psychiatry, 18*(5), 394–397.

Solar, O., & Irwin, A. (2010). *A Conceptual Framework for Action on the Social Determinants of Health: Social Determinants of Health Discussion Paper 2 (Policy and Practice).* WHO Document Production Services. http://hdl.handle.net/1903/23135

Solmi, M., Radua, J., Olivola, M., Croce, E., Soardo, L., Salazar de Pablo, G., Il Shin, J., Kirkbride, J. B., Jones, P., Kim, J. H., Kim, J., Y., Carvalho, A. F., Seeman, M. V., Correll, C. U., & Fusar-Poli, P. (2021). Age at onset of mental disorders world-wide: Large-scale meta-analysis of 192 epidemiological studies. *Molecular Psychiatry,* https://doi.org/10.1038/s41380-41021-01161-41387.

Welsh, J., Ford, L., Strazdins, L., & Friel, L. (2015). *Evidence review: Addressing the social determinants of inequities in mental well-being of children and adolescents.* https://www.vichealth.vic.gov.au/~/media/resourcecentre/publicationsandresources/health%20inequalities/fair%20foundations/full%20reviews/healthequity_mental-wellbeing-evidence-review.pdf?la=en

World Economic Forum. (2020). *A Global Framework for Youth Mental Health: Investing in Future Mental Capital for Individuals, Communities and Economies.* Word Economic Forum. https://www.orygen.org.au/About/Orygen-Global/Files/Orygen-WEF-global-framework-for-youth-mental-healt.aspx

World Health Organization. (2012a). *Making Health Services Adolescent Friendly. Developing national quality standards for adolescent friendly health services.* https://www.who.int/publications/i/item/9789241503594

World Health Organization. (2001). *The World Health Report 2001: Mental Health: New understanding, new hope.* https://apps.who.int/iris/bitstream/handle/10665/42390/WHR_2001.pdf?sequence=1&isAllowed=y

World Health Organization. (2012b). *Draft resolution on mental health: global burden of mental disorders and the need for a comprehensive, co-ordinated response from health and social sectors at the country level (EB 130.R8).* https://apps.who.int/gb/ebwha/pdf_files/EB130/B130_R8-en.pdf

Quotation from the parent of an adolescent who participated in Daráine Murphy's
(2022) Doctoral Dissertation, University College Dublin:

*'I would actually say now after going through all of this I would say we are closer
than ever. I would say it has actually strengthened the relationship between
the two of us but a lot of understanding had to come from me because I really
did not understand what she was going through.'*

Index